Selected Topics

ULTRASOUND CLINICS

www.ultrasound.theclinics.com

April 2009 • Volume 4 • Number 2

SAUNDERS an imprint of ELSEVIER, Inc.

W.B. SAUNDERS COMPANY
A Division of Elsevier Inc.

1600 John F. Kennedy Boulevard ● Suite 1800 ● Philadelphia, Pennsylvania 19103-2899

http://www.theclinics.com

ULTRASOUND CLINICS Volume 4, Number 2
April 2009 ISSN 1556-858X, ISBN-13: 978-1-4377-1405-0, ISBN-10: 1-4377-1405-6

Editor: Barton Dudlick
Developmental Editor: Theresa Collier

Ultrasound Clinics (ISSN 1556-858X) is published quarterly by W.B. Saunders, 360 Park Avenue South, New York, NY 10010-1710. Months of publication are January, April, July, and October. Business and editorial offices: 1600 John F. Kennedy Boulevard, Suite 1800, Philadelphia, Pennsylvania 19103-2899. Accounting and circulation offices: 6277 Sea Harbor Drive, Orlando, FL 32887-4800. Periodicals postage paid at New York, NY, and additional mailing offices. Subscription prices are $189 per year for (US individuals), $274 per year for (US institutions), $94 per year for (US students and residents), $215 per year for (Canadian individuals), $306 per year for (Canadian institutions), $229 per year for (international individuals), $306 per year for (international institutions), and $114 per year for (Canadian and foreign students/residents). To receive student/resident rate, orders must be accompanied by name of affiliated institution, date of term, and the signature of program/residency coordinator on institution letterhead. Orders will be billed at individual rate until proof of status is received. Foreign air speed delivery is included in all Clinics subscription prices. All prices are subject to change without notice. **POSTMASTER:** Send address changes to *Ultrasound Clinics,* Elsevier Health Sciences Division, Subscription Customer Service, 3251 Riverport Lane, Maryland Heights, MO 63043. **Customer Service (orders, claims, online, change of address): Telephone: 1-800-654-2452 (U.S. and Canada); 314-447-8871(outside U.S. and Canada). Fax: 314-447-8029. E-mail: journalscustomerservice-usa@elsevier.com (for print support); journalsonlinesupport-usa@elsevier.com (for online support).**

Reprints: For copies of 100 or more, of articles in this publication, please contact the Commercial Reprints Department, Elsevier Inc., 360 Park Avenue South, New York, NY 10010-1710. Tel.: (+1) 212-633-3812; Fax: (+1) 212-462-1935; E-mail: reprints@elsevier.com.

Contributors

AUTHORS

JACOB ABRAHAM, MD
Fellow in Cardiovascular Medicine, Division
of Cardiology, The Johns Hopkins University,
Baltimore, Maryland

THEODORE P. ABRAHAM, MD
Associate Professor of Medicine, Division
of Cardiology, The Johns Hopkins University,
Baltimore, Maryland

WENDIE A. BERG, MD, PhD, FACR
Breast Imaging Consultant, American
Radiology Services, Johns Hopkins Green
Spring, Lutherville, Maryland

M. ROBERT DeJONG, RDMS, RVT, RCDS
Ultrasound Technical Manager, Russell H.
Morgan Department of Radiology and
Radiological Science, Johns Hopkins
University, School of Medicine, Baltimore,
Maryland

PETER J. DEMPSEY, MD
Professor of Radiology and Section Chief
of Breast Imaging, Division of Diagnostic
Imaging, Department of Diagnostic Radiology,
The University of Texas M.D. Anderson Cancer
Center, Houston, Texas

TERRY S. DESSER, MD
Associate Professor, Department of Radiology,
Stanford University School of Medicine,
Stanford, California

DAVID P. FESSELL, MD
Department of Radiology, University
of Michigan Hospitals and Health Centers,
Taubman Center, Ann Arbor, Michigan

ULRIKE M. HAMPER, MD, MBA
Professor of Radiology, Urology and
Pathology, and Director of Ultrasound, Russell
H. Morgan Department of Radiology and
Radiological Science, Johns Hopkins
University, School of Medicine, Baltimore,
Maryland

JON A. JACOBSON, MD
University of Michigan, Ann Arbor,
Michigan

AYA KAMAYA, MD
Assistant Professor, Department of Radiology,
Stanford University School of Medicine,
Stanford, California

JILL E. LANGER, MD
Associate Professor of Radiology,
Department of Radiology, University of
Pennsylvania School of Medicine, Hospital
of the University of Pennsylvania,
Philadelphia, Pennsylvania

MARK E. LOCKHART, MD, MPH
Associate Professor, Department of Radiology,
University of Alabama at Birmingham,
Birmingham, Alabama

LUCK J. LOUIS, MD, FRCPC
Clinical Assistant Professor of Radiology,
Sections of Musculoskeletal and Emergency
Trauma Radiology, Department of Radiology,
Vancouver General Hospital, University of
British Columbia, Vancouver, British Columbia,
Canada

SUSAN J. MANDEL, MD, MPH
Associate Professor of Medicine, Division of
Endocrinology, Diabetes, and Metabolism,
Department of Medicine, University of
Pennsylvania School of Medicine, Philadelphia,
Pennsylvania

TED PLAPPERT, CVT
Division of Cardiology, Department of
Medicine, University of Pennsylvania Medical
Center, Philadelphia, Pennsylvania

HIND RAHMOUNI, MD
Division of Cardiology, Department of
Medicine, University of Pennsylvania
Medical Center, Philadelphia,
Pennsylvania

MICHELLE L. ROBBIN, MD
Professor, Department of Radiology, University
of Alabama at Birmingham, Birmingham,
Alabama

LESLIE M. SCOUTT, MD
Professor of Radiology and Chief, Ultrasound
Section, Yale University, School of Medicine,
New Haven, Connecticut

**MARTIN G. St. JOHN SUTTON, MBBS,
FRCP**
John Bryfogle Professor of Cardiovascular
Diseases, Division of Cardiology, Department
of Medicine, University of Pennsylvania
Medical Center, Philadelphia, Pennsylvania

THERESE M. WEBER, MD
Professor, Department of Radiology, University
of Alabama at Birmingham, Birmingham,
Alabama

WEI YANG, MD
Associate Professor of Radiology, Division of
Diagnostic Imaging, Department of Diagnostic
Radiology, The University of Texas M.D.
Anderson Cancer Center, Houston, Texas

Contents

Thyroid nodules can be detected in 4% to 8% of the adult population by palpation, but in 40% to 50% of the population by ultrasound. The overwhelming majority of these represent benign hyperplastic nodules or adenomas. Approximately 5% of nodules are malignant, with papillary carcinoma representing approximately 75% to 80% of primary thyroid malignances. Although many sonographic features have been studied as a means of distinguishing benign from malignant nodules, ultrasound- guided fine-needle aspiration with cytologic evaluation remains a mainstay in the management of palpable and incidentally detected nodules. This article reviews the current techniques for sonographic evaluation of the thyroid and the imaging features of the various types of thyroid nodules.

Sonography plays an important role in the evaluation of patients who have thyroid carcinoma by identifying metastatic disease to the regional cervical lymph nodes. The sonographic appearance of lymph node metastases may vary from subtle alterations in echogenicity or vascular patterns to more obvious findings of calcifications and cystic changes within an affected node. Identification of metastatic disease to lateral cervical lymph nodes by sonography may affect the extent of surgical resection at the time of diagnosis. In patients who have had thyroidectomy for cancer, sonographic evaluation has proved to be the most sensitive imaging technique to detect thyroid cancer recurrence in the neck.

This summary of breast ultrasound reviews the current indications for its use, discusses the potential technical and human pitfalls in its performance, and briefly examines possible future applications that currently are works in progress. It also contains an indepth discussion of the use and interpretation of color Doppler and power Doppler imaging, techniques that do not seem to be understood or used fully in daily practice.

This article describes the principles and performance of screening mammography and discusses indications for screening before the age of 40 years and after the age of 69 years. Specific definitions of high risk are provided, and the rationale and performance characteristics to dare of supplemental screening with ultrasound or MR imaging are reviewed.

Echocardiography now is recommended as the most useful diagnostic test for routine evaluation and management of heart failure. This article reviews the role of echocardiography (M-mode, two-dimensional, spectral, and tissue Doppler) for qualitative and quantitative hemodynamic assessment of the patient who has heart failure. It highlights the echocardiographic parameters that have the most diagnostic and/or prognostic relevance for patients who have advanced heart failure. The importance of right heart failure and heart failure with preserved ejection fraction is increasingly recognized, and therefore the echocardiographic evaluation of these conditions is emphasized also.

Echocardiography serves an extremely important role in the diagnosis and management of patients with heart failure. The various stages of structural and functional changes that constitute progressive left ventricle remodeling have all been characterized by two-dimensional echocardiography. In addition, echocardiography has defined the transition from compensated hypertrophy to left ventricle dilatation and progression to end-stage heart failure. Echocardiography has also played an important role in clinical heart failure trials of b-adrenergic blocking agents and angiotensin-converting enzyme inhibitors and angiotensin receptor blockers and demonstrated their efficacy in heart failure.

Ultrasound is the initial imaging modality of choice when evaluating the upper extremity venous system. When sonographic findings are equivocal or nondiagnostic, particularly in evaluating the central deep veins, MR venography or catheter venography correlation may be helpful. Ultrasound provides an accurate, rapid, low-cost, portable, noninvasive method for screening, mapping, and surveillance of the upper extremity venous system.

Over the past 2 decades venous ultrasonography has become the standard primary imaging technique for the initial evaluation of patients for whom there is clinical suspicion of deep venous thrombosis (DVT) of the lower extremity veins. This article addresses the role of duplex ultrasonography and color Doppler ultrasonography in today's clinical practice for the evaluation of patients suspected of harboring a thrombus in their lower extremity veins. It reviews the clinical presentation and differential diagnoses, technique, and diagnostic criteria for acute and chronic DVT. In addition, it addresses the sonographic evaluation of venous insufficiency.

Ultrasound scan is an invaluable tool in the diagnosis and treatment of disorders of the musculoskeletal system. Core concepts that are common to most ultrasoundguided procedures are reviewed, including an in-depth discussion regarding the use of injectable corticosteroids. Various aspects of intra-articular, intratendinous, bursal, and ganglion cyst intervention are discussed and promising advances in the treatment of chronic tendon disorders are presented.

David P. Fessell and Jon A. Jacobson

Ultrasound has demonstrated great utility and accuracy for imaging the hindfoot and midfoot. Its advantages include its capacity to allow evaluation during dynamic maneuvers, imaging of patients who cannot undergo MR imaging, and real-time evaluation of the symptomatic site. It can also reveal abnormalities that are not apparent during static imaging. This article makes the case that radiologists should continue to be experts in all aspects of musculoskeletal imaging, including ultrasound or the business will be taken over by other specialties. If musculoskeletal ultrasound is lost, additional modalities such as MR imaging may be lost as well. Radiologists, with their expertise and years of training, are uniquely suited to apply this versatile modality to foot and ankle pathology.

Ultrasound Clinics

ISSUE OF RELATED INTEREST

Radiologic Clinics of North America, January 2009, Vol 35 Issue 1
Advances in MDCT
Dushyant V. Sahani, MD, and Vahid Yagmai, MD, *Guest Editors*

THE CLINICS ARE NOW AVAILABLE ONLINE!

Access your subscription at:
www.theclinics.com

GOAL STATEMENT

The goal of the *Ultrasound Clinics* is to keep practicing radiologists and radiology residents up to date with current clinical practice in ultrasound by providing timely articles reviewing the state of the art in patient care.

ACCREDITATION

The *Ultrasound Clinics* is planned and implemented in accordance with the Essential Areas and Policies of the Accreditation Council for Continuing Medical Education (ACCME) through the joint sponsorship of the University of Virginia School of Medicine and Elsevier. The University of Virginia School of Medicine is accredited by the ACCME to provide continuing medical education for physicians.

The University of Virginia School of Medicine designates this educational activity for a maximum of 15 *AMA PRA Category 1 Credits*™ for each issue, 60 credits per year. Physicians should only claim credit commensurate with the extent of their participation in the activity.

The American Medical Association has determined that physicians not licensed in the US who participate in this CME activity are eligible for a maximum of 15 *AMA PRA Category 1 Credits*™ for each issue, 60 credits per year.

Credit can be earned by reading the text material, taking the CME examination online at: http://www.theclinics.com/home/cme, and completing the evaluation. After taking the test, you will be required to review any and all incorrect answers. Following completion of the test and evaluation, your credit will be awarded and you may print your certificate.

FACULTY DISCLOSURE/CONFLICT OF INTEREST

The University of Virginia School of Medicine, as an ACCME accredited provider, endorses and strives to comply with the Accreditation Council for Continuing Medical Education (ACCME) Standards of Commercial Support, Commonwealth of Virginia statutes, University of Virginia policies and procedures, and associated federal and private regulations and guidelines on the need for disclosure and monitoring of proprietary and financial interests that may affect the scientific integrity and balance of content delivered in continuing medical education activities under our auspices.

The University of Virginia School of Medicine requires that all CME activities accredited through this institution be developed independently and be scientifically rigorous, balanced and objective in the presentation/discussion of its content, theories and practices.

All authors/editors participating in an accredited CME activity are expected to disclose to the readers relevant financial relationships with commercial entities occurring within the past 12 months (such as grants or research support, employee, consultant, stock holder, member of speakers bureau, etc.). The University of Virginia School of Medicine will employ appropriate mechanisms to resolve potential conflicts of interest to maintain the standards of fair and balanced education to the reader. Questions about specific strategies can be directed to the Office of Continuing Medical Education, University of Virginia School of Medicine, Charlottesville, Virginia.

The faculty and staff of the University of Virginia Office of Continuing Medical Education have no financial affiliations to disclose.

The authors/editors listed below have identified no professional or financial affiliations for themselves or their spouse/partner:
Matthew J. Bassignani, MD (Test Author); M. Robert DeJong, RDMS, RVT, RCDS; Peter J. Dempsey, MD; Terry S. Desser, MD; Vikram S. Dogra, MD (Consulting and Guest Editor); Barton Dudlick (Acquisitions Editor); Ulrike M. Hamper, MD, MBA; Jill E. Langer, MD; Mark E. Lockhart, MD, MPH; Luck J. Louis, MD, FRCPC; Ted Plappert, CVT; Hind Rahmouni, MD; Leslie M. Scoutt, MD; Therese M. Weber, MD; and Wei Yang, MD.

The authors/editors listed below have identified the following professional or financial affiliations for themselves or their spouse/partner:
Jacob Abraham, MD is a consultant for Medica Pharmacy.
Theodore P. Abraham, MD is an industry funded research/investigator for GE Healthcare.
Wendie A. Berg, MD, PhD, FACR received a donated computer from Medi Pattern.
David P. Fessell, MD is a consultant for Bioimaging.
Jon A. Jacobson, MD is a consultant for SonoSite, Hitachi, and BioImaging Technologies, and receives royalties from Elsevier.
Aya Kamaya, MD is an industry funded research/investigator for Canon Inc.
Susan J. Mandel, MD, MPH is a speaker for Abbott Pharmaceuticals and Genzyme Corporation.
Michelle L. Robbin, MD is an industry funded research/investigator for Philips Ultrasound.
Martin G. St. John Sutton, MBBS, FRCP is a consultant for Medtronic Inc.

Disclosure of Discussion of Non-FDA Approved Uses for Pharmaceutical Products and/or Medical Devices.
The University of Virginia School of Medicine, as an ACCME provider, requires that all faculty presenters identify and disclose any off-label uses for pharmaceutical and medical device products. The University of Virginia School of Medicine recommends that each physician fully review all the available data on new products or procedures prior to clinical use.

TO ENROLL

To enroll in the Ultrasound Clinics Continuing Medical Education program, call customer service at 1-800-654-2452 or visit us online at: www.theclinics.com/home/cme. The CME program is available to subscribers for an additional fee of $205.00.

Ultrasound of Thyroid Nodules

Terry S. Desser, MD*, Aya Kamaya, MD

KEYWORDS

- Thyroid nodules • Thyroid carcinoma
- Ultrasound • Sonography

Thyroid nodules are a ubiquitous clinical problem. In years past, when palpation was the sole method of thyroid evaluation, the prevalence of thyroid nodules was estimated at approximately 4% to 8% of the adult population and typically only those nodules 1 cm or larger in diameter were detected.[1] With increasing use of imaging for evaluation of the carotid arteries, cervical spine, and chest, the reported prevalence of thyroid nodules has increased to as high as 40% to 50%,[1-3] approaching the 50% prevalence of nodules found at autopsy. Because the risk for malignancy in these thyroid nodules is low (1.5%–10%), the issue of how best to manage the current epidemic of thyroid nodules in an increasingly cost-constrained environment is a critical one. Furthermore, the vast majority of the cancers detected are papillary carcinomas, which are often clinically occult and virtually never fatal even after spread to regional lymph nodes has occurred.[4-8] A logical strategy for identifying the minority of thyroid nodules that require intervention from among the huge numbers that do not is a topic of much debate among sonographers and endocrinologists.

High-resolution ultrasound is the modality of choice for evaluation of the thyroid gland. It is painless, inexpensive, does not require the use of contrast media, and can display the internal architecture and flow characteristics of nodules as small as 1 to 2 mm. Ultrasound-guided fine-needle aspiration (FNA) with cytologic evaluation is now a mainstay in the management of palpable and incidentally detected nodules. This article reviews the current techniques for sonographic evaluation of the thyroid and the imaging features of the various types of thyroid nodules. We also explore the various strategies for management of thyroid nodules based on clinical and imaging parameters.

ANATOMY AND SCANNING TECHNIQUE

The thyroid gland is an H-shaped organ composed of two lobes joined by a narrow isthmus located just below the laryngeal cartilages. The normal thyroid weighs approximately 15 to 25 g,[9] with each lobe approximately 4 cm in length and 2 cm in thickness. Befitting its vital role in metabolism, it is a highly vascular organ supplied by the superior thyroidal branch of the external carotid artery and the inferior thyroid branch of the subclavian artery. Microscopically, the thyroid parenchyma is organized into follicles, hollow spheres of epithelial cells enclosing a protein-rich material termed colloid. Thin fibrous septations divide the normal thyroid into lobules composed of 20 to 40 follicles each about 50 to 500 μm in size.

To visualize the thyroid gland optimally, the patient is placed in the supine position with a pillow underneath the shoulders to extend the neck slightly, allowing the head to rest on the examination table. In older patients or those who have degenerative changes in the neck, small towels can be placed under the head to the level where the patient is most comfortable while still allowing access to the neck. The thyroid gland is then imaged in transverse and longitudinal views with a high-frequency (10–15 MHz) linear transducer.

This article originally appeared in *Neuroimaging Clinics of North America* 2008;18(3):463–478

Department of Radiology, Stanford University School of Medicine, 300 Pasteur Drive, Mail Code 5621, Stanford, CA 94305, USA

* Corresponding author.

E-mail address: desser@stanford.edu (T.S. Desser).

ultrasound.theclinics.com

The highest frequency is used while still allowing adequate sonographic penetration.

The normal thyroid gland is uniformly echogenic relative to the overlying strap muscles of the neck (**Fig. 1**). A thyroid nodule is defined as a region of parenchyma sonographically distinct from the remainder of the thyroid and located within the confines of the echogenic thyroid capsule. When a nodule is detected, its size should be measured in three dimensions and the location within the thyroid gland (upper pole, mid-gland, lower pole) should be noted by the sonographer. Several sonographic features are helpful for differential diagnosis, including nodule echogenicity, morphology, cystic change, presence of echogenic foci with comet-tail artifact representing colloid, presence and type of calcifications, and flow pattern (peripheral or central). These are discussed in more detail later.

Instrumentation: New Technologies

Several new sonographic technologies have been applied to the imaging of thyroid nodules. Three-dimensional (3D) ultrasound, in which a freehand or automated sweep of the transducer generates an image volume that can be displayed in axial, coronal, or sagittal planes, can generate good-quality images of multinodular thyroids (**Fig. 2**). In a recent study comparing volume measurements of thyroid nodules in 102 children, 3D ultrasound measurements were more accurate, with less intraobserver variability and higher reproducibility, compared with two-dimensional assessment.[10] It may also provide greater workflow efficiency, because entire organs can be scanned in a single transducer sweep.[11] Compound imaging is a signal-averaging technique designed to reduce speckle noise and improve contrast resolution, and has been shown to increase contrast-to-noise ratio in clinical

thyroid images (**Fig. 3**).[12] Tissue harmonic imaging (THI) uses the first harmonic of the transmitted frequency for image formation and results in images with less noise. Its benefits in abdominal and pelvic sonography are dramatic, especially in obese patients. In a study of 144 patients who had thyroid nodules, THI improved lesion conspicuity and gray-scale contrast between lesions;[13] however, the fundamental mode imaging was performed at 7.5 MHz, and therefore the relevance of this work is questionable given that most thyroid ultrasound is performed at 10 MHz or higher. Although these innovations have improved image clarity somewhat, they have not impacted lesion characterization significantly. Similarly, sonographic contrast agents have been used in other organ systems, but to date have not had a significant role in thyroid nodule imaging.

Elastography

By contrast, elastography of thyroid nodules is an evolving technology with early reported promise of differentiating benign nodules from malignant nodules with 96% specificity and 82% specificity.[14] Analogous to palpation, the rationale behind elastography is that a cancerous nodule is stiffer, with less elastic deformation compared with muscle or a benign thyroid nodule. Ultrasound elastography is a dynamic method in which an external compressive force is applied during scanning and the degree of distortion used to estimate the stiffness of the tissue of interest (**Fig. 4**). Ultrasound elastography has already been used to differentiate cancer from benign lesions in the prostate, breast, pancreas, and lymph nodes.[15] Different methods of identifying a stiff thyroid nodule are currently being studied, including manual compression with comparison of the lesion during a cine loop using speckle tracking in two and three dimensions, or with evaluation of the nodule under normal respiratory and cardiac pulsations. One recent study used carotid artery pulsation as the compression source and found that elastography was able to distinguish a papillary carcinoma from a benign nodule located in the same thyroid lobe.[16] Although these implementations of elastography require off-line image processing, some newer machines are capable of real-time image processing. Recent work using a real-time elastography technique in 92 consecutive patients who had solitary thyroid nodules found that elastography scores representing the least strain (stiff lesions with little deformation) were highly predictive of malignancy with sensitivity of 97%, specificity of 100%, and 100% positive predictive value.[15] The patients were highly

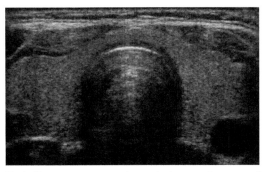

Fig. 1. Transverse gray-scale mode image of a normal thyroid gland, which is uniformly echogenic relative to overlying strap musculature.

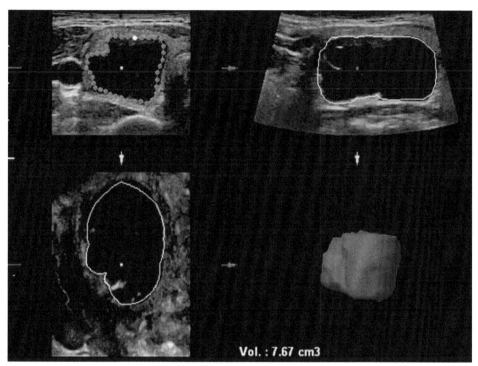

Fig. 2. Volumetric display of cystic thyroid nodule with calculation of nodule volume. A single sweep through the image volume is obtained, and three orthogonal planes are displayed. Upper left image is axial plane, upper right image is sagittal plane, and lower left image is coronal plane. Lower right image shows volume rendering of cystic nodule, with calculated volume beneath. (*Courtesy of* GE Healthcare Technologies.)

selected, however, and cystic nodules, nodules with eggshell calcification, and patients who had multiple nodules were not included in the study. Although promising, elastography needs further study to determine whether the method will prove as robust when used on a larger scale.

THYROID NODULES

Various benign and malignant nodules occur commonly in the thyroid gland (**Box 1**). In the Framingham population study, nodules were found by palpation in 6.4% of women and 1.5% of men.[8] By

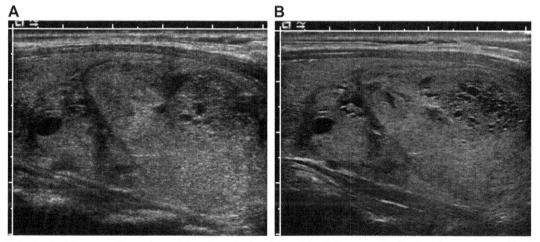

Fig. 3. Sagittal images of complex solid and cystic thyroid nodule. (*A*) Image obtained with conventional high-resolution transducer shows small cystic areas in lower portion of nodule. (*B*) Image obtained at higher frequency and with compounding shows better spatial resolution of tiny cystic areas. (*Courtesy of* Siemens Medical Systems.)

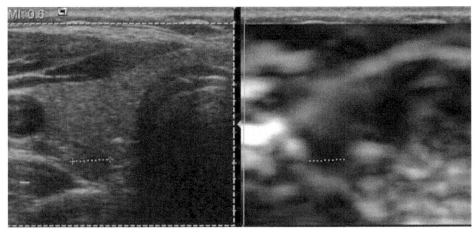

Fig. 4. Simultaneous gray-scale and elastography image of a biopsy-proven benign thyroid nodule. Image on left is a gray-scale image of a thyroid nodule demarcated by calipers. Image on right is corresponding elastography image at same location. On elastography image, the nodule (dark area behind calipers) is smaller in size compared with the nodule seen on gray-scale, which suggests this lesion is more compressible than the adjacent thyroid parenchyma. This finding correlates with a benign pathology.

ultrasound, many more nodules are detected. In one study, 50% of patients who had apparent solitary nodules by palpation had additional nodules detected by ultrasound, and about 25% of those nodules were larger than 1 cm.[17] Location of the nodule (anterior or posterior), size of the patient's neck, and skill of the examiner all affect the likelihood of detection by palpation. With current ultrasound technology, however, even nodules as small as 1 mm may be evident.[18]

Box 1

Types of thyroid nodules

Benign nodules

    Colloid (hyperplastic, adenomatous) nodules

    Hashimoto (chronic lymphocytic) thyroiditis

    Cysts: colloid, simple, or hemorrhagic

    Follicular adenomas

    Hürthle-cell (oxyphil-cell) adenomas (variant of follicular adenoma)

Malignant nodules

    Papillary carcinoma

    Follicular carcinoma

    Medullary carcinoma

    Anaplastic carcinoma

    Primary thyroid lymphoma

    Metastatic carcinoma (breast, renal cell, others)

Hyperplastic Nodules

The most common lesion in the thyroid is the hyperplastic nodule, also termed a colloid or adenomatous nodule. The etiology of thyroid glandular hyperplasia includes iodine deficiency and disorders of hormone synthesis. Production of the thyroid hormones T3 and T4 (thyroxine) by thyroid follicle epithelial cells is regulated by release of thyroid-stimulating hormone (TSH) from the anterior pituitary gland. Impaired or deficient thyroid hormone synthesis causes TSH levels to increase, and increases in TSH then produce follicular cell hypertrophy and hyperplasia. Repetitive cycles of hyperplasia followed by involution may produce irregular thyroid enlargement and multinodular goiter.[9] Otherwise identical-appearing follicular epithelial cells differ in their sensitivity to growth stimuli and in their intrinsic proliferative capabilities, which leads to nodule formation over time.[19] It was formerly believed that hyperplastic nodules could be distinguished from true neoplasms by virtue of their polyclonality. More recent studies, however, suggest that both neoplasms and hyperplastic nodules are monoclonal. Despite their prevalence, therefore, the pathophysiology of thyroid nodule formation remains poorly understood.

On sonography, hyperplastic nodules have a wide spectrum of appearances. They are most often isoechoic, but can also be hypoechoic and commonly undergo cystic and hemorrhagic degeneration (**Fig. 5**). Larger solid masses may be entirely echogenic. Cystic areas may contain either serous fluid or colloid; old hemorrhage and resultant echogenic fluid may also be noted.

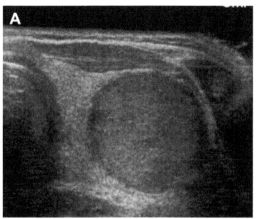
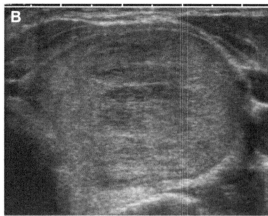

Fig. 5. Hyperplastic nodule. (A) Transverse image shows solid nodule in thyroid with hypoechoic halo, biopsy proven to represent a benign thyroid nodule. (B) Ultrasound 6 months later demonstrates internal cystic degeneration.

Punctuate highly echogenic foci with ring-down artifact represent colloid crystals within colloid cysts (Fig. 6). If residual strands of thyroid tissue remain within the cystic areas, a characteristic honeycomb appearance may result (Fig. 7).[20] Nonuniform patterns of degeneration may produce mural nodules, septations, or internal debris. Degeneration of hyperplastic nodules may also produce dystrophic calcification and manifest as either coarse internal calcification or peripheral "eggshell" calcification (Fig. 8).[18] The term goiter is used when hyperplasia leads to overall increase in the size of the thyroid gland. Multinodular goiter, which is composed of multiple hyperplastic nodules with varying degrees of colloid, necrosis, or hemorrhage, is generally heterogeneous in appearance with multiple masses of varying size and echo texture.

Hashimoto Thyroiditis

Hashimoto thyroiditis is a common autoimmune disease in which patients, predominantly women, develop antibodies to thyroglobulin and the thyroid peroxidase enzyme. It causes a characteristic sonographic pattern of innumerable tiny hypoechoic nodules that may become confluent, interspersed with echogenic fibrous bands (Fig. 9). Vascularity may be increased, decreased, or normal, and FNA is usually not necessary for diagnosis.[20]

THYROID NEOPLASMS

Thyroid cancer is relatively uncommon in the United States. In 2007, an estimated 33,550 cases will be diagnosed, accounting for about 1530 deaths. The incidence of thyroid cancer in the United States has increased from 3.6 per 100,000 in 1973 to 8.7 per 100,000 in 2002, but virtually all of this increase is believed to be attributable to increased detection of small papillary cancers on imaging studies.[21] Thyroid malignancies may arise from follicular epithelium (papillary, follicular, anaplastic) or from parafollicular C-cells (medullary carcinoma) and are classified as differentiated (papillary and follicular), medullary, and undifferentiated (anaplastic) carcinomas. The major risk factor for development of thyroid carcinoma is radiation exposure to the head and neck. Several oncogenes and tumor suppressor genes

RT THYROID TRANS   INF

Fig. 6. Transverse image of right thyroid lobe shows cyst in lower pole of thyroid containing an echogenic focus with ring-down artifact posteriorly. This appearance is diagnostic of a colloid cyst.

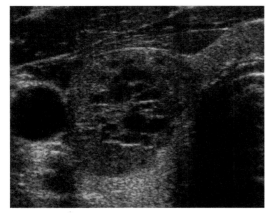

Fig. 7. Transverse image of right thyroid lobe shows innumerable cystic spaces separated by a fine mesh of thin septations. This honeycomb appearance represents a benign thyroid nodule, which was proven by FNA.

have been identified as playing a role in formation of both benign and malignant thyroid nodules.[22]

PAPILLARY CARCINOMA

Papillary cancer is the most common thyroid malignancy, accounting for 75% to 80% of thyroid cancers. Papillary cancers are typically slow-growing tumors with an excellent prognosis. In some autopsy studies, papillary cancers less than 10 mm in size, called papillary microcarcinomas, were found in 22% to 36% of patients who had no known thyroid pathology during life.[5,7] One study of patients who had papillary microcarcinoma found no statistically significant difference in mortality between patients who underwent surgical resection versus a cohort managed by observation alone.[6] Approximately 15% of thyroid

carcinomas behave in an aggressive manner, however.[23] Risk factors for aggressive behavior of papillary microcarcinomas include extracapsular invasion, metastatic lymph node size, hoarseness, and postoperative thyroglobulin levels.[6]

Histologic features of papillary cancer include presence of psammoma bodies and characteristic nuclear changes, such as ground-glass appearance, longitudinal grooves, and inclusions.[24] The most specific sonographic finding of papillary cancer is the presence of punctuate, non-shadowing echogenic foci termed microcalcifications, which are believed to represent dystrophic calcifications associated with psammoma bodies (**Fig. 10**). Although this finding has a high specificity (85%–95%)[1,25] sensitivity is only 25% to 59%.[1] Most papillary cancers are solid (87%) and hypoechoic (86%) compared with the surrounding thyroid parenchyma (**Fig. 11**).[26] Some evidence of intrinsic vascularity is generally seen, though the distribution of vascularity has not been found to be a reliable finding.[26–29] Papillary thyroid cancer metastasizes by way of lymphatics to cervical lymph nodes, which may contain microcalcifications, internal vascularity, and cystic change because of extensive degeneration (**Fig. 12**).

FOLLICULAR NEOPLASMS

Follicular adenomas are encapsulated true neoplasms of the thyroid gland and represent about 5% to 10% of all thyroid nodules. A minority of adenomas may be autonomously hyperfunctioning causing thyrotoxicosis, and thus the initial workup of a palpable thyroid nodule should include measurement of serum TSH levels.[2,3] Low TSH level would be an indication for thyroid scintigraphy, which is otherwise not useful in the

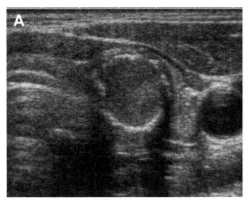
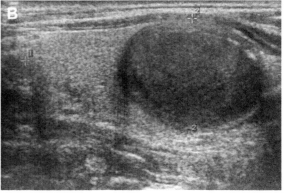

Fig. 8. Eggshell calcification. (A) Transverse image of left thyroid lobe shows complete thin rim of calcification encircling thyroid nodule. (B) Longitudinal image of benign thyroid nodule in a different patient shows incomplete delicate thin rim of calcification at inferior pole of nodule proven to represent a benign hemorrhagic cyst.

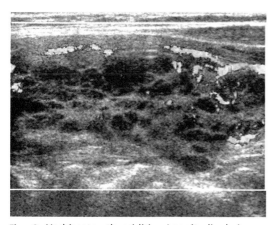

Fig. 9. Hashimoto thyroiditis. Longitudinal image shows innumerable small hypoechoic nodules set against background of echogenic thyroid parenchyma. Vascularity is slightly increased.

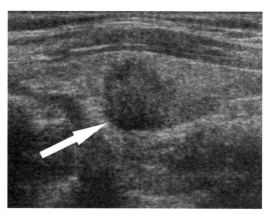

Fig. 11. Longitudinal image of hypoechoic papillary cancer (*arrow*) with irregular margins. The lesion is larger in anteroposterior dimension than in craniocaudal dimension (taller than wide).

evaluation of thyroid nodules. Differentiation of follicular adenoma from a follicular carcinoma is based on the presence of capsular or vascular invasion on histologic examination and thus cannot be made by sonography or by FNA cytology. Like thyroid nodules in general, follicular tumors are more common in women.

On sonography, follicular adenomas and follicular carcinomas are usually solitary encapsulated tumors, often with a well-defined peripheral hypoechoic halo representing the fibrous capsule (**Fig. 13**). Two histologic patterns of growth of follicular carcinomas can be observed. The minimally invasive type is encapsulated, in contrast to the widely invasive type, which extends beyond the tumor capsule into blood vessels and adjacent parenchyma. Echogenicity is variable and follicular neoplasms can be echogenic, isoechoic, or hypoechoic. Echogenic adenomas are often smoothly

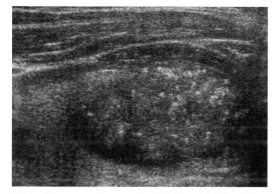

Fig. 10. Transverse image of right thyroid lobe in 39-year-old man who had papillary cancer. Innumerable microcalcifications create a "snowstorm" appearance.

marginated and ovoid in appearance, prompting use of the term "pseudotesticle" to describe their appearance (**Fig. 14**). In contrast to papillary carcinomas, follicular carcinomas metastasize hematogenously to bone, lung, brain, and liver rather than by way of lymphatics. Hürthle (oncocytic) cells may constitute most or all of a follicular tumor, in which case the tumor is classified as a Hürthle cell carcinoma, a variant of follicular carcinoma.[30] Another histologic variant is insular thyroid cancer, which is poorly differentiated and associated with an aggressive clinical course.[24]

MEDULLARY CARCINOMA

Medullary thyroid cancer is a neuroendocrine tumor arising from the parafollicular C cells located in the upper two thirds of the thyroid gland.[31] Although medullary cancer is associated with MEN2A (C cell hyperplasia, pheochromocytoma, hyperparathyroidism), 80% occur sporadically. Ninety-five percent of patients who have MEN2A have C-cell hyperplasia and in 80% of affected patients, medullary thyroid carcinoma is the initial manifestation. Patients who have sporadic medullary carcinoma typically present with a painless palpable nodule in the fifth or sixth decade of life, but the disease is often metastatic to cervical lymph nodes at presentation.[32] There is a slight female preponderance (1.5:1).[31] The value of serum calcitonin screening measurement in patients who have thyroid nodules is dubious because levels are often falsely elevated and FNA is highly accurate; however, calcitonin levels are useful once the diagnosis of medullary thyroid cancer has been established by cytologic evaluation.[32] On sonography, medullary carcinomas are

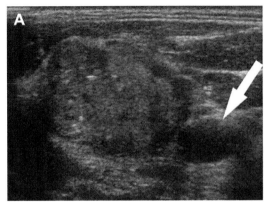
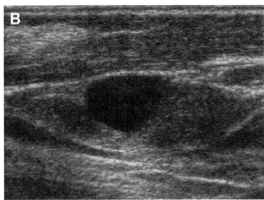

Fig. 12. Metastatic papillary carcinoma involving cervical lymph nodes. (*A*) Transverse gray-scale image of papillary cancer metastatic to a right lateral cervical lymph node containing microcalcifications. The large node is just lateral to the right carotid artery (*arrow*). (*B*) Longitudinal image of metastatic papillary carcinoma with cystic change in cervical lymph node.

typically solid, hypoechoic, and often have coarse central calcifications (**Fig. 15**).

ANAPLASTIC CARCINOMA

Anaplastic carcinoma of the thyroid is a rare tumor of the thyroid, but extremely aggressive, representing the terminal stage in the dedifferentiation of a follicular or papillary carcinoma. Patients are usually elderly with a history of goiter and present with a rapidly growing neck mass. The tumor characteristically invades locally and involves adjacent muscles and blood vessels. Distant metastases most commonly involve the lungs, bones, brain, and liver.[30]

On sonography, anaplastic carcinomas are generally large, at least 5 to 10 cm, fixed, hard, and heterogeneous in appearance (**Fig. 16**). Internal calcifications and cystic or necrotic areas may be seen. Adjacent enlarged lymph nodes are common. Invasion of adjacent structures, such as the carotid sheath, trachea, and muscles,

and the overall extent of tumor are often better assessed on CT or MR imaging.

LYMPHOMA

Primary lymphoma of the thyroid is uncommon, accounting for 2% of extranodal lymphomas and less than 5% of all malignant thyroid tumors. Most thyroid lymphomas are non-Hodgkin lymphomas. Patients present with a rapidly enlarging painless neck mass. Lymphomas may occur in the setting of Hashimoto thyroiditis. On ultrasound, thyroid lymphoma is characteristically very hypoechoic with a pseudocystic pattern (increased through transmission) similar to lymphoma seen in other organs, such as the liver or lymph nodes (**Fig. 17**).[30]

THYROID METASTASIS

Metastatic disease to the thyroid is rare. In a large study of 18,105 thyroidectomies in two Italian pathology databases, only 24 cases (0.13%)

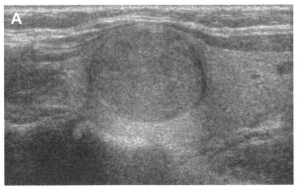
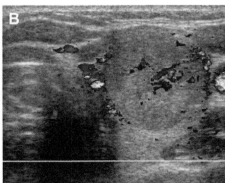

Fig. 13. Follicular adenoma. (*A*) Longitudinal gray-scale image shows well-defined hypoechoic nodule with incomplete halo. (*B*) Transverse image shows flow in peripheral hypoechoic capsule and internally.

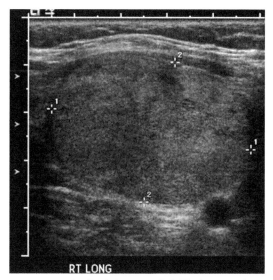

Fig. 14. Longitudinal image of follicular neoplasm (Hürthle cell) with pseudotesticle appearance.

were found to represent metastatic disease to the thyroid with the main sites of origin being lung, esophagus, breast, and kidney.[33] On sonography, metastases to the thyroid have a nonspecific appearance and are usually solid, noncalcified, hypoechoic nodules (**Fig. 18**). With increased use of whole-body fluorodeoxyglucose positron emission tomography (FDG-PET) and PET-CT in patients who have a known primary malignancy, focal areas of hypermetabolism in the thyroid have been identified with increasing frequency, with prevalence ranging from 2.2% to 4.3%. In several studies, the rate of malignancy in these metabolically active thyroid "incidentalomas" ranges from 26.7% to 80%, with the vast majority of malignancies representing primary thyroid carcinomas, not metastatic disease. Although the

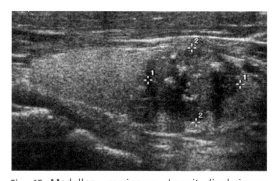

Fig. 15. Medullary carcinoma. Longitudinal image shows hypoechoic nodule at inferior pole of thyroid with coarse central calcifications. (*Courtesy of* Lucy E. Hann, MD, New York, NY.)

standardized uptake values were higher in malignant nodules than benign nodules in most studies, FNA is usually indicated for definitive assessment.[34–40]

The sonographic characteristics of these specific types of thyroid nodules are summarized in **Table 1**.

SONOGRAPHIC FEATURES OF THYROID NODULES

Current management guidelines recommend sonography and FNA for management of thyroid nodules, because no single noninvasive test can reliably distinguish benign from malignant nodules. But with the odds of malignancy only approximately 1 in 20, and thyroid cancer accounting for only 0.5% of all cancer deaths, a sensible strategy for determining which nodules should undergo FNA is essential. Numerous sonographic features of thyroid nodules have been described and studied as a means of triaging nodules for FNA. These include size, multiplicity, echogenicity, presence of calcifications, margins, contour, shape, internal architecture, and vascularity. The most common appearance for papillary thyroid carcinoma is a solitary, solid hypoechoic nodule with ill-defined borders, microcalcifications, and internal vascularity. In one series of 55 papillary carcinomas, however, more than half had at least one feature not commonly associated with malignancy.[26] Conversely, in a series of 68 benign nodules, 69% of them had at least one finding usually associated with malignancy.[41] Although no single feature can distinguish benign from malignant nodules, taking all sonographic features into account can shed some light on which nodules should undergo further testing.

Size and Multiplicity

Thyroid nodules become palpable when they reach approximately 1 cm in size. When palpation was the sole means of identifying nodules, this diameter was the de facto threshold for biopsy. Although the American Association of Clinical Endocrinologists and American Thyroid Association guidelines continue to use 1 to 1.5 cm as a practical threshold for selecting nodules for FNA,[2,3] it has been shown that size is not a good predictor of malignancy. Papini and colleagues[42] evaluated the risk for malignancy in 195 solitary nonpalpable thyroid nodules 8 to 15 mm in size and 207 multinodular goiters, and found that the cancer prevalence was similar in nodules greater or smaller than 10 mm. Rather than a simple size threshold, their study found that a strategy of performing FNA in all hypoechoic solid nodules with irregular margins, intranodular flow, or

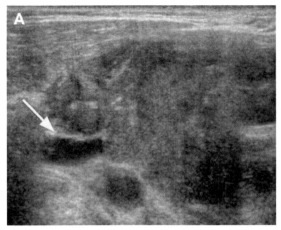
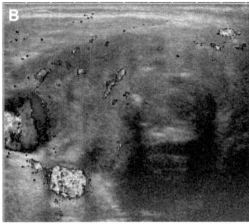

Fig. 16. Anaplastic thyroid cancer in 74-year-old woman. (*A*) Transverse gray-scale image of an enlarged, irregular, heterogeneous thyroid mass with mass effect on the internal jugular vein (*arrow*). Carotid artery is posterior and medial. (*B*) Color Doppler image of the thyroid near the same level. At this level, internal coarse calcifications with shadowing are seen.

microcalcifications would lead to biopsy in only 31% of nodules while still detecting 87% of the cancers. In nodules larger than 1 cm, Frates and colleagues[43] found no significant difference in the rate of malignancy in 1039 solid nodules by size, although there was a trend toward higher rate of malignancy in nodules larger than 3 cm. The recent Society of Radiologists in Ultrasound consensus statement suggests that, rather than a fixed size threshold, sonographic features should be used to guide nodule selection for FNA. More suspicious sonographic features (see later discussion) should trigger biopsy at small nodule size, whereas nearly completely cystic nodules without other suspicious features probably do not require biopsy at any size.[1]

The presence of multiple nodules does not make thyroid carcinoma less likely, contrary to former teaching.[44] In multinodular glands, each nodule should be scrutinized for suspicious features and

selected for FNA on the basis of sonographic features, rather than size alone.

Growth

Interval follow-up is usually recommended for sonographically detected nodules, yet there are no data to suggest which growth rates or patterns are suspicious. Both benign and malignant nodules can increase or decrease in size. Brander and colleagues[45] conducted a 5-year follow-up study of 69 patients who had thyroid abnormalities found incidentally as part of an ultrasound screening study of 253 randomly selected adults. Of the original cohort of 69 patients who had abnormalities, 57 patients participated in the follow-up study. The investigators found that, regardless of echo texture, 35% of the 34 cytologically benign nodules had increased in size at follow-up and remained benign at repeat FNA. Eight (24%) had decreased in size or

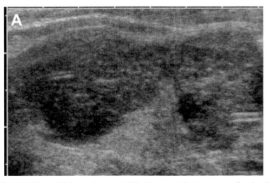
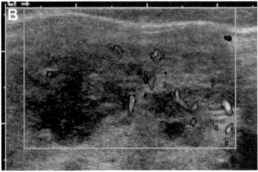

Fig. 17. Thyroid lymphoma. (*A*) Gray-scale image of a bulky, hypoechoic mass with pseudocystic appearance. (*B*) Color Doppler image demonstrates internal vascularity.

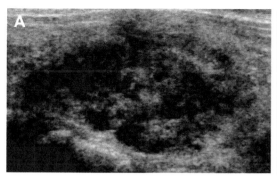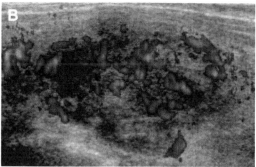

Fig. 18. Thyroid metastasis. (*A*) Gray-scale image of a heterogeneously hypoechoic mass in thyroid, biopsy proven to represent metastases from lung cancer primary. (*B*) Power Doppler demonstrates marked internal vascularity. (*Case courtesy of* R. Brooke Jeffrey MD.)

disappeared altogether. New lesions were detected in 7 subjects, and cytology proved to be benign in the 5 who underwent FNA. The remaining 2 lesions were too small and the patients preferred follow-up. Overall, their results found no malignancies at 5-year follow-up, even among those whose nodules had increased in size. A more recent study of the natural history of 330 benign solid and cystic thyroid nodules showed that 89% of the solid benign thyroid nodules increased in volume by 15% or greater over a 5-year period.[46] Solid nodules were more likely to grow than cystic nodules. At the time of a 9- to 12-month follow-up scan, 39% of benign nodules had increased in volume by 15% or more. Within a higher risk subset of 74 larger nodules with more rapid growth, only one proved to be malignant at re-biopsy.

Calcifications

Calcifications have been found in papillary, medullary, and anaplastic thyroid carcinomas as either psammoma bodies or as amorphous granular deposits. Of all the sonographic features associated with thyroid malignancy, microcalcifications are the most specific. Microcalcifications are defined as punctate echogenic foci without acoustic shadowing or associated comet-tail artifact. The positive predictive value of a finding of microcalcifications in a thyroid nodule ranges from 24.3% to 70%.[1] Other types of calcification may also be present. In one series, microcalcifications were seen in 42% of papillary thyroid cancers, coarse calcifications in 9.1%, and peripheral calcifications in 1.8% (**Fig. 19**).[26] Although formerly considered a benign finding, eggshell calcifications have been reported in thyroid cancers.[47] Coarse central calcifications are a common feature of medullary carcinoma, although this entity represents only 1 of 250 thyroid nodules.[48]

Echogenicity

Most thyroid carcinomas are hypoechoic relative to surrounding thyroid parenchyma. In a series of 55 papillary carcinomas studied by Chan and colleagues,[26] 86% of papillary cancers were hypoechoic. A more recent series of 68 papillary cancers from the same institution found that 78% were hypoechoic, with 12% isoechoic, 9% mixed echogenicity, and 1% hyperechoic.[49] Hypoechogenicity is a sensitive sign but is nonspecific: 30.6% to 55% of benign nodules are also hypoechoic.[25,41] An echogenic appearance is commonly associated with follicular neoplasms, both benign and malignant, but can also be seen in papillary cancers. Kim and colleagues[50] suggested that "marked hypoechogenicity," defined as echogenicity less than that of adjacent musculature, is a more specific appearance for thyroid carcinoma, but others found that this feature had only fair interobserver agreement.

Cystic Change and Ring-Down Artifact

Thyroid cancer is not common in predominantly cystic nodules. In a series of 209 nodules assessed by Frates and colleagues,[27] only 2 of 32 malignant nodules were greater than 50% cystic, as compared with 30 of 177 benign nodules. Nodules that are nearly completely cystic are virtually never cancers in the absence of other concerning features.[1,26] Nevertheless, a cystic component may be seen in 13% to 26% of thyroid cancers.[1,26,51] When FNA is to be performed on a cystic nodule, the biopsy should be targeted to the solid components. Additional features are helpful in assessing cystic nodules. In their series of papillary carcinomas, Chan and colleagues[26] found no cystic carcinomas without internal flow in their solid components. The Mayo Clinic group has observed that a "honeycomb" appearance

Table 1
Summary of sonographic features of thyroid nodules

	Echogenicity	Rim	Vascularity	Calcifications	Cyst Component	Special Distinguishing Findings
Papillary cancer	Usually hypoechoic	Ill defined more worrisome; can be well defined	Usually hypervascular compared with rest of thyroid; pattern not reliable indicator	May see coarse calcifications or microcalcifications	Usually less than 50%	Microcalcifications
Follicular cancer	Usually hypoechoic	Well defined	—	—	No	Pseudotesticle
Medullary cancer	—	—	—	Central coarse calcification	—	May see central coarse calcification
Anaplastic cancer	Heterogeneous	Ill defined	Internal vascularity	Various types	May see internal necrotic change	Invasion of adjacent structures
Lymphoma	Hypoechoic	—	Hypovascular	No	May see cystic necrosis	Increased through transmission
Degenerating adenoma: hemorrhagic degeneration	Variable	Well defined	Yes	May see thin rim eggshell calcification	May be present	Colloid crystals (echogenic foci with ring down)
Cystic degeneration	Variable	Well defined	Variable	—	>75% cystic	—

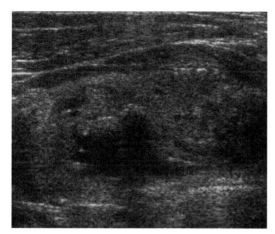

Fig. 19. Longitudinal image of a papillary cancer with coarse, shadowing calcifications. (*Case courtesy of R. Brooke Jeffrey, MD.*)

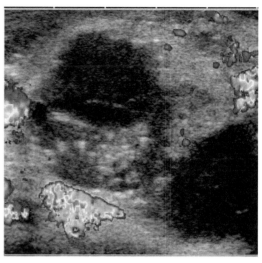

Fig. 20. Transverse image of benign cystic nodule with dependent internal colloid as evidenced by comet-tail artifacts.

of multiple cystic spaces bordered by numerous thin septations virtually always correlates with benign cytology on FNA.[20] Punctate echogenic foci associated with comet-tail artifact representing inspissated colloid seems to be present only in benign cystic nodules. Ahuja and colleagues[52] reviewed the histologies of 100 cystic nodules containing comet-tail artifact, and found they all represented benign hyperplastic (colloid) nodules. During the same time period, they found 70 malignancies on sonography and FNA, none of which were associated with the artifact (**Fig. 20**).

Vascularity

Almost all solid nodules display some flow on color Doppler interrogation with current generation ultrasound equipment. Initial optimism that color Doppler flow patterns could differentiate benign from malignant nodules quickly faded as larger studies were performed. In general, a peripheral flow pattern tends to be a feature of benign nodules, and malignant nodules tend to have internal vascularity (**Fig. 21**), but there is considerable overlap. Among 254 nodules biopsied by Frates and colleagues,[27] a pattern of marked internal vascularity was seen in 14 of 32 malignant nodules (42%) but also in 26 of 177 benign ones (14.7%). Although marked internal vascularity was more often present in malignant than benign nodules, more than half of nodules with internal hypervascularity were benign. Furthermore, 14% of their solid hypovascular nodules were malignant. Another series of 68 papillary thyroid cancers found that 19% were hypovascular.[4] In the study by Chan and colleagues,[26] 9.1% of 55 papillary cancers were hypovascular, but none were entirely

avascular. A cystic nodule without any internal flow therefore is unlikely to be a papillary carcinoma.

Shape and Margins

By analogy with breast carcinomas, Kim and colleagues[50] studied the shape of thyroid carcinomas and found that a shape taller than wide was 92.5% specific for malignancy (see **Fig. 11**). This feature had fairly low (32.7%) sensitivity, however, and was not definitively confirmed in a series by Iannuccilli and colleagues[25] The latter found only 2 "tall" nodules on retrospective review of 70 thyroid nodules (34 malignant and 36 benign), and both were benign. Spherical shape was also found to be predictive of malignancy in a study of 993 thyroid nodules that had undergone

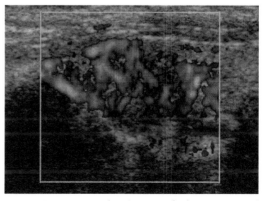

Fig. 21. Power Doppler image of chaotic internal vasculature in a papillary carcinoma.

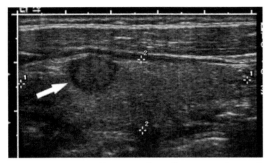

Fig. 22. Longitudinal image of small upper pole papillary carcinoma (*arrow*) with hypoechoic halo.

FNA. The overall rate of thyroid malignancy in their series was 11%, but the incidence in the most spherical nodules was 18% versus only 5% in the least spherical. In the same study, a ratio of long axis to short axis length of greater than 2.5 was 100% predictive of benignity, although this shape was relatively rare.[53]

A sonolucent halo, previously believed to be a feature of benign nodules, can be seen in 10% to 24% of papillary cancers (**Fig. 22**).[25,26,51] The finding of an irregular margin has widely varying sensitivity for malignancy (7% to 97%)[1,26,50,54] and the highest interobserver variability of several sonographic features (see **Fig. 11**).[41]

Local Invasion and Lymphadenopathy

Extension of a mass beyond the thyroid capsule into adjacent trachea or muscle is highly suggestive of an aggressive malignancy (see **Fig. 12**). Likewise, the presence of local lymphadenopathy with any suspicious features, such as rounded shape, loss of fatty hilum, cystic change, microcalcifications, or irregular internal hypervascularity, should prompt FNA of the node and any associated thyroid nodules.[3]

Multivariate Analyses

Clearly no single sonographic feature predicts malignancy, but some features are better than others. Microcalcifications are more commonly associated with papillary cancer than with benign disease and should trigger biopsy at relatively small nodule size. Several groups have tried to develop multivariate predictors of malignancy. Kim and colleagues[50] studied four predictors of malignancy in solid nodules—microcalcifications, irregular margins, hypoechogenicity, and shape more tall than wide—and performed FNA if any of these features were present. In their hands, this system yielded 93.8% sensitivity and 66% specificity with a positive predictive value of 56.1%. But in a follow-up study of 68 benign and 2 malignant nodules assessed using the same method, Wienke found that 69% of benign nodules had at least one finding associated with malignancy.[41] Finally, Koike and colleagues[54] devised a regression formula to predict malignancy using five sonographic features as variables—margin, shape, internal architecture, echogenicity, and calcification—and used it to predict malignancy in follicular and nonfollicular neoplasms. Using the model, the sensitivity of ultrasound was 86.5% for nonfollicular neoplasms, with specificity of 92.3%. Selecting a probability of malignancy of 0.2 with the regression formula yielded sensitivity of 94% and specificity of 87%. They found that

Table 2
Management recommendations for thyroid nodules 1 cm or larger in maximal diameter[1]

Sonographic Feature	Recommendation
Solitary nodule	
Microcalcifications	Strongly consider US-guided FNA if ≥1 cm
Solid or coarse calcification	Strongly consider US-guided FNA if ≥1.5 cm
Mixed cystic and solid or almost entirely cystic with solid mural component	Consider US-guided FNA if ≥2 cm
None of the above but substantial growth since prior US	Consider US-guided FNA
Almost completely cystic and without significant growth or features above	US-guided FNA probably not necessary
Multiple nodules	Consider US-guided FNA of one or more nodules, prioritizing selection based on criteria for solid nodules in order listed above

Abbreviation: US, ultrasound.

follicular neoplasms were not reliably assessed with their formula, however.

SELECTION CRITERIA FOR FINE NEEDLE ASPIRATION OF THYROID NODULES

Given the relative lack of specificity of many ultrasound findings of thyroid malignancy, it can be difficult to determine which nodules should undergo FNA. Guidelines for the selection of nodules for FNA is the subject of a separate article in this issue. Briefly, the recent consensus conference statement of the Society of Radiologists in Ultrasound provides recommendations for management of thyroid nodules 1 cm or larger in maximum diameter (**Table 2**), which are based on the predictive value of different sonographic features, with microcalcifications being most suspicious and a predominantly cystic appearance having least likelihood of malignancy.

SUMMARY

Thyroid nodules can be identified by ultrasound in almost half the adult population of the United States. Approximately 95% of these are benign, and most malignancies are indolent if not altogether clinically occult. Nevertheless, some malignant lesions can be associated with an aggressive course. Risk factors for malignancy include age younger than 20 or greater than 60 years, history of neck irradiation, and family history of thyroid cancer. No single ultrasound feature can distinguish benign from malignant nodules, but the presence of microcalcifications should prompt FNA at smaller nodule sizes than other features. FDG-avid thyroid nodules detected on PET scans performed for cancer staging in patients who have other primary malignancies have a high rate of malignancy and are more likely to represent thyroid carcinomas than metastatic disease. The presence of multiple nodules does not decrease the likelihood of malignancy, and the features of each nodule should be scrutinized to determine which nodules should undergo biopsy.

REFERENCES

1. Frates MC, Benson CB, Charboneau JW, et al. Management of thyroid nodules detected at US: society of radiologists in ultrasound consensus conference statement. Radiology 2005;237: 794–800.
2. Cooper DS, Doherty GM, Haugen BR, et al. Management guidelines for patients with thyroid nodules and differentiated thyroid cancer. Thyroid 2006;16: 109–42.
3. Gharib H, Papini E, Baskin H, et al. American Associazione di Clinical Endocrinologists and Associazione Medici Endocrinologi medical guidelines for clinical practice for the diagnosis and management of thyroid nodules. Endocr Pract 2006;12:63–78.
4. Bramley MD, Harrison BJ. Papillary microcarcinoma of the thyroid gland. Br J Surg 1996;83:1674–83.
5. Harach HR, Franssila KO, Wasenius VM. Occult papillary carcinoma of the thyroid. A "normal" finding in Finland. A systematic autopsy study. Cancer 1985;56:531–8.
6. Ito Y, Uruno T, Nakano K, et al. An observation trial without surgical treatment in patients with papillary microcarcinoma of the thyroid. Thyroid 2003;13:381–7.
7. Martinez-Tello FJ, Martinez-Cabruja R, Fernandez-Martin J, et al. Occult carcinoma of the thyroid. A systematic autopsy study from Spain of two series performed with two different methods. Cancer 1993;71:4022–9.
8. Ross DS. Nonpalpable thyroid nodules—managing an epidemic. J Clin Endocrinol Metab 2002;87: 1938–40.
9. Maitra A, Abbas A. The endocrine system. In: Kumar V, Fausto N, Abbas A, editors. Robbins & Cotran pathologic basis of disease. 7th edition. Philadelphia: Elsevier Saunders; 2004. p. 1155–226.
10. Lyshchik A, Drozd V, Schloegl S, et al. Three-dimensional ultrasonography for volume measurement of thyroid nodules in children. J Ultrasound Med 2004;23:247–54.
11. Hagel J, Bicknell SG. Impact of 3D sonography on workroom time efficiency. AJR Am J Roentgenol 2007;188:966–9.
12. Dahl JJ, Guenther DA, Trahey GE. Adaptive imaging and spatial compounding in the presence of aberration. IEEE Trans Ultrason Ferroelectr Freq Control 2005;52:1131–44.
13. Szopinski KT, Wysocki M, Pajk AM, et al. Tissue harmonic imaging of thyroid nodules: initial experience. J Ultrasound Med 2003;22:5–12.
14. Lyshchik A, Higashi T, Asato R, et al. Thyroid gland tumor diagnosis at US elastography. Radiology 2005;237:202–11.
15. Rago T, Santini F, Scutari M, et al. Elastography: new developments in ultrasound for predicting malignancy in thyroid nodules. J Clin Endocrinol Metab 2007;92(8):2917–22.
16. Bae U, Dighe M, Dubinsky T, et al. Ultrasound thyroid elastography using carotid artery pulsation: preliminary study. J Ultrasound Med 2007;26:797–805.
17. Tan GH, Gharib H. Thyroid incidentalomas: management approaches to nonpalpable nodules discovered incidentally on thyroid imaging. Ann Intern Med 1997;126:226–31.
18. Tessler FN, Tublin ME. Thyroid sonography: current applications and future directions. AJR Am J Roentgenol 1999;173:437–43.

19. Hegedus L, Gerber H, Bonnema SJ. Multinodular goiter. In: Degroot L, Jameson LJ, editors. Endocrinology. Philadelphia: Saunders; 2005. p. 2113–27.

20. Reading CC, Charboneau JW, Hay ID, et al. Sonography of thyroid nodules: a "classic pattern" diagnostic approach. Ultrasound Q 2005;21:157–65.

21. Davies L, Welch HG. Increasing incidence of thyroid cancer in the United States, 1973–2002. JAMA 2006;295:2164–7.

22. Malchoff CD. Oncogenes and tumor suppressor genes in thyroid nodules and nonmedullary thyroid cancer. Available at: http://www.uptodate.com. Accessed October 6, 2007.

23. Ross DS. Overview of thyroid nodule formation. Available at: www.uptodate.com. Accessed October 6, 2007.

24. Lee SL, Ananthakrishnan S. Overview of follicular thyroid cancer. Available at: http://www.uptodate.com. Accessed October 6, 2007.

25. Iannuccilli JD, Cronan JJ, Monchik JM. Risk for malignancy of thyroid nodules as assessed by sonographic criteria: the need for biopsy. J Ultrasound Med 2004;23:1455–64.

26. Chan BK, Desser TS, McDougall IR, et al. Common and uncommon sonographic features of papillary thyroid carcinoma. J Ultrasound Med 2003;22:1083–90.

27. Frates MC, Benson CB, Doubilet PM, et al. Can color Doppler sonography aid in the prediction of malignancy of thyroid nodules? J Ultrasound Med 2003;22:127–31, quiz 132–4.

28. Rago T, Vitti P, Chiovato L, et al. Role of conventional ultrasonography and color flow-Doppler sonography in predicting malignancy in "cold" thyroid nodules. Eur J Endocrinol 1998;138:41–6.

29. Shimamoto K, Endo T, Ishigaki T, et al. Thyroid nodules: evaluation with color Doppler ultrasonography. J Ultrasound Med 1993;12:673–8.

30. Schlumberger M, Caillou B. Miscellaneous tumors of the thyroid. In: Braverman LE, Utiger RD, editors. Werner and Ingbar's the thyroid: a fundamental and clinical text. 7th edition. Philadelphia: Lippincott-Raven; 1996. p. 961–5.

31. Ball DW, Baylin SB, de Bustros AC. Medullary thyroid carcinoma. In: Braverman LE, Utiger RD, editors. Werner and Ingbar's the thyroid: a fundamental and clinical text. 7th edition. Philadelphia: Lippincott-Raven; 1996. p. 946–60.

32. Sherman SI. Clinical manifestations and staging of medullary thyroid carcinoma. Available at: http://www.uptodate.com. Accessed October 6, 2007.

33. Papi G, Fadda G, Corsello SM, et al. Metastases to the thyroid gland: prevalence, clinicopathological aspects and prognosis: a 10-year experience. Clin Endocrinol (Oxf) 2007;66:565–71.

34. Bogsrud TV, Karantanis D, Nathan MA, et al. The value of quantifying 18F-FDG uptake in thyroid nodules found incidentally on whole-body PET-CT. Nucl Med Commun 2007;28:373–81.

35. Van den Bruel A, Maes A, De Potter T, et al. Clinical relevance of thyroid fluorodeoxyglucose-whole body positron emission tomography incidentaloma. J Clin Endocrinol Metab 2002;87:1517–20.

36. Are C, Hsu JF, Schoder H, et al. FDG-PET detected thyroid incidentalomas: need for further investigation? Ann Surg Oncol 2007;14:239–47.

37. Choi JY, Lee KS, Kim HJ, et al. Focal thyroid lesions incidentally identified by integrated 18F-FDG PET/CT: clinical significance and improved characterization. J Nucl Med 2006;47:609–15.

38. Cohen MS, Arslan N, Dehdashti F, et al. Risk of malignancy in thyroid incidentalomas identified by fluorodeoxyglucose-positron emission tomography. Surgery 2001;130:941–6.

39. Kang KW, Kim SK, Kang HS, et al. Prevalence and risk of cancer of focal thyroid incidentaloma identified by 18F-fluorodeoxyglucose positron emission tomography for metastasis evaluation and cancer screening in healthy subjects. J Clin Endocrinol Metab 2003;88:4100–4.

40. Yi JG, Marom EM, Munden RF, et al. Focal uptake of fluorodeoxyglucose by the thyroid in patients undergoing initial disease staging with combined PET/CT for non-small cell lung cancer. Radiology 2005;236:271–5.

41. Wienke JR, Chong WK, Fielding JR, et al. Sonographic features of benign thyroid nodules: interobserver reliability and overlap with malignancy. J Ultrasound Med 2003;22:1027–31.

42. Papini E, Guglielmi R, Bianchini A, et al. Risk of malignancy in nonpalpable thyroid nodules: predictive value of ultrasound and color-Doppler features. J Clin Endocrinol Metab 2002;87:1941–6.

43. Frates MC, Benson CB, Doubilet PM, et al. Likelihood of thyroid cancer based on sonographic assessment of nodule size and composition. Presented at the Radiological society of North America scientific assembly and annual meeting program. Chicago, November 28–December 3, 2004.

44. Utiger RD. The multiplicity of thyroid nodules and carcinomas. N Engl J Med 2005;352:2376–8.

45. Brander AE, Viikinkoski VP, Nickels JI, et al. Importance of thyroid abnormalities detected at US screening: a 5-year follow-up. Radiology 2000;215:801–6.

46. Alexander EK, Hurwitz S, Heering JP, et al. Natural history of benign solid and cystic thyroid nodules. Ann Intern Med 2003;138:315–8.

47. Cheng SP, Lee JJ, Lin J, et al. Eggshell calcification in follicular thyroid carcinoma. Eur Radiol 2005;15:1773–4.

48. Hegedus L. Clinical practice. The thyroid nodule. N Engl J Med 2004;351:1764–71.

49. Jun P, Chow LC, Jeffrey RB. The sonographic features of papillary thyroid carcinomas: pictorial essay. Ultrasound Q 2005;21:39–45.

50. Kim EK, Park CS, Chung WY, et al. New sonographic criteria for recommending fine-needle aspiration biopsy of nonpalpable solid nodules of the thyroid. AJR Am J Roentgenol 2002;178:687–91.

51. Watters DA, Ahuja AT, Evans RM, et al. Role of ultrasound in the management of thyroid nodules. Am J Surg 1992;164:654–7.

52. Ahuja A, Chick W, King W, et al. Clinical significance of the comet-tail artifact in thyroid ultrasound. J Clin Ultrasound 1996;24:129–33.

53. Alexander EK, Marqusee E, Orcutt J, et al. Thyroid nodule shape and prediction of malignancy. Thyroid 2004;14:953–8.

54. Koike E, Noguchi S, Yamashita H, et al. Ultrasonographic characteristics of thyroid nodules: prediction of malignancy. Arch Surg 2001;136:334–7.

Sonographic Imaging of Cervical Lymph Nodes in Patients with Thyroid Cancer

Jill E. Langer, MD[a,*], Susan J. Mandel, MD, MPH[b]

KEYWORDS

- Ultrasound • Thyroid cancer • Lymph nodes

Sonographic evaluation of the neck plays an important role in the evaluation of patients who have thyroid carcinoma at the time of initial diagnosis and in the assessment of recurrent disease. Most patients diagnosed with differentiated thyroid cancer have lesions that are confined to the thyroid or are minimally invasive into the adjacent soft tissues of the neck, yet often these cancers have already metastasized to the regional cervical nodes.[1,2] Sonography has been established as the most sensitive imaging test to diagnose these nodal metastases.[3–7] Detection of metastatic cervical lymph nodes by sonography at the time of initial presentation may alter the surgical approach to include a modified lateral neck dissection at the time of thyroidectomy.[4,8–10] Ultrasonography of the neck also offers an inexpensive and readily available means to detect recurrent thyroid cancer following thyroidectomy. Furthermore, when abnormalities are identified by neck sonography, they can be biopsied under direct sonographic visualization.[3,11]

ANATOMY

It is helpful for the imager evaluating the patient for metastatic thyroid cancer to have familiarity with the nomenclature used to describe the location of cervical nodes. The classic description of nodal location based on superficial anatomic landmarks has been replaced by imaging-based classifications.[12,13] The cervical lymph node classification most widely used by clinicians who specialize in head and neck cancer is that established by The American Joint Committee on Cancer Staging and the American Academy of Otolaryngology–Head and Neck Surgery, which groups the cervical nodes by regions (levels) to more closely reflect the clinical staging of head and neck tumors. Level I refers to nodes in the submental and submandibular regions. Levels II, III, and IV refer to nodes along the anterior cervical and internal jugular chains. Level II encompasses those nodes from the base of the skull to the lower border of the hyoid bone, Level III from the hyoid to the lower margin of the cricoid cartilage, and level IV from the cricoid to the clavicle. Level V nodes are those in the posterior compartment of the neck, along the course of the spinal accessory nerve, and are divided into upper (VA) and lower (VB) levels by the cricoid cartilage. Level VI nodes, the paratracheal nodes, are in the visceral or central compartment of the neck. This compartment extends from the hyoid bone superiorly to the suprasternal notch inferiorly. On each side of the neck, the lateral border of the central neck compartment is formed by the medial border of the carotid sheath. Level VII nodes are in the superior mediastinum (**Fig. 1**).

This article originally appeared in *Neuroimaging Clinics of North America* 2008;18(3):479–489

[a] Department of Radiology, University of Pennsylvania School of Medicine, Hospital of the University of Pennsylvania, 3400 Spruce Street, Philadelphia, PA 19104, USA

[b] Division of Endocrinology, Diabetes, and Metabolism, Department of Medicine, University of Pennsylvania School of Medicine, 700 CRB, 415 Curie Boulevard, Philadelphia, PA 19104, USA

* Corresponding author.

E-mail address: jill.langer@uphs.upenn.edu (J.E. Langer).

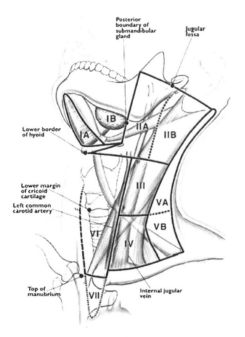

TECHNIQUE

In general, higher-frequency, linear transducers offer the best spatial resolution, whereas lower frequencies give better tissue penetration of the emitted sound waves. Because the findings of metastatic thyroid cancer may be subtle, the examination should be performed with the highest frequency possible. The superficial neck nodes should be evaluated with a linear, high-frequency transducer of at least 7.5 MHz, preferably greater than 10 MHz.[14] Evaluation of the deep lymph nodes of the neck and the superior mediastinal nodes may require a lower frequency (5 to 7.5 MHz), small footprint curvilinear or sector probe that allows deeper sound penetration and can be positioned in the narrow suprasternal notch. Transducers with color Doppler capability are also preferred because assessment of the vascularity of lymph nodes is often helpful in identifying metastatic disease.

The patient should be in a supine position, with a pillow or rolled towel under the upper back to allow maximal extension of the neck. This technique is particularly important to examine the lower level IV and level VI nodes and the upper mediastinum. The examination should be systematic, imaging all the lymph node levels in the transverse plane. The longitudinal plane should also be used to examine levels II through V. Gray-scale sonography is used to identify the size, shape, and nodal architecture. Color Doppler sonography, or the more sensitive power Doppler sonography, is then performed to assess the presence and distribution of intranodular vessels.[15–18]

NORMAL LYMPH NODES

Normal cervical lymph nodes are typically imaged during high-frequency sonography examination of the neck. Normal nodes are most commonly seen in the submandibular region, the upper cervical chain, and the posterior triangle (Levels IB, II, III, and V, respectively).[19,20] There is a tendency for nodes to be larger with advancing age, perhaps because of increased fat deposition.[20] The normal node is typically flat, oval, or kidney bean shaped (**Fig. 2**). Nodes in the submandibular region and

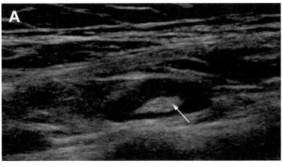
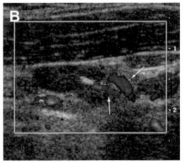

Fig. 2. Normal lateral cervical lymph nodes. (*A*) Sagittal view of a mid cervical lymph node (level III) demonstrates the sonographic appearance of a normal lymph node with a uniformly hypoechoic periphery and a central echogenic hilum (*arrow*). (*B*) Transverse color Doppler shows central vascularity within the feeding artery and vein (*arrow*) entering the hilum.

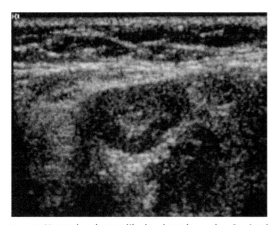

Fig. 3. Normal submandibular lymph node. Sagittal view of a submandibular (level IB) node demonstrates a rounded configuration but normal echogenic hilum. Although a rounded shape may raise concern for nodal pathology, submandibular nodes maybe rounded in the absence of pathology.

parotid region may be rounded without underlying pathology (**Fig. 3**). Each lymph node is encased in a dense connective tissue known as the capsule. The periphery of the lymph node is known as the cortex and contains most of the lymphoid follicles. This dominant portion of the lymph node is typically hypoechoic, less commonly isoechoic to the surrounding soft tissues.[14,19] The inner part of the node or the medulla is made up of fluid-filled sinuses and medullary cords from which the lymph flows from the afferent lymphatic vessels into the node. The feeding artery and vein are located in the hilum of the node along with the efferent draining lymphatic vessels.[15–17] On sonography, the central nodal hilus is typically an echogenic structure caused by sound reflecting off the multiple fluid-filled sinuses.[15,21,22] Normal nodes typically demonstrate only hilar vessels or are avascular,

with the ability to detect vascularity by sonography paralleling the size of the node **Figure 2**.[15,16]

METASTATIC LYMPH NODES

Various sonographic features have been described to aid in the differentiation of metastatic lymph nodes from normal ones, including increased lymph node size, rounded shape, absence of the echogenic hilus, hyper echogenicity, cystic change, presence of calcifications, and increased vascularity. Cervical lymph node size is unreliable as the sole criterion of metastatic thyroid carcinoma because hyperplastic nodes may be large and metastatic nodes may be normal in size (**Fig. 4**).[7,23,24] In general, lymph nodes are considered to be enlarged when the short axis exceeds 8 mm in the submandibular region (Level II) and 5 mm in other cervical regions.[25,26] Malignant infiltration typically transforms nodes from an oval to a rounded shape (**Fig. 5**). This change in shape is quantified by an increase in the short axis/long axis (S:L) ratio to a value greater than 0.5 (**Figs. 5, 6**).[14,24,27,28] An elevated S:L ratio carries a false-positive rate of approximately 10% to 15%, however, reflecting the common occurrence of lateral cervical node enlargement attributable to benign inflammatory conditions of the oropharynx,[29,30] and a false-negative rate of 20% reflecting the propensity for microscopic nodal metastases to occur without enlarging the node, particularly with papillary thyroid carcinomas.[1,2]

Absence of the echogenic hilus of a lymph node raises concern for tumor infiltration, obliterating the central sinuses[14,21,31] and has been reported to carry a positive predictive value of 92% for the presence of metastatic thyroid cancer (see **Fig. 6**).[30] It is worth noting that the detection of a normal hilum does not exclude metastatic

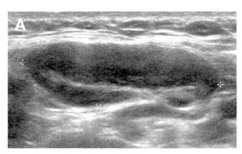
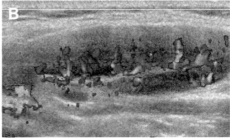

Fig. 4. Hyperplastic lymph node. (*A*) Sagittal gray-scale image of a 2.2 cm long level IIA node in a 22-year-old patient who had a history of thyroid cancer. Although the node is enlarged, the sonographic morphology was otherwise normal with a uniformly hypoechoic periphery and a regular, linear central echogenic hilum. (*B*) Color Doppler image of this node shows slightly increased central flow. Fine needle aspiration of this node demonstrated only reactive hyperplasia.

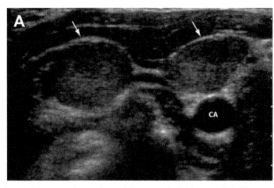
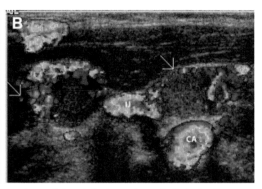

Fig. 5. Metastatic nodes with rounded shape. (A) Transverse view of the right lateral cervical chain shows two abnormal lymph nodes (arrows) that are rounded without a visible echogenic hilum. (B) Both nodes show marked periphery vascularity on color Doppler examination.

disease to that node.[14] The hilar vessels may still be identified with color or power Doppler sonography even in the setting of a non-visualized hilum secondary to metastatic disease.[15,18] Malignant nodes may demonstrate abnormal vascular patterns, including increased peripheral or capsular flow either diffusely or focally, with or without increased central vascularity.[7,15] Tumor deposits within a node may displace hilar vessels, produce avascular areas, or demonstrate focal regions with tortuous and aberrant vessels.[15,18] These vascular patterns help to differentiate metastatic nodes from enlarged hyperplastic nodes, which tend to preserve nodal architecture with only increased central flow (see Fig. 4).

Hyperechogenicity, calcifications, and cystic change are features that highly predict the presence of metastatic thyroid cancer, particularly papillary thyroid cancer to affected nodes. Hyperechogenicity of a node relative to the adjacent musculature is a finding noted in up to 86% of metastatic lymph nodes from papillary thyroid cancer and is a rarely noted in benign nodes.[7,27,28,30] The increased echogenicity is believed to be secondary to malignant follicular cells and colloid deposition within the metastatic node, which alters the normal hypoechoic appearance of cortex to the increased echogenicity typical of thyroid tissue (Fig. 7).[30] Initially the metastatic tumor deposits may be noted as tiny, focal hyperechoic regions in the periphery of the node or near the hilum. The sonographic detection of these often subtle metastatic foci to otherwise normal-appearing nodes can be improved by the use of color Doppler examination, which demonstrates focal increased vascularity in the suspect areas (Fig. 8). As the node becomes progressively infiltrated with tumor, it demonstrates more diffuse regions of hyperechogenicity and increased vascularity, and typically other features of

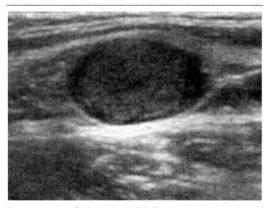

Fig. 6. Lack of the normal hilum. Sagittal view of a right lateral lymph node shows absence of the normal fatty hilum. Additionally this node is rounded in configuration and measured 8 × 14 mm for an S:L ratio of 0.57.

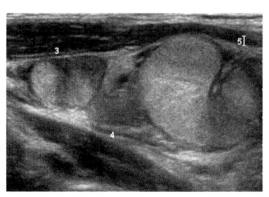

Fig. 7. Hyperechoic lymph nodes. Multiple enlarged and hyperechoic lateral cervical lymph nodes are seen (numbers 3–5) on this sagittal view of the left lateral neck in this 36-year-old patient who had metastatic follicular variant of papillary cancer.

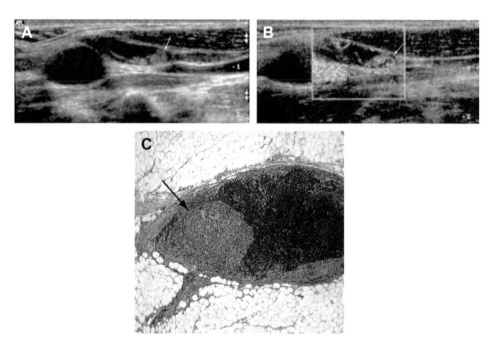

Fig. 8. Small hyperechoic foci. (A) Sagittal view of a lateral cervical lymph node demonstrates a subtle region of hyperechogenicity in the lower aspect of this node (arrow) corresponding to a small metastatic focus. (B) Color vascular examination shows focally increased flow in the same region (arrow). Fine needle aspiration of the focal area was positive for papillary thyroid carcinoma. (C) Pathology specimen obtained from a different patient shows a metastatic focus (arrow) of thyroid cancer within the periphery of the otherwise normal node. (Courtesy of Dr Zubair Baloch, Philadelphia, PA.)

metastatic disease, such as enlarged size, rounded shape, obliteration of the hilum, calcifications, and cystic necrosis.[7]

Intranodal calcifications have been noted in 46% to 69% of metastatic nodes from papillary thyroid carcinoma (Fig. 9).[7,30,32] Although intranodal calcifications may be seen in nodes affected by tuberculosis, sarcoidosis, and following radiotherapy, they are rare in non-thyroid metastases.[27]

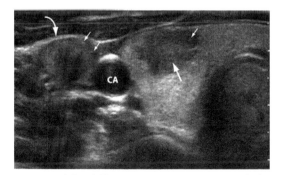

Fig. 9. Nodal calcifications. Transverse view of the right lobe of the thyroid shows a 1.5-cm papillary thyroid cancer (large arrow) that contains subtle punctuate microcalcifications (small arrow). A metastatic right lateral cervical lymph node (curved arrow) lateral to the carotid artery (CA) is also seen to contain these calcifications (small arrows).

The calcifications are typically fine or punctate and are located in the periphery of the node.[27,30]

Perhaps the most specific feature of metastatic papillary thyroid cancer is the tendency of these nodes to undergo cystic degeneration. Affected nodes may contain a small solitary cystic area or multiple scattered cystic areas, or may undergo near complete replacement of the parenchyma by cystic fluid.[7,27,33–35] Often another characteristic feature, such as calcifications, increased echogenicity, or increased vascularity, is noted with the solid component of partially cystic nodes (Fig. 10).[7] In some patients, particularly children, cystic nodal metastases may become large or may be the sole presentation of the underlying malignancy.[34,35] These cystic metastases should be differentiated from branchial cleft cysts, which are rare and tend to occur just medial to the border of the sternocleidomastoid muscle in the upper neck, whereas cystic nodes are more common in the lower neck. In confusing cases, aspiration of the lesion for cytologic evaluation and thyroglobulin assay is recommended.[29,33,34]

EVALUATION OF THE POST-THYROIDECTOMY BED

Following near-total thyroidectomy and remnant ablation, only a minimal amount of echogenic tissue, likely reflecting a combination of normal

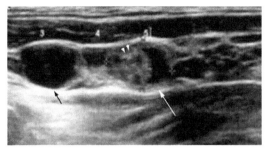

Fig. 10. Cystic nodes. Sagittal view of the right neck shows a chain of metastatic lymph nodes with varying degrees of cystic change. The most superior node (*short black arrow*) is nearly entirely cystic. The most inferior node (*long white arrow*) has both cystic regions and solid elements that contain calcifications.

connective tissue and scar tissue, is noted in the thyroidectomy bed (**Fig. 11**). Recurrent thyroid cancer in the bed typically appears as a solid or mixed cystic and solid soft tissue mass, often with marked vascularity (**Fig. 12**).[3,11,36] If large masses or posteriorly positioned masses are noted in the central compartment of the neck, cross-sectional imaging with CT or MR may be necessary to evaluate for invasive disease into the trachea, esophagus, retropharyngeal space, or skull base, because sonography is limited in evaluating these areas.[29,37] Following thyroidectomy, metastatic disease to the paratracheal lymph nodes can be detected by identifying enlarged, cystic, calcified, or vascular paratracheal lymph nodes (**Figs. 13 and 14**).

MIMICS OF RECURRENT DISEASE

Various benign soft tissue findings may be noted in the postoperative neck that may be confused with

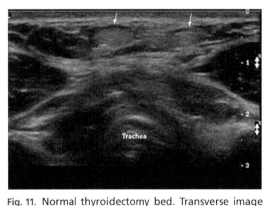

Fig. 11. Normal thyroidectomy bed. Transverse image at the level of the thyroid cartilage shows a small amount of heterogeneous soft tissue in the thyroidectomy bed. There are echogenic areas in the overlying musculature (*arrow*) consistent with expected postoperative change.

metastatic disease. Often the sternocleidomastoid muscle is partially resected causing it to have irregular echogenic regions representing scar often with fatty atrophy. The geometric shape, absence of vascular flow, and location of the echogenic areas in the muscle belly may be helpful features in minimizing concern that the soft tissue abnormalities reflect recurrent disease (see **Fig. 11**).

Other benign focal nonmalignant soft tissue lesions detected by sonography include foreign body granulomas and postoperative neuromas.[38,39] Granulomas may form in the operative bed because of foreign body reaction to suture material or as a nonspecific inflammatory response.[39] Some may have a characteristic appearance of a hypoechoic solid lesion with central curvilinear lines representing the suture material or a complex cystic lesion.[38,39] These granulomas are typically avascular or may be minimally vascular in the periphery and often are relatively superficial in location or within the sternocleidomastoid muscle (**Fig. 15**). Some granulomas require fine needle aspiration (FNA) to exclude a postoperative abscess or recurrence.

Approximately 1% to 2% of patients may develop a traumatic neuroma following neck dissection. Typically these are firm subcutaneous nodules located near the second cranial nerve.[40] About 40% of patients note characteristic sensitivity or pain during palpation of the lesion; in others, the diagnosis is presumptively established when exquisite pain is produced during attempted biopsy to exclude malignancy. These lesions tend to be long and narrow (low S:L ratio) and are solid with minimal vascularity. Similar to granulomas, they often have a central hyperechoic focus, which corresponds to dense collagenous material. Another feature that is helpful in the distinction of these lesions from lymphadenopathy is the their location posterior to but not immediately adjacent to the carotid artery (**Fig. 16**).[40]

The cervical esophagus, which lies posterior to the thyroid, or a pharyngoesophageal diverticulum, which most commonly occurs at the level of thyroid, may be noted during neck sonography.[41,42] Although air within the esophagus may be echogenic with shadowing and simulate a calcified lesion, the real-time examination demonstrates these foci to be mobile pockets of air within the esophagus particularly during swallowing (**Fig. 17**).

ULTRASOUND-GUIDED FINE NEEDLE ASPIRATION

Ultrasound-guided FNA of abnormal-appearing lymph nodes or other soft tissue abnormalities in

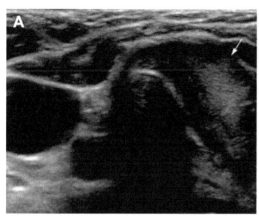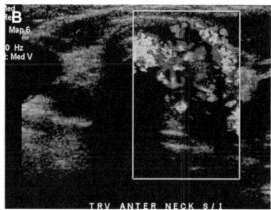

Fig. 12. Central neck recurrence. (A) Transverse image of the thyroidectomy bed shows a hypoechoic soft tissue mass (arrow) in the left bed representing recurrence at the site of tumor resection in this 42-year-old who had positive tumor margins. (B) Color Doppler image shows marked vascularity within the mass.

the neck may be necessary to document the presence of metastatic disease to one or more compartments of the neck. Ultrasound-guided FNA is typically performed with a 25-gauge needle using real-time ultrasound monitoring and aseptic technique, similar to FNA of thyroid nodules.[43] One or more passes can be performed into the node targeting the most suspicious-appearing region. The reported sensitivities for this technique range from 80% to 90%.[44,45] Nondiagnostic aspirates are most common in predominantly cystic nodes and those with a small burden of metastatic disease. In these patients, the sample can be analyzed for the presence of thyroglobulin, a protein produced only by thyroid tissue and most thyroid cancers. The presence of thyroglobulin within an FNA specimen the presence of metastatic disease to that node.[46]

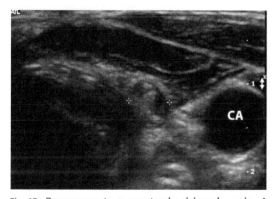

Fig. 13. Recurrence to a paratracheal lymph node. A calcified 5-mm lymph node, surgically proved to be a metastatic paratracheal node, was the only region of recurrence in this 37-year-old woman. CA, common carotid artery.

CLINICAL SCENARIOS FOR ULTRASOUND LYMPH NODE EVALUATION
Preoperatively

Imaging of the neck before surgery for thyroid carcinoma is necessary to determine the appropriate extent of surgical resection. In patients who present with symptoms such as hoarseness, airway compromise, or a rapidly enlarging neck mass, cross-sectional imaging may be necessary to assess for invasion of the tumor into the trachea, esophagus, and adjacent soft tissue structures.[37] Fortunately the vast majority of patients have less aggressive lesions that are confined to the thyroid or have limited extension into the adjacent soft tissue, often with regional lymph node metastases. Sonography has been established as the most sensitive imaging test to diagnose these nodal metastases.[3-7]

At initial diagnosis of differentiated thyroid cancer (DTC), up to 30% of patients have lymph node metastases detected by palpation or imaging.[47,48] Lymph node metastases are noted in up to 60% of patients on histologic review in centers performing ipsilateral and central neck dissections in all patients.[1,8,49] Palpation alone of the lateral neck compartments is not adequate and does not substitute for sonographic evaluation. Although the thyroid itself limits sonographic visualization of central neck lymph nodes before thyroidectomy, the lateral neck compartments can be assessed. In a recent series, ultrasound evaluation identified nonpalpable lateral compartment lymph nodes in 14% of patients undergoing initial surgery.[10] Even when lymph nodes were palpable, sonographic assessment of the extent of lymph node involvement altered 40% of the operative procedures by changing the extent of

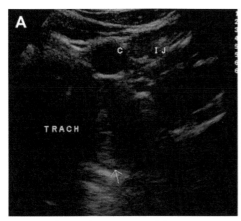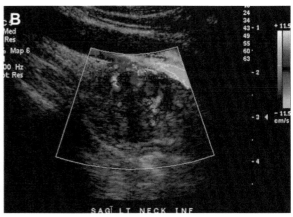

Fig. 14. Mediastinal recurrence. (A) Transverse image of the superior mediastinum obtained by using a curved 8-MHz transducer in the suprasternal notch detected this 2-cm soft tissue mass immediately adjacent to the trachea. (B) Sagittal color image demonstrates marked vascularity to this metastatic level VII node. C, carotid artery; IJ, internal jugular vein.

resection.[9,10] At the time of initial surgery, metastatic lateral lymph nodes are usually located ipsilateral to the primary tumor.[1,8] In fact, if a cancer is unilateral, it is unusual (18%) to have contralateral involvement of the lateral neck compartment.[1] Modified lateral neck dissection in these patients who have clinical (palpation or ultrasound) evidence of lateral lymph node metastases improves survival.[48] Before thyroidectomy, therefore, sonographic evaluation of the lateral compartment and the central compartment as limited by the thyroid is recommended by the recently published guidelines of the American Thyroid Association and the American Association of Clinical Endocrinologists.[50,51]

Surveillance for Recurrent Disease

The primary goal of follow-up in patients who have DTC is the early discovery of recurrent disease. The overall risk for local recurrence of papillary thyroid cancer, either in cervical lymph nodes or in the thyroid bed, is up to 30%.[47] Most recurrences appear in the first decade after initial therapy; however, a small number emerge decades after diagnosis.

In the past, a radioiodine whole-body scan was considered the main tool for disease detection during surveillance, but this has recently been discredited because of failure to identify metastatic lymph nodes even when documented by

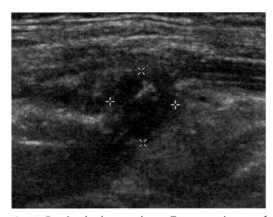

Fig. 15. Foreign body granuloma. Transverse image of the left neck showed this soft tissue lesion with a markedly echogenic central focus in the superficial tissues of the left neck (marked by electronic calipers). Although the fine needle aspiration was negative for malignancy, the patient underwent resection of this lesion, which proved to be a granuloma.

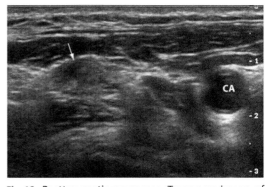

Fig. 16. Posttraumatic neuromas. Transverse image of the right lateral neck in a 53-year-old man who had a history of papillary thyroid cancer and previous right lateral neck dissection shows a heterogeneous soft tissue abnormality (arrow) remote from the carotid artery (CA). The patient experienced a sharp and radiating pain when FNA was attempted. It has been stable for more than 4 years and is presumed neuroma.

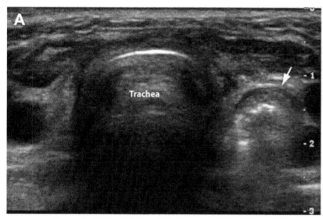
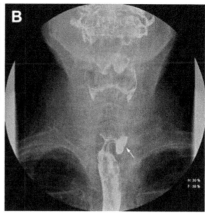

Fig. 17. Esophageal diverticulum. (A) Transverse view of the neck in a 70-year-old woman who had an undetect-able serum thyroglobulin 3 years after thyroidectomy. A rounded, air-containing soft tissue structure was noted just lateral to the trachea (arrow). (B) Frontal radiograph from a barium swallow confirms the presence of an esophageal diverticulum immediately adjacent to the trachea.

ultrasound.[52] For patients who have undetectable serum thyroglobulin levels on levothyroxine suppression, the combination of a detectable stimulated serum thyroglobulin level with neck sonography identifies 95% of patients who have metastatic lymph nodes and has a negative predictive value of 99%.[5,53,54] The American Thyroid Association guidelines therefore support the use of only stimulated thyroglobulin and cervical ultrasound rather than the use of radioio-dine scanning for surveillance in low-risk patients who have DTC.[50]

The timing and interval for performance of neck ultrasound depend on the risk status of the patient. The American Thyroid Association DTC guidelines suggest that "cervical ultrasound to evaluate the thyroid bed and central and lateral cervical nodal compartments should be performed at 6 and 12 months and then annually for at least 3 to 5 years, depending on the patient's risk for recurrent disease and thyroglobulin status."[50] If the serum thyroglobulin level remains detectable and other structural body imaging is negative, cervical ultra-sound should continue to be done on regular interval. If the stimulated serum thyroglobulin level is undetectable and a cervical ultrasound is nega-tive, however, the usefulness of subsequent ultra-sound imaging is low.[55]

The distribution of persistent or recurrent lymph node metastases is most commonly the central compartment (35%–50%), followed by the ipsilat-eral lateral neck (20%–30%). Only rarely (8%–15%) is the contralateral lateral neck area involved.[8,9] Within the levels of the lateral neck, a recent study reported that the pattern of meta-static lymph node involvement was 50% for levels II and III, 40% for level IV, and only 20% for level

V.[56] Palpation is insensitive for detection of recur-rent or residual disease and sonographic identifi-cation of nonpalpable metastatic lymph nodes alters the extent of surgical resection in up to 70% of patients undergoing reoperation.[9,10]

SUMMARY

Sonography has been established as the most sensitive imaging modality to assess the neck for metastatic thyroid carcinoma. Lymph node metas-tases may vary from subtle alterations in echoge-nicity or vascular patterns to more obvious findings of calcifications and cystic changes within an affected node. Identification of metastatic disease by sonography may affect the extent of surgical resection at the time of diagnosis. Sono-graphic surveillance and sonographic-guided FNA offers to the ability to detect and document early thyroid cancer recurrence in the neck.

REFERENCES

1. Mirallie E, Visset J, Sagan C, et al. Localization of cervical node metastasis of papillary thyroid carci-noma. World J Surg 1999;23(9):970–3 [discussion: 973–4].
2. Mazzaferri EL, Kloos RT. Clinical review 128: current approaches to primary therapy for papillary and follicular thyroid cancer. J Clin Endocrinol Metab 2001;86(4):1447–63.
3. Antonelli A, Miccoli P, Ferdeghini M, et al. Role of neck ultrasonography in the follow-up of patients operated on for thyroid cancer. Thyroid 1995;5(1):25–8.
4. Schlumberger M, Berg G, Cohen O, et al. Follow-up of low-risk patients with differentiated thyroid

carcinoma: a European perspective. Eur J Endocrinol 2004;150(2):105–12.

5. Torlontano M, Attard M, Crocetti U, et al. Follow-up of low risk patients with papillary thyroid cancer: role of neck ultrasonography in detecting lymph node metastases. J Clin Endocrinol Metab 2004;89(7):3402–7.

6. Torlontano M, Crocetti U, Augello G, et al. Comparative evaluation of recombinant human thyrotropin-stimulated thyroglobulin levels, 131I whole-body scintigraphy, and neck ultrasonography in the follow-up of patients with papillary thyroid microcarcinoma who have not undergone radioiodine therapy. J Clin Endocrinol Metab 2006;91(1):60–3.

7. Leboulleux S, Girard E, Rose M, et al. Ultrasound criteria of malignancy for cervical lymph nodes in patients followed up for differentiated thyroid cancer. J Clin Endocrinol Metab 2007;92(9):3590–4.

8. Machens A, Hinze R, Thomusch O, et al. Pattern of nodal metastasis for primary and reoperative thyroid cancer. World J Surg 2002;26(1):22–8.

9. Kouvaraki MA, Shapiro SE, Fornage BD, et al. Role of preoperative ultrasonography in the surgical management of patients with thyroid cancer. Surgery 2003;134(6):946–55.

10. Stulak JM, Grant CS, Farley DR, et al. Value of preoperative ultrasonography in the surgical management of initial and reoperative papillary thyroid cancer. Arch Surg 2006;141(5):489–96.

11. Sutton RT, Reading CC, Charboneau JW, et al. US-guided biopsy of neck masses in postoperative management of patients with thyroid cancer. Radiology 1988;168(3):769–72.

12. Som PM, Curtin HD, Mancuso AA. An imaging-based classification for the cervical nodes designed as an adjunct to recent clinically based nodal classifications. Arch Otolaryngol Head Neck Surg 1999;125(4):388–96.

13. Som PM, Curtin HD, Mancuso AA. Imaging-based nodal classification for evaluation of neck metastatic adenopathy. AJR Am J Roentgenol 2000;174(3):837–44.

14. Vassallo P, Wernecke K, Roos N, et al. Differentiation of benign from malignant superficial lymphadenopathy: the role of high-resolution US. Radiology 1992;183(1):215–20.

15. Ahuja A, Ying M, King A, et al. Lymph node hilus: gray scale and power Doppler sonography of cervical nodes. J Ultrasound Med 2001;20(9):987–92, quiz 994.

16. Ying M, Ahuja A, Brook F, et al. Power Doppler sonography of normal cervical lymph nodes. J Ultrasound Med 2000;19(8):511–7.

17. Ahuja AT, Ying M, Ho SS, et al. Distribution of intra-nodal vessels in differentiating benign from metastatic neck nodes. Clin Radiol 2001;56(3):197–201.

18. Wu CH, Chang YL, Hsu WC, et al. Usefulness of Doppler spectral analysis and power Doppler

sonography in the differentiation of cervical lymphadenopathies. AJR Am J Roentgenol 1998;171(2):503–9.

19. Ying M, Ahuja A, Brook F, et al. Sonographic appearance and distribution of normal cervical lymph nodes in a Chinese population. J Ultrasound Med 1996;15(6):431–6.

20. Ying M, Ahuja A, Brook F. Sonographic appearances of cervical lymph nodes: variations by age and sex. J Clin Ultrasound 2002;30(1):1–11.

21. Rubaltelli L, Proto E, Salmaso R, et al. Sonography of abnormal lymph nodes in vitro: correlation of sonographic and histologic findings. AJR Am J Roentgenol 1990;155(6):1241–4.

22. Bruneton JN, Balu-Maestro C, Marcy PY, et al. Very high frequency (13 MHz) ultrasonographic examination of the normal neck: detection of normal lymph nodes and thyroid nodules. J Ultrasound Med 1994;13(2):87–90.

23. van den Brekel MW, Stel HV, Castelijns JA, et al. Cervical lymph node metastasis: assessment of radiologic criteria. Radiology 1990;177(2):379–84.

24. Ying M, Ahuja A, Metreweli C. Diagnostic accuracy of sonographic criteria for evaluation of cervical lymphadenopathy. J Ultrasound Med 1998;17(7):437–45.

25. Bruneton JN, Roux P, Caramella E, et al. Ear, nose, and throat cancer: ultrasound diagnosis of metastasis to cervical lymph nodes. Radiology 1984;152(3):771–3.

26. Ying M, Ahuja A. Sonography of neck lymph nodes. Part I: normal lymph nodes. Clin Radiol 2003;58(5):351–8.

27. Ahuja A, Ying M. Sonography of neck lymph nodes. Part II: abnormal lymph nodes. Clin Radiol 2003;58(5):359–66.

28. Ahuja AT, Chow L, Chick W, et al. Metastatic cervical nodes in papillary carcinoma of the thyroid: ultrasound and histological correlation. Clin Radiol 1995;50(4):229–31.

29. Gor DM, Langer JE, Loevner LA. Imaging of cervical lymph nodes in head and neck cancer: the basics. Radiol Clin North Am 2006;44(1):101–10, viii.

30. Rosario PW, de Faria S, Bicalho L, et al. Ultrasonographic differentiation between metastatic and benign lymph nodes in patients with papillary thyroid carcinoma. J Ultrasound Med 2005;24(10):1385–9.

31. Chan BK, Desser TS, McDougall IR, et al. Common and uncommon sonographic features of papillary thyroid carcinoma. J Ultrasound Med 2003;22(10):1083–90.

32. Kuna SK, Bracic I, Tesic V, et al. Ultrasonographic differentiation of benign from malignant neck lymphadenopathy in thyroid cancer. J Ultrasound Med 2006;25(12):1531–7, quiz 1538–40.

33. Kessler A, Rappaport Y, Blank A, et al. Cystic appearance of cervical lymph nodes is

characteristic of metastatic papillary thyroid carcinoma. J Clin Ultrasound 2003;31(1):21–5.

34. Wunderbaldinger P, Harisinghani MG, Hahn PF, et al. Cystic lymph node metastases in papillary thyroid carcinoma. AJR Am J Roentgenol 2002; 178(3):693–7.

35. Verge J, Guixa J, Alejo M, et al. Cervical cystic lymph node metastasis as first manifestation of occult papillary thyroid carcinoma: report of seven cases. Head Neck 1999;21(4):370–4.

36. Simeone JF, Daniels GH, Hall DA, et al. Sonography in the follow-up of 100 patients with thyroid carcinoma. AJR Am J Roentgenol 1987;148(1):45–9.

37. King AD, Ahuja AT, To EW, et al. Staging papillary carcinoma of the thyroid: magnetic resonance imaging vs ultrasound of the neck. Clin Radiol 2000;55(3):222–6.

38. Gritzmann N, Hollerweger A, Macheiner P, et al. Sonography of soft tissue masses of the neck. J Clin Ultrasound 2002;30(6):356–73.

39. Langer JE, Luster E, Horii SC, et al. Chronic granulomatous lesions after thyroidectomy: imaging findings. AJR Am J Roentgenol 2005;185(5):1350–4.

40. Yabuuchi H, Kuroiwa T, Fukuya T, et al. Traumatic neuroma and recurrent lymphadenopathy after neck dissection: comparison of radiologic features. Radiology 2004;233(2):523–9.

41. Mercer D, Blachar A, Khafif A, et al. Real-time sonography of Killian-Jamieson diverticulum and its differentiation from thyroid nodules. J Ultrasound Med 2005;24(4):557–60.

42. Kwak JY, Kim EK. Sonographic findings of Zenker diverticula. J Ultrasound Med 2006;25(5):639–42.

43. Takashima S, Sone S, Nomura N, et al. Nonpalpable lymph nodes of the neck: assessment with US and US-guided fine-needle aspiration biopsy. J Clin Ultrasound 1997;25(6):283–92.

44. Frasoldati A, Valcavi R. Challenges in neck ultrasonography: lymphadenopathy and parathyroid glands. Endocr Pract 2004;10(3):261–8.

45. Boi F, Baghino G, Atzeni F, et al. The diagnostic value for differentiated thyroid carcinoma metastases of thyroglobulin (Tg) measurement in washout fluid from fine-needle aspiration biopsy of neck lymph nodes is maintained in the presence of circulating anti-Tg antibodies. J Clin Endocrinol Metab 2006;91(4):1364–9.

46. Cignarelli M, Ambrosi A, Marino A, et al. Diagnostic utility of thyroglobulin detection in fine-needle aspiration of cervical cystic metastatic lymph nodes from papillary thyroid cancer with negative cytology. Thyroid 2003;13(12):1163–7.

47. Schlumberger M. Papillary and follicular thyroid carcinoma. N Engl J Med 1998;338:297–306.

48. Noguchi S, Maurakami N, Yamashita H, et al. Papillary thyroid carcinoma: modified radical neck dissection improves prognosis. Arch Surg 1998; 133:276–80.

49. Ito Y, Tomoda C, Uruno T, et al. Ultrasonographically and anatomopathologically detectable node metastases in the lateral compartment as indicators of wrose relapse-free survival in patients with papillary thyroid carcinoma. World J Surg 2005;29:917–20.

50. Cooper DS, Doherty GM, Haugen BR, et al. Management guidelines for patients with thyroid nodules and differentiated thyroid cancer. Thyroid 2006;16(2):109–42.

51. American Association of Clinical Endocrinologists and Associazone Medici Endocrinologi medical guidelines for clinical practice for the diagnosis and management of thyroid nodules. Endocr Pract 2006;12:63–99.

52. Mazzaferri EL, Kloos RT. Is diagnostic iodine-131 scanning with recombinant human TSH useful in the follow-up of differentiated thyroid cancer after thyroid ablation. J Clin Endocrinol Metab 2002;87: 1490–8.

53. Frasoldati A, Pesent M, Gallo M, et al. Diagnosis of neck recurrences in patients with differentiated thyroid carcinoma. Cancer 2003;97:90–6.

54. Pacini F, Molinaro E, Castagna MG, et al. Recombinant human thyrotropin-stimulated serum thyroglobulin combined with neck ultrasonography has the highest sensitivity in monitoring differentiated thyroid carcinoma. J Clin Endocrinol Metab 2003;88:3668–73.

55. Kloos RT, Mazzaferri EL. A single recombinant human thyrotropin-stimulated serum thyroglobulin measurement predicts differentiated thyroid carcinoma metastases three to five years later. J Clin Endocrinol Metab 2005;90(9):5047–57.

56. Kupferman ME, Patterson M, Mandel SJ, et al. Patterns of lateral neck metastasis in papillary thyroid carcinoma. Arch Otolaryngol Head Neck Surg 2004;130:857–60.

Diagnostic Breast Ultrasound: Current Status and Future Directions

Wei Yang, MD*, Peter J. Dempsey, MD

KEYWORDS

- Ultrasound • Positron emission tomography
- Mammogram • Elastography • Sonography

As with many modalities eventually used in medicine, the basic technology of diagnostic medical ultrasound became available after being released by the military after the end of World War II. High-frequency ultrasound had been used to detect flaws in metal surfaces. Almost 60 years later, it has matured into an integral facet of the breast imaging armamentarium. Despite developments in MR imaging and positron emission tomography (PET), ultrasound remains the most cost effective, accurate, and useful of the adjunctive breast imaging tools and is available in virtually every practice. It clearly is the instrument of choice for image-guided breast biopsies and preoperative needle localizations and has revolutionized diagnostic breast evaluation by providing rapid, cheap, and accurate guidance for breast intervention. Mindful of the range of breast imaging practices throughout the United States, Europe, and Asia, this article documents the currently accepted uses for breast ultrasound and suggests fruitful areas for further development and application. Particular emphasis is given to potentially useful aspects of breast ultrasound, color Doppler, and power Doppler imaging, that are seldom highlighted in the clinical literature.

ESTABLISHED AREAS OF PROGRESS
Breast Imaging Reporting and Data System Nomenclature

To assimilate the impact of the expanded role of breast ultrasound and to underscore the integral role breast ultrasound plays in evaluating clinical breast problems, the Breast Imaging Reporting and Data System (BI-RADS) lexicon for reporting breast ultrasound findings was developed to correlate exactly with the terms that have been used for several years in radiographic mammography. This lexicon provides a unified method for reporting all breast imaging findings, highlighting for clinicians the overall impression of the study and clearly indicating the clinical management recommended. Several recent studies have evaluated the sensitivity and positive and negative predictive values of the BI-RADS lexicon for ultrasound.[1–3] The general consensus is that it creates a uniform platform for communication of important information regarding sonographic findings among breast radiologists and primary physicians including surgeons, medical oncologists, family practitioners, and gynecologists. One of the most important features of the BI-RADS lexicon for lesion characterization is margin analysis.

LIMITATIONS
Operator Dependency

Despite several attempts during the past 25 years to automate the image acquisition process, the standard throughout the country remains the use of hand-held transducers, relying on the operator's experience, technical proficiency, and clinical acumen to differentiate true abnormalities from normal structures.[4] With this practice it is easy to

This article originally appeared in *Radiologic Clinics of North America* 2007;45(5):845–861
Division of Diagnostic Imaging, Department of Diagnostic Radiology, The University of Texas, M.D. Anderson Cancer Center, P.O. Box 301439 – Unit 1350, Houston, TX 77230, USA
* Corresponding author.
E-mail address: wyang@di.mdacc.tmc.edu (W. Yang).

Ultrasound Clin 4 (2009) 117–133
doi:10.1016/j.cult.2009.04.011

create false-positive findings, leading to misinterpretation and misdiagnosis. Some companies are seeking to minimize this operator dependency by automating the process with a high-frequency, multidetector sweep-scanning device that permits precise localization and correlation in two planes within the breast and allows reconstruction of the images in the coronal plane, similar to methods available in CT and MR imaging.

Equipment Dependency

The initial rudimentary machines did not have scan converters, and not until approximately 1974 was true gray-scale imaging technically possible. Resolution was limited by transducer technology. Initial units used for breast employed transducers using frequencies of 3.5 or 5 mHz, which, although allowing deep tissue penetration, severely limited resolution. Technical advances found newer ways to achieve the necessary depth of penetration while improving resolution capability. Currently, 10- to 15-mHz transducers are the norm and achieve excellent resolution without sacrificing the necessary depth of penetration. Extended-field-of-view imaging, available on most current ultrasound scanners, allows simple and elegant demonstration and measurement of large lesions that extend beyond the width of the transducer footprint (**Fig. 1**).

Need for a Recent Mammogram

Although an American College of Radiology Imaging Network trial to assess the possibilities of breast ultrasound as a screening instrument is in progress, to date breast ultrasound has been used as an adjunctive tool, not as a screening modality.[5–8] The exception is in young patients (in their teens or early 20s); in these patients breast ultrasound often can reach a definitive diagnosis for a clinically palpable finding. As a general rule for daily clinical practice, performing a breast ultrasound without an accompanying mammogram is dangerous and can lead to erroneous conclusions and missed cancer diagnoses.

Erroneous Conclusions Resulting from the Use of Image-processing Algorithms Without Understanding the Electronic Principles

Recently, various manufacturers have developed several different image-processing methods (eg, tissue harmonic imaging, spatial compound imaging) in the laudable effort to make diagnosis of lesions easier for the breast imager.[9–11] Employing these methods without understanding their basis

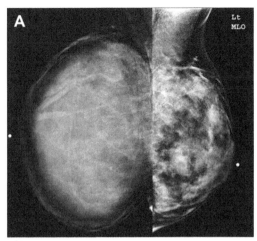

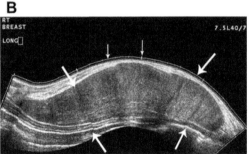

Fig. 1. (*A*) A 17-year-old-female presents with an enlarging mass in her right breast. Bilateral mediolateral oblique mammograms show global asymmetry of the right breast. (*B*) Sagittal extended-field-of-view ultrasound image demonstrates a solid homogeneously hypoechoic mass with circumscribed margins and a pseudocapsule (*thick arrows*). The centimeter markers superficial to the mass (*thin arrow*) allow a simple estimate of the dimensions of this mass. Surgical excision with reconstruction confirmed a giant fibroadenoma.

in physics, however, is dangerous. The goal has been to improve the conspicuity of real lesions while reducing the possibility for false-positive findings.

CHANGING INDICATIONS FOR BIOPSY

In earlier years, biopsies were done to avoid the risk of a false-negative result when the imaging findings were inconclusive or indeterminate. With the marked improvement in resolution coupled with a greater understanding of breast pathology, imaging findings often are sufficient to make a confident diagnosis of a benign lesion, thus avoiding an unnecessary biopsy.[12] A common example is the detection and diagnosis of small and perhaps multiple fibroadenomas in younger patients. Ultrasound often can depict them confidently as circumscribed, ovoid lesions

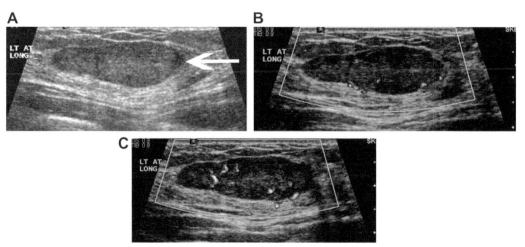

Fig. 2. (*A*) A 19-year-old female presents with a palpable mass in the left axillary tail. Transverse gray-scale ultrasound shows typical features of a fibroadenoma, comprising an oval solid hypoechoic circumscribed mass with a pseudocapsule (*arrow*). (*B*) Color Doppler ultrasound image shows weak peripheral and central vascularity associated with this mass. (*C*) Power Doppler ultrasound image shows longer segments of vessels in the periphery and center of this mass.

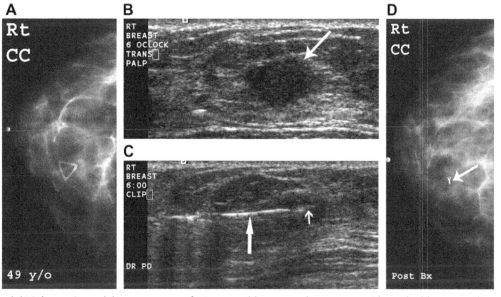

Fig. 3. (*A*) Right craniocaudal mammogram of a 44-year-old woman who presents with a palpable mass and a negative diagnostic mammogram. The triangle skin marker demonstrates the site of the palpable mass. (*B*) A transverse sonogram shows an irregular, solid, hypoechoic nodule corresponding to the palpable mass at the right 6 o'clock position (*arrow*). (*C*) A transverse ultrasound image during ultrasound guided clip placement within this mass. The long arrow indicates the needle shaft, and the short arrow indicates the clip. (*D*) Postbiopsy right craniocaudal mammogram shows clip marking the site of mammographically occult palpable cancer (*arrow*).

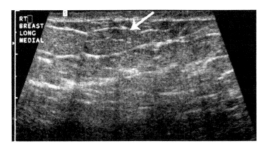

Fig. 4. Transverse sonogram of the medial right breast at a site of palpable concern in a 60-year-old woman demonstrates a benign fat lobule (*arrow*), without suspicious findings.

with specular echoes typical of fibroadenomas (**Fig. 2**). With an experienced sonographer using good equipment and technique, further invasive procedures often are unnecessary.

CURRENT INDICATIONS
Adjunct to Mammography and Clinical Breast Examination

Although entities such as summation artifacts seen on one view of a screening mammogram are always best investigated first by work-up mammography, diagnostic breast ultrasound is effective in the clarification of many positive findings on both mammography and clinical examination. Except for summation artifacts, the ultrasound examination can establish whether a lesion is present at all or if the finding previously noted is simply a normal parenchymal variation. The combination of a negative diagnostic mammogram and a negative diagnostic ultrasound has a sufficiently high negative predictive

value that biopsy of a low-suspicion palpable lesion is not indicated.[13–16] If a lesion does exist, ultrasound is capable of further characterization and, more importantly, of indicating whether an ultrasound-guided biopsy is appropriate. **Fig. 3** shows a clinically palpable finding not seen mammographically that was imaged easily and biopsied under ultrasound guidance and proved to be a cancer. On the other hand, one of the common benign findings of a clinically palpable area is a prominent fat lobule (**Fig. 4**). A physician can use the real-time sonographic image viewed on the screen as an effective display tool for the patient and allay the patient's fears quite effectively.

Primary Methodology for Young Patients

Quite frequently a palpable finding in a young patient is a fibroadenoma (see **Fig. 2**) (and its variants), a breast abscess (**Fig. 5**), or changes best described as "developmental anomalies" (macromastia, micromastia).[17–21] Healthy adolescent girls, rarely, may present with painless discharge from around the nipple and a periareolar mass. Ultrasound is a useful tool in the diagnosis of this condition (**Fig. 6**)[22] and in this clinical setting is the primary imaging tool. Ultrasound intuitively seems advantageous in this group of patients because of the homogeneously dense parenchyma and the reported increased radiosensitivity of breast tissue in these young women.[23] Technically well-performed ultrasound in young girls can be the key to preventing the devastating mistake of excision of a normally developing breast bud (**Fig. 7**) resulting in the complete lack of development of that breast.

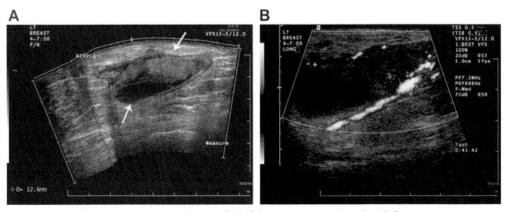

Fig. 5. (*A*) 56-year-old woman presents with a painful left breast mass associated with fever. Transverse sonogram shows a complex oval mass with mixed solid and cystic components and a partially defined capsule (*arrows*), highly suggestive of abscess formation. (*B*) Power Doppler sonography in the same patient shows peripheral rimlike vascularity in this biopsy-proven abscess that later underwent ultrasound-guided drainage and catheter placement.

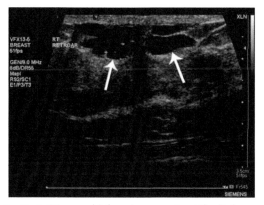

Fig. 6. A 13-year-old female presents with discharge from the Montgomery tubercles and a palpable right periareolar mass. Transverse right sonogram shows prominent retroareolar ducts (*arrows*) consistent with fibrocystic change. No suspicious findings were noted. The patient's symptoms resolved spontaneously after 3 months.

Initial imaging Modality for Pregnant Patients who have Clinical Symptoms

Unfortunately, young women, and especially young pregnant women, are not immune to breast cancer. Because of the patient's young age and the hormonal environment in pregnancy, these cancers tend to be high grade and rapidly growing, so prompt and accurate diagnosis is critical for therapy to be initiated. These cancers may be mammographically occult because of dense parenchyma, but they can be detected and evaluated effectively with sonography (**Fig. 8**).[24] With recently documented advances, pregnant women who have breast cancer can be treated effectively

with specific chemotherapy regimens and have a full-term, successful outcome of the pregnancy.[25,26] After delivery, definitive surgery can be performed.

Fortunately, in most pregnant patients referred for ultrasound examination of palpable findings, findings are benign; entities such as fibroadenomas enlarging in the hormonal environment of pregnancy, lactating adenomas, and galactoceles are common (**Fig. 9**).

Infection

Infection happens frequently in the postoperative and the postpartum setting, when the patient may present with an enlarged, red, and tender breast with or without associated overlying skin changes. The clinical dilemma is to exclude an underlying abscess that requires intervention (either imaging-guided or surgically guided) or an early inflammatory breast carcinoma.[27,28] Ultrasound is the imaging modality of choice because the breast frequently is too tender for compression with mammography. Careful and gentle scanning provides valuable information regarding the presence or absence of an underlying fluid collection (including abscess or galactocele in the postpartum setting or abscess or progressive tumor after surgical treatment of breast cancer). When an abscess is identified (see **Fig. 6**), imaging-guided drainage is swift and efficacious.

Ultrasonography of the Male Breast

Although male breast cancer is uncommon, there are multiple indications for imaging the male breast with sonography. These indications include a palpable mass in the breast or axilla, particularly in males who have a known primary tumor, including melanoma, prostate cancer, or lymphoma. Ultrasound often can characterize such masses and offer immediate pathologic confirmation using ultrasound-guided fine-needle aspiration biopsy. Men who have chronic liver disease and men taking long-term antihypertensive medication who present with palpable swelling of the breast(s) have a clinical diagnosis of gynecomastia. The sonographic features of gynecomastia include prominent glandular tissue in the acute nodular hypoechoic form (**Fig. 10**) or the chronic hyperechoic dendritic form.[29] This finding is distinct from the solid or complex cystic mass in the subareolar position that is typical for male breast carcinoma (**Fig. 11**).[30,31]

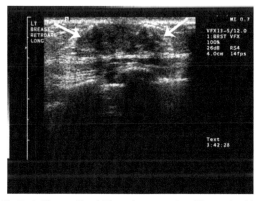

Fig. 7. A 13-month-old female presents with a palpable asymmetric right breast mass. Transverse sonogram demonstrates a normal breast bud in the retroareolar position with normal fibroglandular parenchyma (*arrows*).

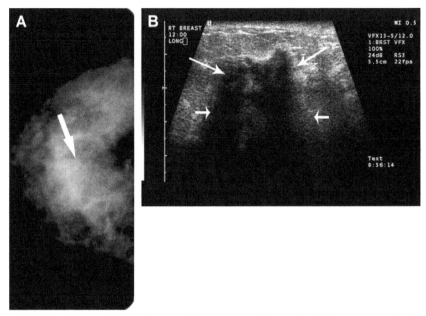

Fig. 8. (A) A33-year-old woman at 26 weeks' gestation presents with a palpable breast mass in the right breast. Right craniocaudal mammogram demonstrates a vague focal asymmetry in the central 12 o'clock position (*arrow*). (B) Transverse sonogram of the right 12 o'clock position demonstrates an irregular solid hypoechoic mass (*long arrows*) with an echogenic boundary and posterior acoustic shadowing (*short arrows*). Core-needle biopsy showed high-grade invasive ductal carcinoma.

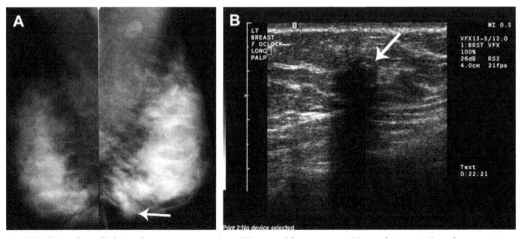

Fig. 9. (A) Bilateral mediolateral mammograms in a 33-year-old woman at 32 weeks' gestation demonstrates an oval mass in the inferior left breast (*arrow*) corresponding to a palpable finding. Global increased breast density bilaterally is consistent with gestational and lactation change. (B) Transverse sonogram demonstrates an irregular solid hypoechoic mass (*arrow*) that was avascular (not shown) and demonstrates marked posterior acoustic shadowing. Core biopsy showed galactocele with inflammatory change and no evidence of malignancy. This lesion had resolved spontaneously at 12-month follow-up.

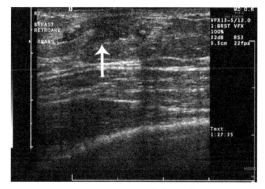

Fig. 10. Transverse sonogram of the right retroareolar region shows hypoechoic nodular gynecomastia (*arrow*) in a 16-year-old male who presented with a palpable mass.

Imaging Guidance for Interventional Procedures

It is now commonplace for needle biopsies using either fine-needle aspiration or core technique to be done with ultrasound guidance, if technically feasible. Even vacuum-assisted biopsies can be done in this fashion, although resorting to this more aggressive method is not always necessary. If a diagnosis of cancer is established, and if preoperative neoadjuvant chemotherapy is to be employed, a metallic (titanium) tumor marker can be placed percutaneously into the epicenter of the tumor at the time of biopsy (see **Fig. 3**; **Fig. 12**).[32–35] Up to 30% of these tumors undergo complete clinical response, and thus the marker would be the only way that an accurate pre-excision localization could be performed.

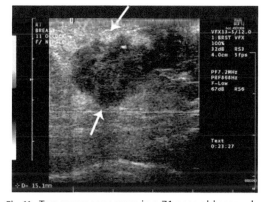

Fig. 11. Transverse sonogram in a 71-year-old man who presented with a palpable mass shows an eccentric mass at 11 o'clock in the right breast that is irregular in shape and has microlobulated margins and internal hypervascularity (*arrows*). Pathology showed grade 2 invasive ductal carcinoma.

Any cancer easily visible on ultrasound is a candidate for preoperative localization by this method. Careful preprocedure scrutiny should be used, however, because any segmental areas of microcalcifications associated with the cancer are better localized mammographically with a bracketing technique.

At a few institutions, such as the University of Texas M.D. Anderson Cancer Center, preoperative localization using ultrasound is actually performed in the operating room after the patient has been anesthetized and positioned for surgery.[36] Some surgeons appreciate the real-time demonstration of the perpendicular distance from the overlying skin to the center of the tumor (**Fig. 13**). This method also obviates the need for an additional procedure requiring local anesthesia and needle placement in the conscious patient.

Second-look Study after a Positive Breast MR Imaging or Positron Emission Tomography Study

At the M.D. Anderson Cancer Center, as at many institutions, ultrasound has been used effectively to investigate possible areas of significance that have been detected on either breast MR imaging or PET/CT scan. Even if the patient has had a previous breast ultrasound, the second-look procedure allows attention to be focused on targeted areas whose localities have been documented on the MR imaging or PET/CT roadmap. If successfully imaged and localized by ultrasound, the area can be biopsied quickly and accurately, and a clip can be placed in both a time-effective and cost-effective manner (**Fig. 14**).[37–39] Otherwise, a separate MR imaging–guided procedure, which is much more expensive and technically more complicated, must be scheduled.

Breast Cancer Imaging

Definitive surgery, as the name indicates, should be a planned curative procedure based on the most accurate anatomic information available concerning the precise area of breast cancer involvement. When the surgery is performed and undiagnosed metastatic nodes are present in the infraclavicular, internal mammary, supraclavicular, or low neck region(s), the ultimate clinical outcome will be less than ideal.

At the M.D. Anderson Cancer Center, ultrasound is used regularly for staging purposes. It is surprising how frequently unsuspected nodal metastases can be easily imaged, biopsied, and histologically proven (by fine-needle

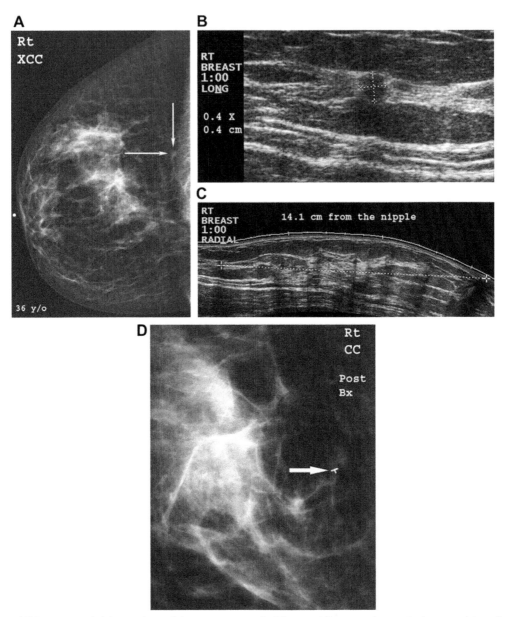

Fig.12. (A) Exaggerated right craniocaudal mammogram of a 36-year-old woman demonstrates a suspicious 4-mm irregular nodule (arrows) detected on screening mammography. (B) Longitudinal ultrasound demonstrates a solid hypoechoic mass (marked by dotted cross) with irregular margins and no posterior acoustic phenomena. (C) Longitudinal extended-field-of-view view ultrasound image accurately documents distance of the lesion from the nipple, confirming sonographic–mammographic correlation of this abnormality. (D) Postbiopsy right cranio-caudal mammogram demonstrates the postbiopsy clip within the mass (arrow).

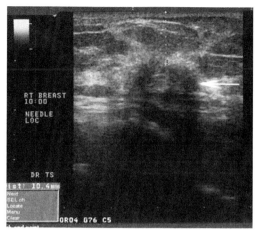

Fig. 13. Transverse intraoperative ultrasound image demonstrates known cancer (*arrow*) at the 10 o'clock position in the right breast, and the perpendicular distance of the cancer from the skin measured by calipers (10.4 mm).

aspiration), thus providing more accurate TNM staging and, ultimately, the best patient care. The authors believe that many cases reported as early recurrences are undoubtedly patients who were treated conservatively and who had unsuspected metastatic disease at the time of initial diagnosis.

Many recent papers cite MR imaging as the best initial staging method for breast cancer.[8,40,41] Although the sensitivity of MR imaging is superb, the detection of additional "enhancing lesions" poses the problem of obtaining quick, inexpensive histologic proof of their significance. Furthermore, assessment of all regional nodal basins is not possible with MR imaging, whereas ultrasound allows assessment of multifocality (**Fig. 15**) and multicentricity (**Fig. 16**); histologic proof can be obtained inexpensively at the time of the study. In addition, all regional nodal basins can be assessed and biopsied as needed with fine-needle aspiration biopsy.[42–45]

At the M.D. Anderson cancer center, patients who have been diagnosed as having breast cancer by needle or excisional biopsy undergo an ultrasound of the ipsilateral breast and axillary, internal mammary, and infraclavicular nodal basins. If suspicious nodes are seen in any of these sites, the supraclavicular area is scanned as well (**Fig. 17**). Histologic verification is achieved by immediate fine-needle aspiration biopsy beginning with the highest-order suspicious node detected. This procedure is appropriate in a primary cancer institution where the N stage affects overall staging and determines eligibility for various chemotherapy protocols.[46] Additionally, these sites of disease can be used to assess response in patients undergoing neoadjuvant chemotherapy.

Older literature focused entirely on the presence of a fatty hilum.[47–50] If it was present, the node was considered benign. More recent experience demonstrates this assumption is not true. Because the afferent lymphatic channels enter the node through the periphery of the cortex, it is in this area that early changes of metastatic disease become manifest. Specifically, very subtle cortical nodularity can be seen as the first sign of metastatic involvement, even when a prominent fatty hilum is still present (**Fig. 18**). These nodular areas may be perceived as somewhat hypoechoic relative to the rest of the nodal cortex, but this observation is predicated on the most meticulous technique. When doing a biopsy, it is critical to direct the needle tip to these nodular areas and not to the hilar regions or the cortical regions as yet unaffected sonographically.

Ultrasound also is used effectively to assess tumor response after the initiation of chemotherapy protocols. Volume measurements of a mass by ultrasound are obtained by taking measurements in three orthogonal planes and applying a volumetric formula for an ellipsoid, thus rendering ultrasound a particularly facile and cost-effective tool. In addition, should a marked positive response to chemotherapy be noted with significant reduction in tumor volume, a metallic tumor marker can be placed at the time of the examination.

BENIGN VERSUS MALIGNANT: THE GOAL OF LESION CHARACTERIZATION

Since the first papers reporting the use of breast ultrasound were published in the early 1950s, one of the principal goals of its use has been distinguishing benign from malignant tumors using a variety of sonographic criteria. A frequently cited article regarding tissue characterization was published in 1995 by Stavros and colleagues.[51] Based on a large volume of data derived from the study of 750 breast nodules, the acoustic characteristics of benign and malignant lesions were enumerated and described in detail. Although the ultimate reference standard for the distinction between benign and malignant lesions remains histologic, this article helped decrease the "gray areas" in interpretation.

USE AND INTERPRETATION OF COLOR DOPPLER AND POWER DOPPLER IMAGING

Neoangiogenesis is believed to be caused by the protein angiogenin that is produced by tumor

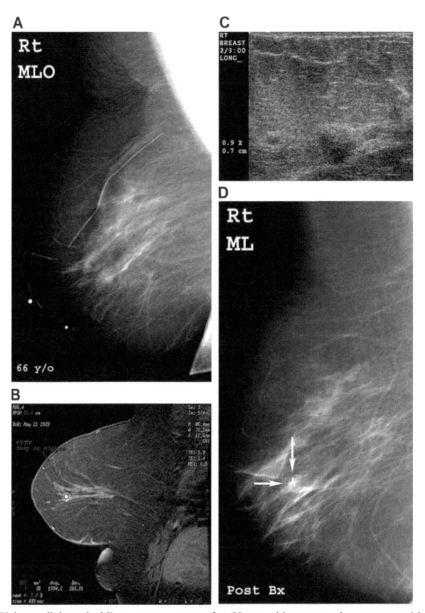

Fig. 14. (*A*) Right mediolateral oblique mammogram of a 66-year-old woman who presents with a palpable nodule denoted by radiopaque skin marker. No definite lesion is seen mammographically. A previous benign surgical biopsy site is marked with an opaque, linear scar marker. The palpable nodule was sonographically occult (not shown). (*B*) Sagittal, dynamic, contrast-enhanced MR image of the right breast demonstrates a small, enhancing lesion with malignant-type washout kinetics (not shown) corresponding to site of the palpable nodule (*purple arrow*). (*C*) A second-look ultrasound demonstrated an irregular, solid, hypoechoic nodule measuring 9 mm by 7 mm. Ultrasound-guided core biopsy showed intermediate-grade invasive ductal carcinoma. (*D*) Post-biopsy lateral right mammogram demonstrates postbiopsy clip (*arrows*) without corresponding mammographic abnormality corresponding to the lesion visualized on MR imaging.

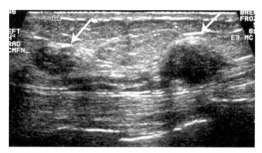

Fig. 15. Transverse sonogram in a 26-year-old woman shows two masses in the left breast (*arrows*) consistent with multifocal invasive carcinoma.

cells[52] and has been shown to correlate with rapid tumor growth and metastasis.[53] Tumoral vessels frequently are irregular, tortuous, and variable in caliber, forming reticular networks with arteriovenous shunts and dichotomous branching.[54] Doppler ultrasound requires a high-frequency transducer; usually, a 7- to 13-MHz annular array or broadband linear array is used. Ideally, the technique should be able to evaluate flow signals of very small vessels with diameters below 0.1 mm and with low flow velocity. Successful Doppler-based assessment requires standardization of technique, evaluation, and analysis.[55–57] The different forms of Doppler imaging include color Doppler, spectral Doppler, and power Doppler. Color Doppler and spectral Doppler imaging employ instruments to visualize the mean intravascular frequency shift caused by Doppler effects of flowing blood corpuscles that are frequency modulated.

Advances in technology and ultrasound equipment have led to improved detection of blood flow with Doppler sonography in all solid masses, benign and malignant, thus improving the sensitivity and specificity.[58,59] The proof of or extent of tumor vascularity alone is no longer a sufficient criterion in the differential diagnosis of breast lesions.[60–64] Additional useful criteria include structural characteristics of tumor vessels correlating to histologic patterns. Characteristics of malignant tumors include hypervascularity (92%–9%), irregular abnormal vascularity (54.2%), and more than one vascular pole[65] (**Fig. 19A–C**). Benign lesions tend to have one vascular pole, weak, peripheral vascularity (**Fig. 20**), and no central vessels (**Fig. 21**).[66] Color Doppler imaging is less helpful in the differential diagnosis of breast lesions, such as mucinous and in situ carcinomas, and of invasive ductal carcinoma less than 9 mm in diameter, which often may show avascularity.[65] Benign lesions that display a false-positive malignant-type hypervascularity include hypervascularized, proliferating, juvenile phyllodes tumors and fibroadenomas (**Fig. 22**). These hypervascularized masses require biopsy.

Spectral Doppler imaging is less useful than color Doppler imaging in differentiating benign from malignant masses.[66,67] The large variation of velocities within cancers presumably is caused by the tortuous vessels and arteriovenous shunts that are typical of malignant neovascularization.[68,69] The formation of arteriovenous shunts and thin-walled vessels lacking smooth muscle, as seen in malignant tumors, results in high-

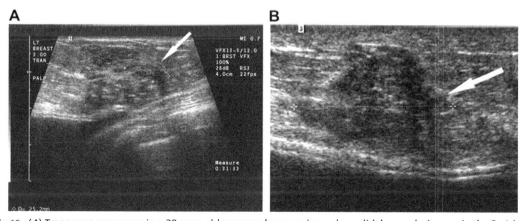

Fig. 16. (*A*) Transverse sonogram in a 29-year-old woman shows an irregular, solid, hypoechoic mass in the 3 o'clock position in the left breast with indistinct margins and internal microcalcifications (*arrow*) corresponding to a palpable finding. Pathology from ultrasound-guided core-needle biopsy showed high-grade ductal carcinoma in situ. (*B*) A second nonpalpable mass with similar features (*arrow*) was detected in the 9 o'clock position in the left breast, consistent with multicentric disease.

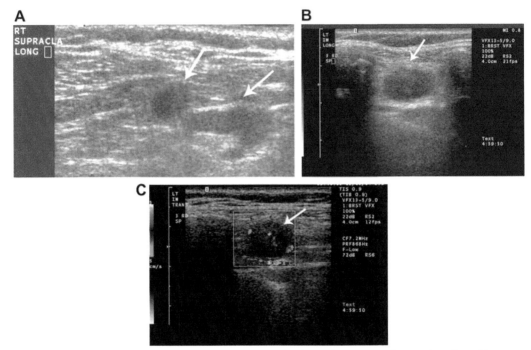

Fig. 17. (A) Transverse sonogram of the right supraclavicular fossa shows two abnormal nodes with eccentric cortical hypertrophy (*arrows*). (B) Transverse sonogram in left third internal mammary lymph node space shows an abnormal oval solid hypoechoic nodule (*arrow*) consistent with internal mammary lymphadenopathy. (C) Color Doppler ultrasound image of this node demonstrates internal hypervascularity (*arrow*).

velocity and high-pulsatility flow[70] with significantly higher peak systolic Doppler frequency shifts in malignant than in benign lesions ($P < .01–<.0001$).[62,71] A wide overlap of parameters prevents spectral Doppler imaging from being a valuable tool in the differentiation of breast lesions.[71,72]

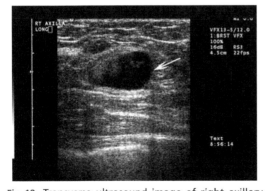

Fig. 18. Transverse ultrasound image of right axillary node in a 36-year-old woman who had documented right breast cancer shows focal eccentric cortical hypertrophy (*arrow*). Ultrasound-guided fine-needle aspiration biopsy confirmed metastatic carcinoma.

Power Doppler imaging depicts the intensity of energy of the Doppler signal and is based on the amplitude of Doppler shift.[73,74] The wider dynamic range of power Doppler imaging makes it more sensitive in detecting small vessels and low flow. Power Doppler imaging is independent of the Doppler angle and therefore is not subject to aliasing; power Doppler also may depict longer segments of smaller vessels because of the increased signal-to-noise ratio (see **Fig. 2**). Disadvantages of power Doppler imaging include reduced temporal resolution, lack of directional or velocity information, a high number of color artifacts, and the inability to differentiate between arteries and veins. Power Doppler imaging has a sensitivity of 74.5% and a specificity of 74.6% that is useful in the depiction of small cancers that are less than 5 mm in size.[75] One study foundthat penetrating vessels were more likely to be present in malignant tumors.[76,77] Typical power Doppler signs of malignancy include central, borderline penetrating, branching, disordered, and intratumoral vessels (see **Figs. 19–21**).[75–77]

Doppler imaging may be useful in differentiating postoperative changes from recurrent tumor. In the first 18 months, nodular scars or granulomas

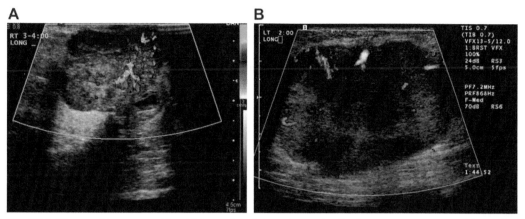

Fig. 19. (A) A 53-year-old woman with a history of ductal carcinoma in situ 5 years ago presents with a palpable finding at the segmentectomy site in the right breast at 4 o'clock position. Color and power Doppler ultrasound images show marked internal hypervascularity within a recurrent invasive ductal cancer that extends to the overlying dermis. Note the chaotic pattern of branching vascularity and vessels of varying caliber. (B) A 57-year-old woman presents with a palpable left breast mass. The power Doppler ultrasound image shows internal hypervascularity (vessels of varied caliber) within an invasive metaplastic cancer.

also may be hypervascularized, although the likelihood of hypervascularity decreases as the age of the scar increases. Criteria include the number and regularity of vessels.[78] Postsurgical scars usually are slightly or not vascularized, whereas all malignant lesions tend to display increased and irregular vascularity.[78]

FUTURE DIRECTIONS
Elastography in Breast Imaging

Because malignant lesions tend to be "harder" than benign lesions, several groups have suggested and investigated the application of elastography to evaluate breast lesions visualized on ultrasound. The major problems have been in the exact quantification of these results. Three distinct

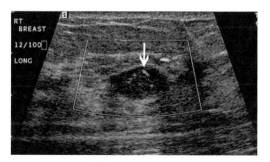

Fig. 20. A 41-year-old woman presents with a palpable finding in the right breast at 12 o'clock position. Transverse power Doppler ultrasound shows a single peripheral vessel (arrow) associated with a biopsy-proven fibroadenoma.

methods of measurement have been proposed and tested, with varying degrees of success: spatial correlation, phase-shift tracking, and combined autocorrelation.

The major drawbacks can be summarized under the general heading of operator dependency. This limitation involves the technique of pressure application, the experience of the investigator(s), and the very involved manual tracing of lesion boundaries. In its present form, the use of elastography in routine clinical practice does not seem feasible.[79–81]

Breast Ablation Techniques

In other organs, such as prostate, liver, and kidney, the possibility of avoiding open surgical intervention by the ablation of small tumors has received much attention. Ablative techniques for benign (fibroadenomas) and malignant breast tumors have reached the stage of clinical testing, and early results seem encouraging. Numerous forms of possible tumor ablation have been examined, including chemical, thermal (radiofrequency, laser, cryoablation), microwave, and ultrasound.[82] The two techniques most widely tested and used thus far are cryoablation and ablation using radiofrequency currents. Both modalities are directed and confined to a highly localized area to avoid collateral tissue damage.

The cryoablation technique that has been used for both benign and malignant tumors employs a disposable, air-gap–insulated cryoablation

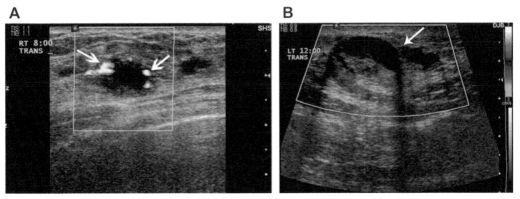

Fig. 21. (A) A 44-year-old woman who had a biopsy-proven left breast cancer presents with an exquisitely tender mass in the right breast. The power Doppler ultrasound image shows marked peripheral hypervascularity (*arrows*) associated with a densely inflamed cyst that was aspirated and showed benign ductal cells, with no evidence of malignancy. Note lack of central vascularity. (B) A 39-year-old woman presents with a palpable finding after transverse rectus abdominus myocutaneous reconstruction of the left breast. The color Doppler ultrasound shows an avascular mixed cystic and solid mass (*arrow*). Fine-needle aspiration biopsy confirmed fat necrosis.

probe 2.4 mm in diameter. In some cases, multiple probes have been used for larger masses. As ablation takes place, an ice ball is formed, the diameter of which is monitored with ultrasound.[83,84]

With radiofrequency ablation, the initial device inserted is a 15-gauge probe through which multi-pronged expandable electrodes are inserted and then deployed. Ablation progress is monitored both by constant temperature recording from the electrode tips as well as with ultrasound imaging.[85]

If ablation is used as the only therapy for potentially malignant neoplasms, without subsequent surgical removal, the greatest potential drawback is the inability to assess tumor margins. This assessment always has been the primary measure of successful cancer surgical therapy, and loss of the ability to document tumor margins carefully will invariably leave an element of doubt.

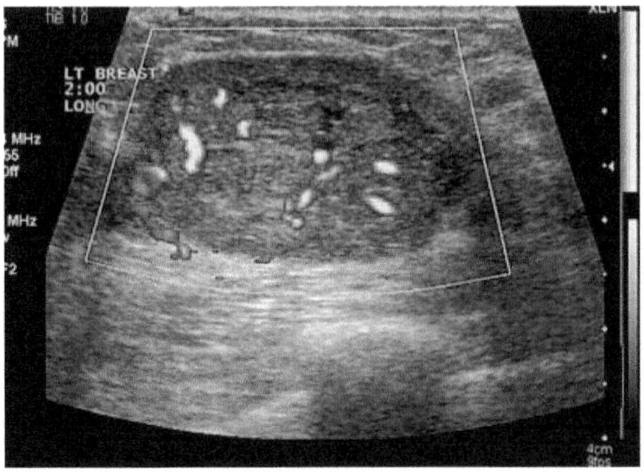

Three-dimensional Sonography

The advantages of three-dimensional sonography compared with those of conventional sonographic imaging remains controversial. Some single-institution studies have demonstrated superior image quality on three-dimensional sonography,[86,87] but the diagnostic accuracy of this method was not statistically significant.[88] Three-dimensional sonography as an adjunct to conventional sonography requires further evaluation in larger clinical trials to determine clinical relevance and efficacy in diagnostic breast imaging.

SUMMARY

Breast ultrasound remains a critical and reliable adjunctive modality in the detection and diagnosis of benign and malignant entities within the breast parenchyma and in the surrounding regional nodal basins. It is established as the first-line guidance modality for percutaneous biopsy, preoperative localization, and tumor marker placement procedures. Although operator-dependent, it nonetheless is accurate, patient friendly, and cost effective when used properly. It is a modality that seems destined for continued growth in both technical innovations and clinical use.

Fig. 22. A 27-year-old woman presents with a palpable mass in the left upper outer quadrant. Power Doppler ultrasound shows multiple internal vessels in a biopsy-proven phyllodes tumor.

REFERENCES

1. Hong AS, Rosen EL, Soo MS, et al. BI-RADS for sonography: positive and negative predictive values of sonographic features. AJR Am J Roentgenol 2005;184(4):1260–5.

2. Lazarus E, Mainiero MB, Schepps B, et al. BI-RADS lexicon for US and mammography: interobserver variability and positive predictive value. Radiology 2006;239(2):385–91.

3. Costantini M, Belli P, Lombardi R, et al. Characterization of solid breast masses: use of the sonographic breast imaging reporting and data system lexicon. J Ultrasound Med 2006;25(5):649–59.

4. Baker JA, Soo MS, Rosen EL. Artifacts and pitfalls in sonographic imaging of the breast. AJR Am J Roentgenol 2001;176(5):1261–6.

5. Kolb TM, Lichy J, Newhouse JH. Occult cancer in women with dense breasts: detection with screening US—diagnostic yield and tumor characteristics. Radiology 1998;207(1):191–9.

6. Berg WA. Rationale for a trial of screening breast ultrasound: American College of Radiology Imaging Network (ACRIN) 6666. AJR Am J Roentgenol 2003; 180(5):1225–8.

7. Berg WA. Supplemental screening sonography in dense breasts. Radiol Clin North Am 2004;42(5): 845–51, vi.

8. Berg WA, Gutierrez L, NessAiver MS, et al. Diagnostic accuracy of mammography, clinical examination, US, and MR imaging in preoperative assessment of breast cancer. Radiology 2004;233(3):830–49.

9. Szopinski KT, Pajk AM, Wysocki M, et al. Tissue harmonic imaging: utility in breast sonography. J Ultrasound Med 2003;22(5):479–87.

10. Haerten R, Lowery C, Becker G, et al. "Ensemble™ Tissue Harmonic Imaging": the technology and clinical utility. Electromedica 1999;1:50–6.

11. Cha JH, Moon WK, Cho N, et al. Differentiation of benign from malignant solid breast masses: conventional US versus spatial compound imaging. Radiology 2005;237(3):841–6.

12. Gordon PB, Gagnon FA, Lanzkowsky L. Solid breast masses diagnosed as fibroadenoma at fine-needle aspiration biopsy: acceptable rates of growth at long-term follow-up. Radiology 2003;229(1):233–8.

13. Harvey JA. Sonography of palpable breast masses. Semin Ultrasound CT MR 2006;27(4):284–97.

14. Mendelson EB. Problem-solving ultrasound. Radiol Clin North Am 2004;42(5):909–18, vii.

15. Soo MS, Rosen EL, Baker JA, et al. Negative predictive value of sonography with mammography in patients with palpable breast lesions. AJR Am J Roentgenol 2001;177(5):1167–70.

16. Shetty MK, Shah YP, Sharman RS. Prospective evaluation of the value of combined mammographic and sonographic assessment in patients with palpable abnormalities of the breast. J Ultrasound Med 2003;22(3):263–8.

17. Hall FM. Mammography and sonography in young symptomatic women. AJR Am J Roentgenol 2003; 181(5):1424 [author reply 1424–5].

18. Morrow M, Wong S, Venta L. The evaluation of breast masses in women younger than forty years of age. Surgery 1998;124(4):634–40 [discussion: 640–1].

19. Jackson VP, Reynolds HE, Hawes DR. Sonography of the breast. Semin Ultrasound CT MR 1996;17(5): 460–75.

20. Brand IR, Sapherson DA, Brown TS. Breast imaging in women under 35 with symptomatic breast disease. Br J Radiol 1993;66(785):394–7.

21. Bock K, Duda VF, Hadji P, et al. Pathologic breast conditions in childhood and adolescence: evaluation by sonographic diagnosis. J Ultrasound Med 2005;24(10):1347–54.

22. Rogerson T, Ingram D, Sterrett G, et al. Areolar discharge and peri-areolar breast cysts in adolescent females. Breast 2002;11(2):181–4.

23. Feig SA. Radiation risk from mammography: is it clinically significant? AJR Am J Roentgenol 1984; 143(3):469–75.

24. Yang WT, Dryden MJ, Gwyn K, et al. Imaging of breast cancer diagnosed and treated with chemotherapy during pregnancy. Radiology 2006;239(1):52–60.

25. Foxcroft LM, Evans EB, Porter AJ. The diagnosis of breast cancer in women younger than 40. Breast 2004;13(4):297–306.

26. Hahn KM, Johnson PH, Gordon N, et al. Treatment of pregnant breast cancer patients and outcomes of children exposed to chemotherapy in utero. Cancer 2006;107(6):1219–26.

27. Whitman GJ, Kushwaha AC, Cristofanilli M, et al. Inflammatory breast cancer: current imaging perspectives. Seminars in Breast Disease 2001;4:122–31.

28. Gunhan-Bilgen I, Ustun EE, Memis A. Inflammatory breast carcinoma: mammographic, ultrasonographic, clinical, and pathologic findings in 142 cases. Radiology 2002;223(3):829–38.

29. Caruso G, Ienzi R, Piovana G, et al. High-frequency ultrasound in the study of male breast palpable masses. Radiol Med (Torino) 2004;108(3):185–93.

30. Yang WT, Whitman GJ, Yuen EH, et al. Sonographic features of primary breast cancer in men. AJR Am J Roentgenol 2001;176(2):413–6.

31. Chen L, Chantra PK, Larsen LH, et al. Imaging characteristics of malignant lesions of the male breast. Radiographics 2006;26(4):993–1006.

32. Edeiken BS, Fornage BD, Bedi DG, et al. US-guided implantation of metallic markers for permanent localization of the tumor bed in patients with breast cancer who undergo preoperative chemotherapy. Radiology 1999;213(3):895–900.

33. Dash N, Chafin SH, Johnson RR, et al. Usefulness of tissue marker clips in patients undergoing

neoadjuvant chemotherapy for breast cancer. AJR Am J Roentgenol 1999;173(4):911–7.

34. Alonso-Bartolome P, Ortega Garcia E, Garijo Ayensa F, et al. Utility of the tumor bed marker in patients with breast cancer receiving induction chemotherapy. Acta Radiol 2002;43(1):29–33.

35. Nurko J, Mancino AT, Whitacre E, et al. Surgical benefits conveyed by biopsy site marking system using ultrasound localization. Am J Surg 2005; 190(4):618–22.

36. Snider HC Jr, Morrison DG. Intraoperative ultrasound localization of nonpalpable breast lesions. Ann Surg Oncol 1999;6(3):308–14.

37. Obdeijn IM, Brouwers-Kuyper EM, Tilanus-Linthorst MM, et al. MR imaging-guided sonography followed by fine-needle aspiration cytology in occult carcinoma of the breast. AJR Am J Roentgen 2000; 174(4):1079–84.

38. LaTrenta LR, Menell JH, Morris EA, et al. Breast lesions detected with MR imaging: utility of histopathologic importance of identification with US. Radiology 2003;227(3):856–61.

39. Sim LS, Hendriks JH, Bult P, et al. US correlation for MRI-detected breast lesions in women with familial risk of breast cancer. Clin Radiol 2005;60(7):801–6.

40. Pavic D, Koomen MA, Kuzmiak CM, et al. The role of magnetic resonance imaging in diagnosis and management of breast cancer. Technol Cancer Res Treat 2004;3(6):527–41.

41. Blair S, McElroy M, Middleton MS, et al. The efficacy of breast MRI in predicting breast conservation therapy. J Surg Oncol 2006;94(3):220–5.

42. Krishnamurthy S, Sneige N, Bedi DG, et al. Role of ultrasound-guided fine-needle aspiration of indeterminate and suspicious axillary lymph nodes in the initial staging of breast carcinoma. Cancer 2002; 95(5):982–8.

43. Khan A, Sabel MS, Nees A, et al. Comprehensive axillary evaluation in neoadjuvant chemotherapy patients with ultrasonography and sentinel lymph node biopsy. Ann Surg Oncol 2005;12(9):697–704.

44. Mathijssen IM, Strijdhorst H, Kiestra SK, et al. Added value of ultrasound in screening the clinically negative axilla in breast cancer. J Surg Oncol 2006;94(5): 364–7.

45. Somasundar P, Gass J, Steinhoff M, et al. Role of ultrasound-guided axillary fine-needle aspiration in the management of invasive breast cancer. Am J Surg 2006;192(4):458–61.

46. Greene FL, Page DL, Fleming ID, et al. American Joint Cancer Committee cancer staging manual. 6th edition. New York: Springer-Verlag; 2002. p. 221–40.

47. Yang WT, Ahuja A, Tang A, et al. High resolution sonographic detection of axillary lymph node metastases in breast cancer. J Ultrasound Med 1996;15(3):241–6.

48. Pamilo M, Soiva M, Lavast EM. Real-time ultrasound, axillary mammography, and clinical examination in the detection of axillary lymph node metastases in breast cancer patient. J Ultrasound Med 1989;8(3): 115–20.

49. Yang WT, Ahuja A, Tang A, et al. Ultrasonographic demonstration of normal axillary lymph nodes: a learning curve. J Ultrasound Med 1995;14(11): 823–7.

50. Feu J, Tresserra F, Fabregas R, et al. Metastatic breast carcinoma in axillary lymph nodes: in vitro US detection. Radiology 1997;205(3):831–5.

51. Stavros AT, Thickman D, Rapp CL, et al. Solid breast nodules: use of sonography to distinguish between benign and malignant lesions. Radiology 1995; 196(1):123–34.

52. Hartmann A, Kunz M, Kostlin S, et al. Hypoxia-induced up-regulation of angiogenin in human malignant melanoma. Cancer Res 1999;59(7):1578–83.

53. Srivastava A, Hughes LE, Woodcock JP, et al. Vascularity in cutaneous melanoma detected by Doppler sonography and histology: correlation with tumour behaviour. Br J Cancer 1989;59(1):89–91.

54. Less JR, Skalak TC, Sevick EM, et al. Microvascular architecture in a mammary carcinoma: branching patterns and vessel dimensions. Cancer Res 1991; 51(1):265–73.

55. Foster FS, Burns PN, Simpson DH, et al. Ultrasound for the visualization and quantification of tumor microcirculation. Cancer Metastasis Rev 2000; 19(1–2):131–8.

56. Donnelly EF, Geng L, Wojcicki WE, et al. Quantified power Doppler US of tumor blood flow correlates with microscopic quantification of tumor blood vessels. Radiology 2001;219(1):166–70.

57. Cosgrove D, Eckersley R, Blomley M, et al. Quantification of blood flow. Eur Radiol 2001;11(8):1338–44.

58. Ozdemir A, Ozdemir H, Maral I, et al. Differential diagnosis of solid breast lesions: contribution of Doppler studies to mammography and gray scale imaging. J Ultrasound Med 2001;20(10):1091–101.

59. Mehta TS, Raza S, Baum JK. Use of Doppler ultrasound in the evaluation of breast carcinoma. Semin Ultrasound CT MR 2000;21(4):297–307.

60. Peters-Engl C, Frank W, Leodolter S, et al. Tumor flow in malignant breast tumors measured by Doppler ultrasound: an independent predictor of survival. Breast Cancer Res Treat 1999;54(1):65–71.

61. Lee WJ, Chu JS, Huang CS, et al. Breast cancer vascularity: color Doppler sonography and histopathology study. Breast Cancer Res Treat 1996;37(3): 291–8.

62. Madjar H, Sauerbrei W, Prompeler HJ, et al. Color Doppler and duplex flow analysis for classification of breast lesions. Gynecol Oncol 1997;64(3):392–403.

63. McNicholas MM, Mercer PM, Miller JC, et al. Color Doppler sonography in the evaluation of palpable breast masses. AJR Am J Roentgenol 1993;161(4): 765–71.

64. del Cura JL, Elizagaray E, Zabala R, et al. The use of unenhanced Doppler sonography in the evaluation of solid breast lesions. AJR Am J Roentgenol 2005;184(6):1788–94.

65. Giuseppetti GM, Baldassarre S, Marconi E. Color Doppler sonography. Eur J Radiol 1998;27(Suppl 2): S254–8.

66. Lee WJ, Chu JS, Houng SJ, et al. Breast cancer angiogenesis: a quantitative morphologic and Doppler imaging study. Ann Surg Oncol 1995;2(3):246–51.

67. Chao TC, Lo YF, Chen SC, et al. Color Doppler ultrasound in benign and malignant breast tumors. Breast Cancer Res Treat 1999;57(2):193–9.

68. Schor AM, Schor SL. Tumour angiogenesis. J Pathol 1983;141(3):385–413.

69. Strickland B. The value of arteriography in the diagnosis of bone tumours. Br J Radiol 1959;32:705–13.

70. Taylor KJ, Ramos I, Carter D, et al. Correlation of Doppler US tumor signals with neovascular morphologic features. Radiology 1988;166(1 Pt 1):57–62.

71. Sahin-Akyar G, Sumer H. Color Doppler ultrasound and spectral analysis of tumor vessels in the differential diagnosis of solid breast masses. Invest Radiol 1996;31(2):72–9.

72. Rettenbacher T, Hollerweger A, Macheiner P, et al. Color Doppler sonography of normal breasts: detectability of arterial blood vessels and typical flow patterns. Ultrasound Med Biol 1998;24(9):1307–11.

73. Rubin JM, Bude RO, Carson PL, et al. Power Doppler US: a potentially useful alternative to mean frequency-based color Doppler US. Radiology 1994;190(3):853–6.

74. Bude RO, Rubin JM. Power Doppler sonography. Radiology 1996;200(1):21–3.

75. Kook SH, Park HW, Lee YR, et al. Evaluation of solid breast lesions with power Doppler sonography. J Clin Ultrasound 1999;27(5):231–7.

76. Raza S, Baum JK. Solid breast lesions: evaluation with power Doppler US. Radiology 1997;203(1):164–8.

77. Milz P, Lienemann A, Kessler M, et al. Evaluation of breast lesions by power Doppler sonography. Eur Radiol 2001;11(4):547–54.

78. Baz E, Madjar H, Reuss C, et al. The role of enhanced Doppler ultrasound in differentiation of benign vs. malignant scar lesion after breast surgery for malignancy. Ultrasound Obstet Gynecol 2000; 15(5):377–82.

79. Moon WK, Chang RF, Chen CJ, et al. Solid breast masses: classification with computer-aided analysis of continuous US images obtained with probe compression. Radiology 2005;236(2):458–64.

80. Regner DM, Hesley GK, Hangiandreou NJ, et al. Breast lesions: evaluation with US strain imaging – clinical experience of multiple observers. Radiology 2006;238(2):425–37.

81. Itoh A, Ueno E, Tohno E, et al. Breast disease: clinical application of US elastography for diagnosis. Radiology 2006;239(2):341–50.

82. Goldberg SN, Grassi CJ, Cardella JF, et al. Image-guided tumor ablation: standardization of terminology and reporting criteria. Radiology 2005; 235(3):728–39.

83. Littrup PJ, Freeman-Gibb L, Andea A, et al. Cryotherapy for breast fibroadenomas. Radiology 2005; 234(1):63–72.

84. Roubidoux MA, Sabel MS, Bailey JE, et al. Small (<2.0-cm) breast cancers: mammographic and US findings at US-guided cryoablation—initial experience. Radiology 2004;233(3):857–67.

85. Fornage BD, Sneige N, Ross MI, et al. Small (< or = 2-cm) breast cancer treated with US-guided radiofrequency ablation: feasibility study. Radiology 2004;231(1):215–24.

86. Watermann DO, Foldi M, Hanjalic-Beck A, et al. Three-dimensional ultrasound for the assessment of breast lesions. Ultrasound Obstet Gynecol 2005; 25(6):592–8.

87. Cho KR, Seo BK, Lee JY, et al. A comparative study of 2D and 3D ultrasonography for evaluation of solid breast masses. Eur J Radiol 2005;54(3):365–70.

88. Cho N, Moon WK, Cha JH, et al. Differentiating benign from malignant solid breast masses: comparison of two-dimensional and three-dimensional US. Radiology 2006;240:26–32.

Beyond Standard Mammographic Screening: Mammography at Age Extremes, Ultrasound, and MR Imaging

Wendie A. Berg, MD, PhD, FACR

KEYWORDS

- Mammogram • Screening • Lymph node
- Ultrasound • MR imaging

The basic principles of screening are as follows: (1) earlier detection of disease will reduce mortality; (2) healthy individuals who are screened will not be harmed; (3) the screening test must be widely available and well tolerated; and (4) screening should be cost effective. Randomized, controlled trials have proven mammographic screening to be effective by each of these criteria. Across seven randomized, controlled trials, in women aged 50 to 69 years, a 22% reduction in mortality was observed among women screened at 14 years of observation (95% confidence interval [CI], 13%–30%).[1] Among women aged 40 to 49 years, the summary risk reduction was 15% (95% CI, 1%–27%). Among women aged 40 to 69 who actually were screened by service screening from 1988 through 1996 in the Swedish Two County trial, a 63% reduction in mortality was observed, which represented a 50% reduction in mortality compared with the period between 1968 and 1977 when no mammographic screening was available.[2] Improved treatment can be credited with a 12% to 13% reduction in mortality during the same period.[2]

Randomized, controlled trials of mammographic screening have not included women younger than 40 years of age or older than 69 years, nor have they analyzed outcomes specifically in women at increased risk of developing breast cancer. This article explores the status of screening in such women and, in particular, the use of supplemental screening with ultrasound (US) and/or MR imaging for screening high-risk women.

Policy decisions to begin screening at age 40 or 50 years are derived largely from the prevalence of disease, which is less than 40 cases per 100,000 population below age 35 years across all ethnic groups and increases moderately beginning in the forties.[3] One in 2500 women without any known risk factors will develop breast cancer by age 30 years, one in 200 by age 40 years, and one in 50 by age 50 years. Rates peak from ages 75 to 79 years and decrease after age 80 years; one in eight women who live to age 85 will develop breast cancer.[3]

HIGH RISK

Definitions of "high risk" vary. Generally, women with the risk factor who are at least three times more likely to develop breast cancer than those without the risk factor (ie, relative risk ≥ 3.0) are considered at "high risk." High risk often is defined by use of models that incorporate family history

This article originally appeared in *Radiologic Clinics of North America* 2007;45(5):895–906
WAB is supported by grants from The Avon Foundation and the National Cancer Institute (CA89008) through the American College of Radiology Imaging Network.
American Radiology Services, Johns Hopkins Green Spring, 301 Merrie Hunt Dr., Lutherville, MD 21093, USA
E-mail address: wendieberg@gmail.com

Ultrasound Clin 4 (2009) 135–147
doi:10.1016/j.cult.2009.04.006

and prior biopsies. A lifetime risk of breast cancer of 20% or 25% by the models of Gail and colleagues[4,5] or Claus and colleagues[6] or at least a 1.7% 5-year risk of breast cancer by the Gail model[7] is considered high risk. Fibrocystic changes, even when proliferative, confer only minimal increased risk of 1.5 to 2.0, as do early menarche (< age 13) or late menopause (> age 55).

The age at which to begin screening women who are at increased risk would reasonably derive from the age at which the risk is equal to that for an average woman of age 40 or 50 years, depending on national policy. **Table 1** summarizes risk factor data. A family history of male breast cancer and/or a relative who had both breast and ovarian cancer increases the likelihood of a *BRCA* mutation, and many high-risk screening programs enroll women who have either or both of these criteria.[8,9] The BRCAPRO model calculates the risk of carrying a *BRCA* gene mutation as well as the subsequent risk of breast or ovarian cancer for individuals in families with known or suspected carriers.[10] It has been estimated that 2% of Ashkenazi Jewish women are *BRCA*-mutation carriers, and genetic testing should be considered.[11] For women who have a known or suspected *BRCA* mutation, most studies begin screening at age 25 years. For women who have an intermediate family history of breast cancer (see **Table 1**), screening usually begins 10 years before the age of diagnosis of the first-degree relative who had breast cancer or at least by age 40 years.[12]

Earlier studies of women who had mantle radiation therapy to the breasts (eg, for Hodgkin's disease) after age 18 years and before age 30 years showed a very high risk of breast cancer beginning 8 years after treatment and peaking at 15 years after treatment.[13] When treatment began after 1974 and used lower doses of radiation and more limited fields, no such increased risk has been found.[14]

No studies have addressed specifically the reduction in mortality from screening high-risk women. Therefore this article considers surrogate end points.

SURROGATE END POINTS AND MORTALITY

Lymph node status is the single most important prognostic factor for predicting disease-free and overall survival in breast cancer.[15,16] The decrease in mortality from randomized, controlled trials of mammographic screening is almost entirely attributable to earlier detection. The decrease in mortality parallels the reduction in size distribution of cancers depicted[17] and closely parallels the reduction in rates of node-positive breast

cancer.[18] Many screening programs have performed only biannual screening in women 40 to 49 years of age, and there has been relatively little reduction in the size distribution or rates of node-positive cancers compared with women aged 50 to 69 years who were screened annually.[19] The single most important predictor of the success of a screening program, independent of the type of intervention or imaging, is likely to be the reduction in node-positive cancers. Absent a control group, this article considers the percentage of cancers that are node positive at diagnosis as a surrogate measure of the efficacy of various screening strategies.

Although mortality is not considered specifically in most of this discussion, it is important to recognize that the benefit from mammographic screening in terms of reduction in mortality is not seen until 5 to 7 years after the onset of screening. As such, a woman who has a life expectancy of less than 5 years is not expected to benefit from screening. The cost effectiveness of screening usually is measured in cost per year of life saved. There is a higher cost to screening younger women, especially women younger than 40 years of age, due to lower prevalence of disease. This may be justifiable because of the increased number of years of life that can be saved. In young women at high risk for breast cancer, it may even be cost effective to screen with more expensive technologies, such as MRI. For women older than 69 years, life expectancy is relatively shorter, and comorbidities are frequent, but the yield of screening is higher because of the higher prevalence of disease. In women older than 69 years, the cost effectiveness of screening needs to be considered in terms of potential years of life saved based on the individual woman's life expectancy.

DIGITAL MAMMOGRAPHY AND DENSE BREASTS

Dense breast tissue itself is a risk factor for breast cancer. The risk is four- to sixfold higher in women who have extremely dense breasts than in matched controls who have fatty breasts,[20–23] and breast cancer is more likely to develop in denser areas of the breast.[24] Extremely dense (> 75% dense) or heterogeneously dense (51%–75% dense) parenchyma[25] is present in more than half of women younger than age 50 years and in one third of women age 50 years and older.[26]

Mammography has reduced sensitivity in dense breast tissue, with sensitivity as low as 30% to 48% in extremely dense parenchyma.[27,28] There is a correspondingly high rate of interval cancers (cancers coming to clinical attention between screening intervals) among women who have dense breasts, and more than half of interval cancers have a poor prognosis.[29] The multicenter Digital Mammographic Imaging Screening Trial showed improved performance of digital mammography in women who had dense breasts, with 70% sensitivity compared with 55% sensitivity for film-screen mammography.[30] False negatives were identified by a single annual mammographic follow-up or by cancers coming to clinical attention although no systematic clinical breast examination program was included. [30] The true sensitivity of digital mammography in dense breasts may be far lower than 70%, but digital mammography, when available, is recommended in such women. A similar detection benefit was observed for digital mammography in screening women younger than 50 years and in pre- or perimenopausal women, with substantial overlap among the groups attributable largely to denser parenchyma in younger women.

SCREENING ULTRASOUND

Supplemental screening with US and MR imaging is being studied in women who are at increased risk of breast cancer because of increased breast density, family or personal history, or both. Across seven published series of whole-breast US screening, using only film-screen mammography for comparison, 178 cancers were identified only sonographically in 49,586 women, for a yield of 0.36% (Table 2). In all but one series,[28] only a single prevalence screen was performed; an estimate of the yield from annual screening sonography is not available. Women who have fatty breast tissue were excluded from screening US, and more than 90% of cancers seen only sonographically have been in heterogeneously dense or extremely dense parenchyma (hereafter collectively termed "dense" breast tissue).[31] Ductal carcinoma in situ (DCIS) is difficult to visualize on US; 94% of cancers seen only on US were invasive.[31] More than 70% of cancers seen only on US were 1 cm in size or smaller,[31] and, when reported, 63 of 73 (86%) of cancers seen only on US were node negative[28,32-34] (with update by S. Ciatto, personal communication, 2006). In the recently published Italian multicenter study, screening US more than doubled the rate of breast cancer detection in women who had dense breasts, with 34 cancers seen in 7615 women on mammography and 36 seen only on US[34] (update by S. Ciatto, personal communication, 2006). Eighteen of 36 (50%) cancers seen only on US were visible in retrospect on mammography[34]

(update by S. Ciatto, personal communication, 2006).

On average, 3% of patients who have screening breast US have been recommended for an US-guided biopsy (see Table 2). In some of the series, additional patients were recommended for US-guided cyst aspiration, but the numbers of such patients are not always identified easily from the reports. Although the positive predictive value of biopsy has been low for lesions seen only on US (averaging 11%, see Table 2), US-guided biopsy is not considered particularly onerous by patients (M. Schleinitz, MD, personal communication and American College of Radiology Imaging Network [ACRIN] 6666, unpublished data, 2006) or practitioners. Recall for additional work-up from screening US is not specifically reported in the studies to date, because most screening US has been physician performed (see Table 2), with results given to the patient at the time of the examination; this practice may change with use of automated devices and potential resulting batch reading. Short-interval follow-up has been recommended in another 3% to 10% (averaging 6%) of women screened with US.[28,32,35,36]

Although screening US seems to allow detection of cancers that are clinically significant at an early stage, an important but heretofore missing piece of information is the rate of interval cancers and number of such cancers that are node positive: even combined US and mammography on an annual basis may not detect the cancers that clinically are most significant. The ongoing ACRIN 6666 protocol[37,38] is a prospective, multicenter study of three rounds of annual screening US and mammography. The rate of interval cancers and the node status of both interval and screen-detected cancers will be important outcomes.

Screening US is well tolerated by patients and is inexpensive. If results of the studies in Table 2 are maintained, and three cancers are found per 1000 women screened with US, at the age of 45 years, preliminary cost effectiveness analysis shows a $50,000 to $70,000 cost per year of life saved (MD Schleinitz, MD, personal communication, 2003). This cost is within the accepted range for seat belts, mammography, and other public health interventions.[39] As of a 2005 report from survey of Fellows of the Society of Breast Imaging, supplemental screening sonography was offered at approximately 35% of United States facilities.[40] Current reimbursement (used to calculate costs) probably does not cover the true costs of this examination if performed by a physician. Automated whole-breast US may improve the practical implementation of screening US.

Table 1
Summary of relative risk and absolute risk of breast cancer by family history and other high-risk factors

Risk Factor	Relative Risk (95% CI)	Absolute Risk (95% CI)	References
No known risk factors	1	12% by age 80 years	66
		0.04% in next 10 years if age 20 years	
		0.4% in next 10 years if age 30 years	
		1.4% in next 10 years if age 40 years	
		1.9% in next 10 years if age 50 years	
		2.3% in next 10 years if age 60 years	
		2.5% in next 10 years if age 70 years	
BRCA-1 or *-2* mutation	—	33% by age 50 years	11
		56% by age 70 years	
BRCA-1 mutation	—	18% by age 39 years	67
		59% by age 49 years	
		65% (44–78%) by age 70 years	
BRCA-2 mutation	—	15% by age 39 years	67
		34% by age 49 years	
		45% (31–56%) by age 70 years	
Li-Fraumeni syndrome (*TP53* mutation)	—	90% lifetime risk	68
CHEK2 mutation	—	<20% lifetime risk	69
First-degree relative with breast cancer before age 40 years	5.7 (2.7–11.8) for a woman < age 40 years; 3.0 (1.8–4.9) for a woman aged 40–49 years	—	66
Mother diagnosed before age 50 years	2.4 (1.86–3.12)	—	70

Risk factor	Relative risk	Absolute risk	References
Sister diagnosed before age 50 years	3.18 (2.15–4.72)	—	70
Two family members with breast cancer, at least one diagnosed before age 40 years	13.5 (3.4–53.9) for a woman < age 50 years; 3.9 (1.8–8.6) for a woman ≥ age 50 years	—	66
Two or more family members with breast cancer	2.9 (2.4–3.6)	2% in next 10 years if age 30 years; 5.2%–5.7% in next 10 years if age 40–70 years	66
Three or more family members with breast cancer	3.9 (2.0–7.5)	—	66,70
Personal history of breast cancer[a]	8–10 overall; 3–4 for second primary	10% risk of recurrence within 12 years if radiation given; 14% risk of recurrence within 20 years	71–73
Personal history of lobular carcinoma in situ	8–12	18–37% lifetime risk	74
Personal history of atypical ductal hyperplasia[a]	4–5	—	75
Personal history of atypical lobular hyperplasia	3	—	76
Age greater than 60 years	—	> 1.7% 5-year risk	Gail model[4]
Extremely dense breast tissue[b]	4–6	—	20–24

Relative risk is the risk of developing breast cancer for women with the risk factor compared with risk of developing breast cancer for women without any known risk factors (95% confidence interval). Note: "High risk" is usually defined as an absolute risk which is ≥three-fold that of an average woman in her 40s (ie, ≥4.2% in the next 10 years) or 50s (ie, ≥5.7% in the next 10 years), depending on national policy for the age to begin routine screening. In women who are at high risk, supplemental screening with ultrasound or MR imaging may be considered in addition to routine mammography. In general, risks from various risk factors are multiplicative.[70]

[a] Chemoprevention with tamoxifen or aromatase inhibitors decreases relative risk by 0.47–0.74.

[b] For women who have known *BRCA* mutations, the effect of increasing breast density is similar in magnitude to the effect in controls without known mutations.[77] Relative risks associated with other risk factors, such as nulliparity, alcohol use, early menarche, late menopause, and hormone use are similar in women who have a family history of breast cancer and women without a family history.[66]

Table 2
Results with screening breast ultrasound

Author	# in Study	# Biopsies (%)	# Cancers (% of Biopsies)	Details
Gordon and Goldenberg 1995[35]	12,706	279 (2.2)	44 (16)	Screening and diagnostic patients, physician performed
Buchberger et al 2000[36]	8103[a]	362 (4.5)[b]	32 (8.8)	Screening, physician performed
Kaplan 2001[32]	1862	102 (5.5)	6 (6.6)	Screening, technologist performed
Kolb et al 2002[28]	13,547[c]	358 (2.6)[b]	37 (10)	Screening over several years, physician performed
Crystal et al 2003[33]	1517	38 (2.5)	7 (18)	Screening, physician performed
Leconte et al 2003[78]	4236	NS	16	Screening, physician performed
Corsetti et al 2006,[34] with update by S. Ciatto, personal communication, 2006	7615	NS[d]	36	Multicenter, screening, physician performed
Total	49,586	1139/37,735 (3.0)	178	

Abbreviation: NS, not stated.
[a] Not included are another eight cancers found in another 867 examinations performed in the diagnostic setting.
[b] Biopsies as stated do not include cyst aspirations.
[c] Number of examinations performed in 5418 women; in all other series, the number of women evaluated is the same as the number of examinations.
[d] In the published series,[34] 15 core biopsies, 66 surgical biopsies, and 405 aspirations were performed in 6449 women examined with screening US.

MR IMAGING

MR imaging is limited as a screening test because of its high cost and requirement for intravenous contrast injection. Claustrophobia further reduces patient tolerance of MR imaging. As of the 2005 survey previously mentioned, 51% of United States facilities offered diagnostic breast MR imaging, and 12% offered screening MR imaging.[40] As a result of these limitations, MR imaging is being considered only for screening women at high risk of breast cancer. MR imaging screening of the contralateral breast in women who have newly diagnosed cancer has been shown to depict mammographically and clinically occult cancer in 3–6% of women but is not discussed further in this article.[41–45]

Tables 3 and 4 summarize results from five studies of screening of women at high risk using MR imaging. Series in which patients were selected for MR imaging on the basis of negative mammography have been excluded from this analysis,[46] and insufficient data are available on use of MR imaging to screen women at increased risk because of lobular carcinoma in situ or atypical hyperplasias.[47] With normalizing for the number of MR imaging screening rounds, on average 8.3 cancers were depicted only on MR imaging for every 1000 examinations performed (70 cancers per 8426 examinations, 0.83%, **Table 4**). The higher yield observed in these studies than reported for screening US is explained, at least in part, by differences in the patient populations studied. In four of the MR imaging series,[8,48–50] women were enrolled because they were known or suspected carriers of BRCA-1 or -2 mutations, and rates of cancers detected only on MR imaging (normalized per screening round) were 1.0% to 1.5%.[8,48–50] In the series of Kriege and colleagues,[51,52] 358 women were proven mutation carriers, and the other 1551 enrolled women had a risk of breast cancer as low as 15% or greater by the Claus model;[6] the rate of cancer detected only on MR imaging (normalized per screening round) was 0.48%. In the US series, where reported, the rate of breast cancer detected only on US in the subset of women at higher risk because of personal or family history of breast cancer, was 0.48% to 1.3%, versus 0.18% to 0.26% in women at average risk.[28,33,36]

On average, 7.8% of women who had screening by MR imaging were recalled for additional evaluation or biopsy (see **Table 4**). Of those recalled, 19% proved to have cancer (see **Table 4**). In several series,[8,51] a relatively high proportion of cancers detected on MR imaging were classified initially as Breast Imaging Reporting and Data

System category 3, probably benign.[53] Only 16% of cancers were node positive at detection, and only 8 of 164 cancers (4.9%) were interval cancers (see **Table 4**). DCIS is readily depicted on MR imaging; 11 of 70 (17%) of cancers seen only on MR imaging were DCIS.[8,48–51] The relatively low specificity of MR imaging improved with subsequent rounds of screening, although the rate of cancer detection by annual MR imaging remained relatively constant.[8,48,52] Both the low observed interval cancer rate and the relatively constant rate of detection with annual MR imaging screening suggest that the annual interval is appropriate.

In three of these series,[8,48,50] mammography, US, and MR imaging were performed and interpreted independently. Across those three series,[8,48,50] only 2 of 81 (2.5%) of cancers were seen only on US, compared with 31 of 81 (38%) seen only on MR imaging. Screening with US seems to have little value after combined mammography and MR imaging, although targeted US often is successful in guiding biopsy of suspicious findings seen on MR imaging even when the initial survey US is negative.[43] Even after combined mammography and US, across these series, only 53% of cancers were depicted, whereas combined mammography and MR imaging depicted 92% of cancers (see **Table 3**). Thus it would seem that even the combination of mammography and US is inadequate in screening women at high risk. This assumption may not be true, however. It may be that cancers seen only on MR imaging would be detected at the next annual screening with combined mammography and US and would still be node negative at detection. The ACRIN 6666 protocol will provide the rate of interval cancers and node-positive cancers at each round of combined mammography and US screening, and at 24 months a subset of patients will undergo screening with MR imaging.[38] The difference in rates of node-positive cancers at 36 months in the subgroup of ACRIN 6666 participants who have had MR imaging and the group that has not will be important information. In the series of Kriege and colleagues,[51] 21% of cases of invasive cancer were node positive in the group screened with MR imaging, compared with 52% to 56% in two control groups. These findings suggest that, compared with mammography alone, supplemental screening with MR imaging should reduce mortality caused by breast cancer in high-risk women.

Based on Medicare reimbursement, breast MR imaging costs about 10 times as much as film-screen mammography. The cost effectiveness of screening with MR imaging has been studied in

Table 3
Detection of cancers with mammography, ultrasound, MR imaging, or a combination of mammography with ultrasound or MR imaging across five series of high-risk women

Study	# Women[a]	# Cancers	# cancers Seen on Mammography (% of Cancers)	# Cancers Seen on Ultrasound (%)	# Cancers Seen on Ultrasound Plus Mammography (%)	# Cancers Seen on MR Imaging (%)	# Cancers Seen on Mammography Plus MR Imaging (%)
Warner et al 2004[48]	236	22	8 (36)	7 (32)	12 (55)	17 (77)	20 (91)
Kriege et al 2004[51]	1909	45[b]	15 (33)	ND	ND	29 (64)	40 (89)
Kuhl et al 2005[8]	529	43	14 (33)	17 (40)	21 (49)	39 (91)	40 (93)
Leach et al 2005[49]	649	35	14 (40)	ND	ND	27 (77)	33 (94)
Sardanelli et al 2007[50]	278	14[c]	8 (57)	8 (57)	9 (64)	13 (93)	14 (100)
Total	3601	159	59 (37)	32/79 (41)	42/79 (53)	125 (79)	147 (92)

Abbreviation: ND, not determined.
[a] Women were screened annually for multiple rounds in each of these studies.
[b] A total of 50 cancers were found in this study, with results summarized for the 45 cancers found in women who had been imaged by both mammography and MR imaging.
[c] A total of 18 cancers were found in this study, with results summarized for the 14 cancers found in women who had been imaged by all screening modalities.

Table 4
Results of high-risk screening with MR imaging across five series

Study	# Patients	# Cancers	# Invasive Cancers (%)	# Node-Positive Cancers (%)[a]	Cancers Seen Only on MR Imaging (% of Cancers)	MR Imaging Recalls/# MR Imaging Examinations (%)	PPV MR Imaging Recall (%)	# Interval Cancers (%)
Warner 2004[48]	236	22	16 (73)	2 (13)	7 (32)	37/457 (8.1)	17 (46)	1 (4.5)
Kriege 2004[51]	1909	50	44 (88)	9 (20)	20 (40)	177/4169 (4.2)	29 (16)	4 (8.0)
Kuhl 2005[8]	529	43	34 (79)	5 (15)	19 (44)	78/1542 (5.1)	39 (50)	1 (2.3)
Leach 2005[49]	649	35	29 (83)	5 (17)	19 (54)	344/1881 (18.3)	27 (7.8)	2 (5.7)
Sardanelli 2007[50b]	278	14	10 (71)	1 (10)	5 (36)	24/377 (6.4)	15 (63)	0 (0)
Total	3601	164	133 (81)	22 (16)	70 (43)	660/8426 (7.8)	127 (19)	8 (4.9)

Abbreviation: PPV, positive predictive value.
[a] % = Percentage of invasive cancers that are node positive.
[b] A total of 18 cancers were found in this study, with results summarized for the 14 cancers found in women who had been imaged by all screening modalities.

BRCA-1 and *-2* carriers and varies substantially with patient age at screening.[54] Addition of annual screening with MR imaging after mammography between the ages of 35 and 54 years yielded a cost per quality-adjusted year of life saved of $55,420 for all *BRCA-1* carriers and of $98,454 for the subset of *BRCA-2* carriers who had dense breasts.[54] Based on cost effectiveness estimates from the United Kingdom study,[55] MR imaging screening will be offered to women aged 30 to 39 years at familial risk who have a 10-year risk greater than 8% and to women aged 40 to 49 years who have at a 10-year risk greater than 20% or greater than 12% if the breast parenchyma is dense.[56]

The latest guidelines from the American Cancer Society[56] endorse annual screening with both MR imaging and mammography of all women with who have a *BRCA* mutation, Li-Fraumeni, Cowden, or Bannayan-Riley-Ruvalcaba syndromes, of untested first-degree (mother, sister, daughter) relatives of a *BRCA* carrier or those who have the listed syndromes, and of those who have lifetime risk of 20% to 25% or greater by validated risk-assessment models. The American Cancer Society recommends against MR imaging screening in women who have less than a 15% lifetime risk of breast cancer.[56] For women at intermediate risk, including those for whom dense breast tissue is the only risk factor, the American Cancer Society states payment should not be a barrier and that further study is warranted.[56]

SCREENING IN WOMEN OLDER THAN AGE 69 YEARS

Because of the high prevalence of breast cancer in this population, all women over age 69 years are considered to be at high risk and to have a 5-year risk of developing breast cancer of at least 1.7% (see **Table 1**). Mammographic sensitivity is as high as 98% in fatty breasts,[57] and fatty replacement increases with age (in the absence of hormone replacement therapy). Thus, there is reason to expect success with mammographic screening in older women.

As stated, the mortality benefit to screening mammography begins to be seen from 5 to 7 years after the onset of screening.[1] Therefore patients who have life expectancies of less than 5 years are unlikely to benefit from screening. Further, there may be harm from detecting cancers that would never have become clinically important. The risk of detecting nonprogressive cancer is estimated at 37% of DCIS on the prevalence (first) screen and only 4% on subsequent incidence screens,[58] although it may take 7 to 10 years for most DCIS to become clinically significant. The average life expectancy of a woman reaching age 80 years is 8.6 years and of a woman reaching age 85 years is 5.9 years.[59] The upper quartile of women reaching age 90 years still has a life expectancy of 6.8 years.[59] Smith-Bindman and colleagues[60] showed a reduced risk of metastatic breast cancer among California Medicare beneficiaries aged 66 to 79 years who underwent screening mammography (relative risk, 0.57; 95% CI, 0.45–0.72) and a corresponding increase of in situ, local, and regional breast cancer among those screened. McPherson and colleagues[61] analyzed the relative risk of all-cause mortality among women diagnosed as having invasive breast cancer from the Upper Midwest Tumor Registry System as a function of age and comorbidities. Patients who had mammographically detected tumors had a significantly lower risk of death among all age groups over age 69 years, even when mild-to-moderate comorbidities were present. They found that only women over age 74 years who had severe or multiple comorbidities were unlikely to benefit from screening.[61]

Currently the American Cancer Society does not set an upper age limit in guidelines for mammographic screening, with the caveats that a woman should be in reasonably good health and would be a candidate for treatment should cancer be detected.[62] Nonetheless, most organized screening programs throughout the world currently restrict screening to women younger than 70 years, or 75 years at most.[63]

SUMMARY

The reduction in mortality achieved by mammographic screening is proven for women between the ages of 40 and 69 years, and more limited data suggest a benefit in women older than 69 years. At the same time, there is increasing awareness of the limitations of mammography, particularly in women who have dense breast tissue. Indeed, dense breast tissue itself has been validated increasingly as a marker of a high risk of developing breast cancer. In women who have dense breast tissue, several steps should be considered. When available, digital mammography has better performance in dense breast tissue. Having the mammogram interpreted by a radiologist who specializes in breast imaging improves the likelihood of cancer detection[64] and diagnosis.[65] Substantial data have shown improved detection of breast cancer with a single screening US examination. Data are needed to support the use of supplemental US in annual screening, and results from the ongoing ACRIN

6666 protocol will help inform such a policy. At present, there is a lack of trained personnel to offer widespread US screening. There is a need for whole-breast automated devices and their validation.

Because of its high cost, limited availability, and reduced patient tolerance, supplemental screening using MR imaging probably will remain more selective, on a case-by-case basis, for the foreseeable future. In women known or suspected to be carriers of a known mutation in *BRCA-1* or *-2*, it seems appropriate to consider screening beginning as early as age 25 years with both mammography and MR imaging. Although data support using supplemental MR imaging in other women at high risk, specific performance characteristics of MR imaging in many subgroups merits further evaluation.

REFERENCES

1. Humphrey LL, Helfand M, Chan BK, et al. Breast cancer screening: a summary of the evidence for the U.S. Preventive Services Task Force. Ann Intern Med 2002;137:347–60.
2. Tabar L, Vitak B, Tony HH, et al. Beyond randomized controlled trials: organized mammographic screening substantially reduces breast carcinoma mortality. Cancer 2001;91:1724–31.
3. National Cancer Institute. Surveillance, Epidemiology, and End Results. Available at: www.seer.gov/. Accessed July 4, 2007.
4. Gail MH, Brinton LA, Byar DP, et al. Projecting individualized probabilities of developing breast cancer for white females who are being examined annually. J Natl Cancer Inst 1989;81:1879–86.
5. Gail MH, Costantino JP. Validating and improving models for projecting the absolute risk of breast cancer. J Natl Cancer Inst 2001;00:004–5.
6. Claus EB, Risch N, Thompson WD. Autosomal dominant inheritance of early-onset breast cancer. Implications for risk prediction. Cancer 1994;73:643–51.
7. National Cancer Institute. Available at: http://www.cancer.gov/bcrisktool/. Accessed on July 4, 2007.
8. Kuhl CK, Schrading S, Leutner CC, et al. Mammography, breast ultrasound, and magnetic resonance imaging for surveillance of women at high familial risk for breast cancer. J Clin Oncol 2005;23:8469–76.
9. Cortesi L, Turchetti D, Marchi I, et al. Breast cancer screening in women at increased risk according to different family histories: an update of the Modena Study Group experience. BMC Cancer 2006;6:210.
10. Berry DA, Iversen ES Jr, Gudbjartsson DF, et al. BRCAPRO validation, sensitivity of genetic testing of BRCA1/BRCA2, and prevalence of other breast cancer susceptibility genes. J Clin Oncol 2002;20:2701–12.
11. Struewing JP, Hartge P, Wacholder S, et al. The risk of cancer associated with specific mutations of BRCA1 and BRCA2 among Ashkenazi Jews. N Engl J Med 1997;336:1401–8.
12. Dershaw DD. Are there any indications for routine breast cancer screening of asymptomatic women who are less than 40 years old? AJR Am J Roentgenol 1999;172:1136–7.
13. Aisenberg AC, Finkelstein DM, Doppke KP, et al. High risk of breast carcinoma after irradiation of young women with Hodgkin's disease. Cancer 1997;79:1203–10.
14. Tinger A, Wasserman TH, Klein EE, et al. The incidence of breast cancer following mantle field radiation therapy as a function of dose and technique. Int J Radiat Oncol Biol Phys 1997;37:865–70.
15. Russo J, Frederick J, Ownby HE, et al. Predictors of recurrence and survival of patients with breast cancer. Am J Clin Pathol 1987;88:123–31.
16. Fisher ER, Anderson S, Redmond C, et al. Pathologic findings from the National Surgical Adjuvant Breast Project protocol B-06. 10-year pathologic and clinical prognostic discriminants. Cancer 1993;71:2507–14.
17. Michaelson JS, Silverstein M, Sgroi D, et al. The effect of tumor size and lymph node status on breast carcinoma lethality. Cancer 2003;98:2133–43.
18. Smith RA, Duffy SW, Gabe R, et al. The randomized trials of breast cancer screening: what have we learned? Radiol Clin North Am 2004;42:793–806, v.
19. Zabicki K, Colbert JA, Dominguez FJ, et al. Breast cancer diagnosis in women < or = 40 versus 50 to 60 years: increasing size and stage disparity compared with older women over time. Ann Surg Oncol 2006;13:1072–7.
20. Wolfe JN, Saftlas AF, Salane M. Mammographic parenchymal patterns and quantitative evaluation of mammographic densities: a case-control study. AJR Am J Roentgenol 1987;148:1087–92.
21. Boyd NF, Byng JW, Jong RA, et al. Quantitative classification of mammographic densities and breast cancer risk: results from the Canadian National Breast Screening Study. J Natl Cancer Inst 1995;87:670–5.
22. Harvey JA, Bovbjerg VE. Quantitative assessment of mammographic breast density: relationship with breast cancer risk. Radiology 2004;230:29–41.
23. McCormack VA, dos Santos Silva I. Breast density and parenchymal patterns as markers of breast cancer risk: a meta-analysis. Cancer Epidemiol Biomarkers Prev 2006;15:1159–69.
24. Boyd NF, Guo H, Martin LJ, et al. Mammographic density and the risk and detection of breast cancer. N Engl J Med 2007;356:227–36.
25. D'Orsi CJ, Bassett LW, Berg WA, et al. Breast imaging reporting and data system, BI-RADS: mammography.

4th edition. Reston (VA): American College of Radiology; 2003.

26. Stomper PC, D'Souza DJ, DiNitto PA, et al. Analysis of parenchymal density on mammograms in 1353 women 25-79 years old. AJR Am J Roentgenol 1996;167:1261–5.

27. Mandelson MT, Oestreicher N, Porter PL, et al. Breast density as a predictor of mammographic detection: comparison of interval- and screen-detected cancers. J Natl Cancer Inst 2000;92:1081–7.

28. Kolb TM, Lichy J, Newhouse JH. Comparison of the performance of screening mammography, physical examination, and breast US and evaluation of factors that influence them: an analysis of 27,825 patient evaluations. Radiology 2002;225:165–75.

29. Tabar L, Vitak B, Chen HH, et al. The Swedish Two-County Trial twenty years later. Updated mortality results and new insights from long-term follow-up. Radiol Clin North Am 2000;38:625–51.

30. Pisano ED, Gatsonis C, Hendrick E, et al. Diagnostic performance of digital versus film mammography for breast-cancer screening. N Engl J Med 2005;353: 1773–83.

31. Berg WA. Supplemental screening sonography in dense breasts. Radiol Clin North Am 2004;42: 845–51, vi.

32. Kaplan SS. Clinical utility of bilateral whole-breast US in the evaluation of women with dense breast tissue. Radiology 2001;221:641–9.

33. Crystal P, Strano SD, Shcharynski S, et al. Using sonography to screen women with mammographically dense breasts. AJR Am J Roentgenol 2003; 181:177–82.

34. Corsetti V, Ferrari A, Ghirardi M, et al. Role of ultrasonography in detecting mammographically occult breast carcinoma in women with dense breasts. Radiol Med (Torino) 2006;111:440–8.

35. Gordon PB, Goldenberg SL. Malignant breast masses detected only by ultrasound. A retrospective review. [see comments]. Cancer 1995;76:626–30.

36. Buchberger W, Niehoff A, Obrist P, et al. Clinically and mammographically occult breast lesions: detection and classification with high-resolution sonography. Semin Ultrasound CT MR 2000;21: 325–36.

37. Berg WA. Rationale for a trial of screening breast ultrasound: American College of Radiology Imaging Network (ACRIN) 6666. AJR Am J Roentgenol 2003; 180:1225–8.

38. American College of Radiology Imaging Network. Available at: http://www.acrin.org/6666_protocol. html. Accessed July 4, 2007.

39. Farria D, Feig SA. An introduction to economic issues in breast imaging. Radiol Clin North Am 2000;38:825–42.

40. Farria DM, Schmidt ME, Monsees BS, et al. Professional and economic factors affecting access to mammography: a crisis today, or tomorrow? Cancer 2005;104:491–8.

41. Liberman L, Morris EA, Kim CM, et al. MR imaging findings in the contralateral breast of women with recently diagnosed breast cancer. AJR Am J Roentgenol 2003;180:333–41.

42. Lee SG, Orel SG, Woo IJ, et al. MR imaging screening of the contralateral breast in patients with newly diagnosed breast cancer: preliminary results. Radiology 2003;226:773–8.

43. Berg WA, Gutierrez L, Nessaiver MS, et al. Diagnostic accuracy of mammography, clinical examination, US, and MR imaging in preoperative assessment of breast cancer. Radiology 2004;233:830–49.

44. Lehman CD, Blume JD, Thickman D, et al. Added cancer yield of MRI in screening the contralateral breast of women recently diagnosed with breast cancer: results from the International Breast Magnetic Resonance Consortium (IBMC) trial. J Surg Oncol 2005;92:9–15 [discussion: 15–6].

45. Lehman CD, Gatsonis C, Kuhl CK, et al. MRI evaluation of the contralateral breast in women with recently diagnosed breast cancer. N Engl J Med 2007;356:1295–303.

46. Morris EA, Liberman L, Ballon DJ, et al. MRI of occult breast carcinoma in a high-risk population. AJR Am J Roentgenol 2003;181:619–26.

47. Port ER, Park A, Borgen PI, et al. Results of MRI screening for breast cancer in high-risk patients with LCIS and atypical hyperplasia. Ann Surg Oncol 2007;14:1051–7.

48. Warner E, Plewes DB, Hill KA, et al. Surveillance of BRCA1 and BRCA2 mutation carriers with magnetic resonance imaging, ultrasound, mammography, and clinical breast examination. JAMA 2004;292: 1317–25.

49. Leach MO, Boggis CR, Dixon AK, et al. Screening with magnetic resonance imaging and mammography of a UK population at high familial risk of breast cancer: a prospective multicentre cohort study (MARIBS). Lancet 2005;365:1769–78.

50. Sardanelli F, Podo F, D'Agnolo G, et al. Multicenter comparative multimodality surveillance of women at genetic-familial high risk for breast cancer (HIBCRIT study): interim results. Radiology 2007; 242:698–715.

51. Kriege M, Brekelmans CT, Boetes C, et al. Efficacy of MRI and mammography for breast-cancer screening in women with a familial or genetic predisposition. N Engl J Med 2004;351:427–37.

52. Kriege M, Brekelmans CT, Boetes C, et al. Differences between first and subsequent rounds of the MRISC breast cancer screening program for women with a familial or genetic predisposition. Cancer 2006;106:2318–26.

53. Ikeda DM, Hylton NM, Kuhl CK, et al. Breast Imaging Reporting and Data System, BI-RADS: magnetic

resonance imaging. Reston (VA): American College of Radiology; 2003.

54. Plevritis SK, Kurian AW, Sigal BM, et al. Cost-effectiveness of screening BRCA1/2 mutation carriers with breast magnetic resonance imaging. JAMA 2006;295:2374–84.

55. Griebsch I, Brown J, Boggis C, et al. Cost-effectiveness of screening with contrast enhanced magnetic resonance imaging vs X-ray mammography of women at a high familial risk of breast cancer. Br J Cancer 2006;95:801–10.

56. Saslow D, Boetes C, Burke W, et al. American Cancer Society guidelines for breast screening with MRI as an adjunct to mammography. CA Cancer J Clin 2007;57:75–89.

57. Kerlikowske K, Grady D, Barclay J, et al. Effect of age, breast density, and family history on the sensitivity of first screening mammography [see comments]. JAMA 1996;276:33–8.

58. Yen MF, Tabar L, Vitak B, et al. Quantifying the potential problem of overdiagnosis of ductal carcinoma in situ in breast cancer screening. Eur J Cancer 2003;39:1746–54.

59. Walter LC, Covinsky KE. Cancer screening in elderly patients: a framework for individualized decision making. JAMA 2001;285:2750–6.

60. Smith-Bindman R, Kerlikowske K, Gebretsadik T, et al. Is screening mammography effective in elderly women? Am J Med 2000;108:112–9.

61. McPherson CP, Swenson KK, Lee MW. The effects of mammographic detection and comorbidity on the survival of older women with breast cancer. J Am Geriatr Soc 2002;50:1061–8.

62. Smith RA, Saslow D, Sawyer KA, et al. American Cancer Society guidelines for breast cancer screening: update 2003. CA Cancer J Clin 2003;53:141–69.

63. Ballard-Barbash R, Klabunde C, Paci E, et al. Breast cancer screening in 21 countries: delivery of services, notification of results and outcomes ascertainment. Eur J Cancer Prev 1999;8:417–26.

64. Sickles EA, Wolverton DE, Dee KE. Performance parameters for screening and diagnostic mammography: specialist and general radiologists. Radiology 2002;224:861–9.

65. Leung JW, Margolin FR, Dee KE, et al. Performance parameters for screening and diagnostic mammography in a community practice: are there differences between specialists and general radiologists? AJR Am J Roentgenol 2007;188:236–41.

66. Collaborative Group on Hormonal Factors in Breast Cancer Familial breast cancer. Collaborative reanalysis of individual data from 52 epidemiological studies including 58,209 women with breast cancer and 101,986 women without the disease. Lancet 2001;358:1389–99.

67. Easton DF, Ford D, Bishop DT. Breast and ovarian cancer incidence in BRCA1-mutation carriers. Breast cancer linkage consortium. Am J Hum Genet 1995;56:265–71.

68. Lux MP, Fasching PA, Beckmann MW. Hereditary breast and ovarian cancer: review and future perspectives. J Mol Med 2006;84:16–28.

69. Wooster R, Weber BL. Breast and ovarian cancer. N Engl J Med 2003;348:2339–47.

70. Easton DF. Familial risks of breast cancer. Breast Cancer Res 2002;4:179–81.

71. Fisher B, Anderson S, Redmond CK, et al. Reanalysis and results after 12 years of follow-up in a randomized clinical trial comparing total mastectomy with lumpectomy with or without irradiation in the treatment of breast cancer. N Engl J Med 1995;333:1456–61.

72. Fisher B, Anderson S, Bryant J, et al. Twenty-year follow-up of a randomized trial comparing total mastectomy, lumpectomy, and lumpectomy plus irradiation for the treatment of invasive breast cancer. N Engl J Med 2002;347:1233–41.

73. American Chemical Society. 2007. Available at: www.acs.org. Accessed July 18, 2007.

74. Frykberg ER. Lobular carcinoma in situ of the breast. Breast J 1999;5:296–303.

75. Dupont WD, Parl FF, Hartmann WH, et al. Breast cancer risk associated with proliferative breast disease and atypical hyperplasia. Cancer 1993;71:1258–65.

76. Page DL, Schuyler PA, Dupont WD, et al. Atypical lobular hyperplasia as a unilateral predictor of breast cancer risk: a retrospective cohort study. Lancet 2003;361:125–9.

77. Mitchell G, Antoniou AC, Warren R, et al. Mammographic density and breast cancer risk in BRCA1 and BRCA2 mutation carriers. Cancer Res 2006;66:1866–72.

78. Leconte I, Feger C, Galant C, et al. Mammography and subsequent whole-breast sonography of nonpalpable breast cancers: the importance of radiologic breast density. AJR Am J Roentgenol 2003;180:1675–9.

The Role of Echocardiography in Hemodynamic Assessment in Heart Failure

Jacob Abraham, MD, Theodore P. Abraham, MD*

KEYWORDS

- Heart failure • Hemodynamics • Echocardiography
- Diastolic function • Contractile indices • RV function

Hemodynamic derangement—the inability of the heart to generate adequate cardiac output at normal filling pressures—is a defining feature of the syndrome of heart failure (HF). HF is not a diagnosis but rather is the clinical expression of hemodynamic and neurohormonal abnormalities initiated by a variety of cardiac insults, including myocardial ischemia, cardiomyopathy, valve disease, congenital lesions, and pericardial disease. Careful clinical assessment remains the cornerstone of management of the patient who has HF. The utility of quantitative hemodynamic measurements for routine HF management is unproven, but invasive hemodynamic evaluation still is needed to guide management of HF in specific settings.[1] In such cases, direct measurement of intra-cardiac pressures, vascular resistances, and cardiac output by catheterization remains the reference standard. For routine evaluation and management of HF, however, echocardiography now is recommended as the most useful diagnostic test.[2] Comprehensive Doppler analysis enables accurate assessment of cardiac output, ventricular filling pressures, and vascular resistances (Table 1). Echocardiography, however, is not merely a noninvasive surrogate for the right heart catheter. Whereas invasive hemodynamic data represent an instantaneous measurement in time, echocardiography provides details of cardiac structure and function that reflect the consequences of chronic hemodynamic disturbances. Furthermore, echocardiography yields unique information that complements hemodynamic data in assessing the clinical significance of hemodynamic abnormalities and in determining prognosis.

This article reviews the role of echocardiography (M-mode, two-dimensional, spectral, and tissue Doppler) for qualitative and quantitative hemodynamic assessment of the patient who has HF. It highlights the echocardiographic parameters that have the most diagnostic and/or prognostic relevance for patients who have advanced HF. The importance of right heart failure and HF with preserved ejection fraction (HFpEF) is increasingly recognized, and therefore the echocardiographic evaluation of these conditions is emphasized also.

CONTRACTILE FUNCTION OF THE LEFT VENTRICLE

Muscle fiber shortening generates the ventricular stroke volume and thus cardiac output. The extent of muscle shortening, or contractility, is best described by pressure–volume loop analysis, but this method is not feasible in routine clinical practice.[3] Clinical assessment of ventricular contractile

This article originally appeared in *Heart Failure Clinics* 2009;5(2):191–208.

The Johns Hopkins University, Baltimore, MD, USA

* Corresponding author. Division of Cardiology, The Johns Hopkins University, 600 North Wolfe Street, Baltimore, MD 21287.

E-mail address: tabraha3@jhmi.edu (T.P. Abraham).

Ultrasound Clin 4 (2009) 149–166
doi:10.1016/j.cult.2009.04.002

Table 1
Hemodynamic parameters and their echocardiographic correlates

Hemodynamic Parameter	Echocardiographic Correlate	Comment	Reference
Right atrial pressure	IVC diameter and respirophasic variation	Not valid in positive pressure ventilation except to exclude high RAP	41
Pulmonary artery systolic pressure	$4(V_{TR})^2$ + RAP	See Table 3 for RAP estimation	
Pulmonary artery diastolic pressure	$4(V_{PR})^2$ + RAP	See Table 3 for RAP estimation	
Pulmonary capillary wedge pressure	E/E_m	E/E_m > 12 (TDE of septal mitral annulus) predicts PCWP > 15 mm Hg in patients who have reduced EF	46
Left atrial pressure	SBP – $4(V_{MR})^2$	Exclude patients with acute MR, prosthetic mitral valve, and LVOT obstruction or peripheral arterial disease of the arm	22
Cardiac output	HR × VTI × area	Accurate measure of LVOT diameter is critical	4
dP/dt	32/Δt	Δt measured from continuous wave Doppler of MR jet	8
Pulmonary vascular resistance	10 × (V_{TR}/RVOT VTI) + 0.16		43

Abbreviation: PCWP, pulmonary capillary wedge pressure.

performance thus has relied on imperfect and indirect measurements that are sensitive to changes in loading conditions, such as ventricular volumes, cardiac output, and ejection fraction (EF). Unique echocardiographic indices of myocardial contractile function also have been derived and validated.

Cardiac Output

Quantitation of cardiac output by echocardiography involves Doppler measurement of flow across an orifice. In the absence of an intracardiac shunt or significant valvular regurgitation, the conservation of mass dictates that the volume of blood (Q) flowing through the heart in the steady state is constant. In general, the rate of blood flow can be determined using the hydraulic orifice formula, dQ/dt = A × V, where dQ/dt is flow rate, A is the cross-sectional area of the orifice, and V is the flow velocity. In the cardiovascular system, flow is pulsatile, and thus V varies during the cardiac cycle. Summing (integrating) the flow velocities at each time point during systole yields

the stroke distance, or the linear distance blood is pumped during ejection. This measure also is called the velocity–time integral (VTI) because it represents the area under the velocity–time curve. Stroke volume (SV) then is given as SV = VTI × A and cardiac output (CO) as CO = heart rate (HR) × SV. Pulsed-wave Doppler interrogation of the left ventricular outflow tract (LVOT) at the aortic annulus typically is used for assessment of stroke volume. If continuous-wave Doppler is used, then A must be assessed at the sinotubular junction, the narrowest portion of the aorta, where peak velocity will be recorded. By measuring the LVOT diameter D and assuming a circular cross section, $A = \pi \times (D/2)^2 = \pi\ 0.785 \times D^2$ (**Fig. 1**). An analogous calculation can made for right ventricular (RV) output from the basal short axis. Doppler-based cardiac output measurements correlate well with invasively measured cardiac output, including in critically ill patients.[4]

Accurate quantification of cardiac output using this method requires that several conditions be

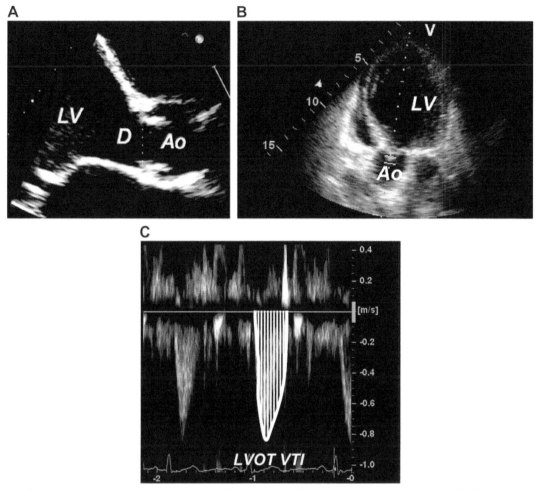

Fig. 1. Measurement of cardiac output using pulse wave Doppler technique. (A) Measurement of the LV outflow tract diameter using the edge-to-edge technique. Ao, aorta; D, diameter. (*From* Vivekananthan K, Kalputa T, Mehra M, et al. Usefulness of the combined index of systolic and diastolic myocardial performance to identify cardiac allograft rejection. Am J Cardiol 2002;90(5):518; with permission.) (*B*) Stroke distance (LVOT VTI) is measured using pulse wave Doppler at the aortic annulus. (*C*) VTI measurement of aortic Doppler velocity profile.

mot. First, precise measurement of the LVOT diameter D is crucial, because any measurement errors are amplified when the term is squared. To avoid this source of error, VTI alone can be used as a surrogate for cardiac output.[5] Second, the diameter and velocity measurements must be made at the same anatomic location and under similar load and HR conditions. For the latter condition to be met, images must be obtained in close sequence during the echocardiographic examination. Finally, the Doppler beam must be aligned parallel with blood flow to avoid underestimation of the velocity signal.

Ejection Fraction

Although the EF is the most widely used index of contractile function in clinical practice and research, it has major limitations. First, in clinical settings the EF is estimated by visual assessment of endocardial excursion and therefore is susceptible to subjectivity and interobserver variability. Even when cardiac volumes are quantified and the EF is computed, as discussed later, geometric assumptions are made that may be prone to error. Second, like most indices of contractile function, the EF is sensitive to changes in preload and afterload. Finally, in the management of patients who have HF, there is little correlation between EF and symptoms, exercise capacity, maximum oxygen consumption, or cardiac filling pressures.[6] Despite these limitations, the EF is ingrained in clinical practice because of its proven prognostic ability and relative ease of measurement.

The EF is calculated as EDV – ESV/EDV, where EDV equals end-diastolic volume, and ESV equals end-systolic volume. Calculation of left ventricular (LV) volumes from linear measurements is inaccurate. Professional guidelines recommend that volumes be measured using the biplane method of discs (modified Simpson's rule).[7] With this method, the endocardial border is traced from two orthogonal apical views. Echocardiographic analysis software automatically generates multiple elliptic disks whose cross-sectional area is based on the diameter measured from two- and four-chamber views. The height of each disk is calculated as a fraction of the LV long axis. The volumes of the disks then are summed to provide ventricular volume (**Fig. 2**). If only a single apical view is available, the cross-section of the heart is assumed to be circular; this assumption is most error prone in the setting of regional wall motion abnormalities. If the endocardium is not well visualized, the area–length method is an alternative (**Fig. 3**). This method assumes a bullet-shaped ventricle and requires planimetry of the mid-ventricle short-axis area and the annulus-to-apex length in the four-chamber view. Volumes in systole and diastole are determined from the equation volume = [5(area) (length)]/6.

Rate of Pressure Change During Contraction

The rate of pressure change during contraction (dP/dt), an index of contractility measured at catheterization, also can be estimated noninvasively from the continuous-wave Doppler mitral regurgitation (MR) velocity curve. During the isovolumic contraction phase of systole, the rate of pressure rise is relatively independent of load. From the Doppler MR spectral signal, the time interval Δt (in milliseconds) between velocities of 1 m/s and 3 m/s on the ascending slope are measured (**Fig. 4**).[8] From the Bernoulli equation ($\Delta P = 4V_{MR}^2$, where ΔP is the LV–LA pressure gradient and V_{MR} is the MR velocity), these MR velocities correspond to a pressure difference of 32 mm Hg (36 − 4 mm Hg), so that dP/dt = 32/Δt. Using this approach, Doppler-derived dP/dt was found to correlate well with catheter-measured dP/dt.[8]

Tei Index

The Tei index, or index of myocardial performance (IMP), is defined as (IRT + ICT)/ET, where IRT equals isovolumic relaxation time, ICT equals isovolumic contraction time, and ET equals ejection

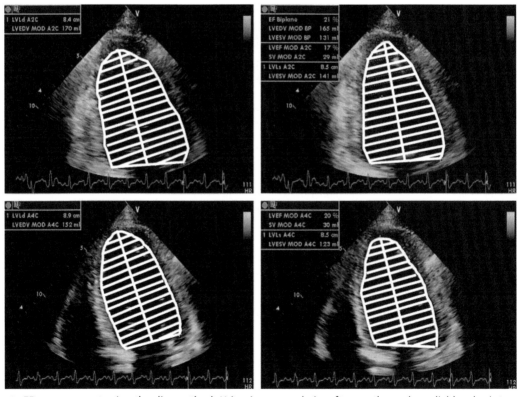

Fig. 2. EF measurement using the disc method. Using image analysis software, the endocardial border is traced manually in systole and diastole in both two- and four-chamber views. The discs technique is applied, yielding EDV and ESV from which EF and SV are computed.

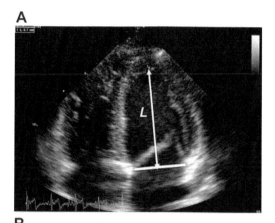

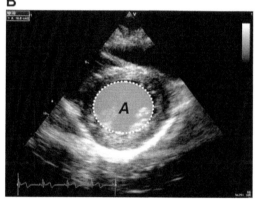

Fig. 3. Area–length method for calculating EF. (*A*) Length L is measured from apex to mitral annulus in the apical four-chamber view. (*B*) Short-axis area *A* is measured at the papillary muscle level. Note that the papillary muscles are excluded from the area calculation.

time. The sum IRT + ICT is computed by subtracting ET from the interval between cessation and onset of mitral inflow (**Fig. 5**). This index was proposed as an integrated measure of global systolic and diastolic function. The correlation of IMP with invasively determined indices of ventricular performance, such as dP/dt_{max}, dP/dt_{min}, and tau (τ), is modest.[9] Moreover, in an animal study, IMP was sensitive to acute changes in loading conditions but insensitive to changes in inotropic state.[10] Despite these limitations, IMP retains strong prognostic value in population-based studies. An IMP higher than 0.75 has been shown to predict survival in patients who have dilated cardiomyopathy and severe LV dysfunction.[11]

Strain Rate

Tissue Doppler echocardiography (TDE) quantifies myocardial tissue velocity. Systolic tissue velocity (S_m) correlates modestly with catheter-derived peak dP/dt and has been proposed as

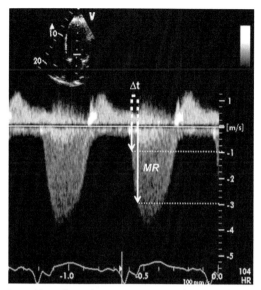

Fig. 4. Use of continuous wave Doppler recording of MR to calculate dP/dt. Time interval (Δt) is measured from 1 m/s to 3 m/s of the velocity curve. dP/dt = $32/\Delta t$.

a noninvasive index of global contractile function.[12] A significant limitation of TDE is that myocardial velocity is measured relative to an external reference frame (the echocardiography probe) and therefore is affected by tissue translation and tethering.

Strain rate (SR) measurement circumvents this limitation by measuring deformation and velocity relative to a myocardial reference frame. Strain rate, measured in seconds^{-1}, is the spatial derivative of velocity at two points in the myocardium: $SR = V_a - V_b/d$, where $V_a - V_b$ is the instantaneous velocity difference between points *a* and *b* separated by distance *d* (**Fig. 6**). Greenburg and colleagues[13] demonstrated in dogs that peak SR measured at the basal septum by TDL color M-mode cardiography correlated robustly with invasive indices of contractility under varying inotropic conditions. Although promising, clinical application of SR imaging for hemodynamic assessment is limited at present to the detection of reduced contractile function in subclinical cardiomyopathy.[14]

CARDIAC MORPHOLOGY AND REMODELING
Chamber Geometry

Hemodynamic assessment by echocardiography should incorporate cardiac morphology. The heart has limited morphologic responses to pressure and volume overload—hypertrophy and/or dilatation. Chamber geometry provides insight into the nature, chronicity, and severity of adverse loading

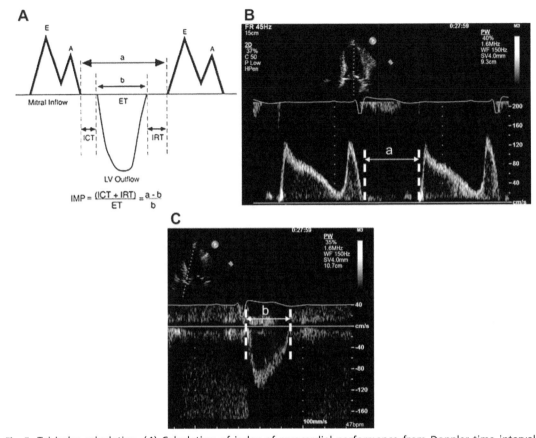

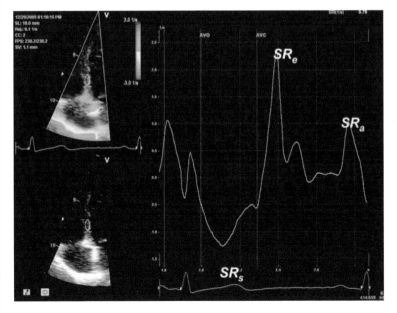

Fig. 5. Tei index calculation. (*A*) Calculation of index of myocardial performance from Doppler time intervals. (*From* Vivekananthan K, Kalputa T, Mehra M, et al. Usefulness of the combined index of systolic and diastolic myocardial performance to identify cardiac allograft rejection. Am J Cardiol 2002;90(5):518; with permission). (*B*) From the apical two-chamber view, the continuous wave Doppler sample volume is placed between the mitral valve leaflet tips to measure the isovolumic contraction time and isovolumic relaxation time, a. (*C*) The ejection time, b, is measured from the outflow ejection time. The Tei index is computed as (a − b)/b.

Fig. 6. Strain rate imaging. Strain rate measures the spatial gradient of velocity. Tissue Doppler echocardiography is performed using a high frame rate and narrow sector width (*top panel, left*). A sample volume is placed in the basal septum (*bottom panel, left*). Systolic (SR$_s$), early diastolic (SR$_e$), and late diastolic (SR$_a$) strain rate peaks are shown in the right panel.

conditions, and the extent of remodeling is a strong determinant of prognosis. In an echocardiographic substudy of the Beta-blocker Evaluation of Survival Trial (BEST), for example, Grayburn and colleagues[15] found that an LV diastolic volume index (ie, LV diastolic volume/body surface area) greater than 120 mL/m² was the only predictor of death in multivariate analysis. Moreover, once ventricular enlargement is severe (LV diastolic dimension > 7 cm), medical treatment is unlikely to reverse remodeling.[16]

Cardiac remodeling also is central to the pathogenesis of HFpEF. Comparing patients who have HFpEF with a matched control group consisting of individuals who had hypertensive LV hypertrophy but without HF, Melanovsky and colleagues[17] found that LV mass index and maximal left atrial volume (LAV) best distinguished patients from controls. Both groups had similar systolic, diastolic, and vascular dysfunction, suggesting that remodeling was a decisive factor in the transition to HF.

Mitral Regurgitation

Functional MR is a common complication of HF that perpetuates LV remodeling, volume overload, diastolic dysfunction, and secondary pulmonary hypertension (PH). Higher grades of MR are an independent predictor of death in HF.[18] In patients who have dilated cardiomyopathy, poor coaptation of mitral leaflets results from apical displacement of the papillary muscles, abnormalities in regional ventricular wall motion, tethering of the mitral chordae, annular dilatation, and weakening of mitral closing forces (**Fig. 7**). Although it often is difficult to determine whether MR is a cause or consequence of HF, it is important to distinguish between functional MR and primary valvular diseases (eg, calcification, perforation, flail leaflet, or prolapse), because these lesions dictate different management strategies. Multiple quantitative Doppler methods should be used to quantify the severity of MR, because over-reliance on color Doppler estimation can be misleading.

This caveat is particularly important in acute MR, because the short duration of regurgitation and normal chamber sizes limit jet area and the rapid equilibration of left atrial pressure (LAP) and LV pressure (LVP) reduces jet velocities. Confronted with an acutely ill patient who has pulmonary edema and seemingly mild MR, a careful examination of vena contracta width, pulse

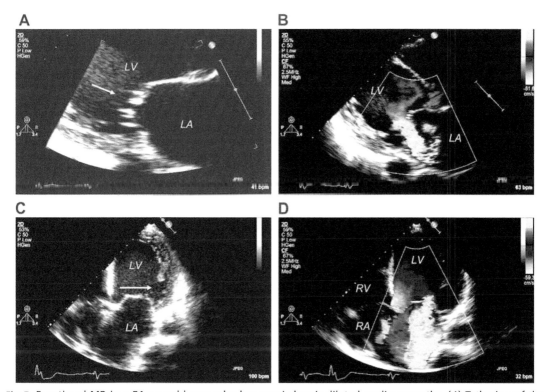

Fig. 7. Functional MR in a 54-year-old man who has non-ischemic dilated cardiomyopathy. (*A*) Tethering of the mitral valve chordae prevents full coaptation of the mitral leaflets in systole. (*B*) Color Doppler demonstrates severe, eccentric MR. (*C*) Apical four-chamber view showing tethering. (*D*) Severe MR with large vena contracta width and jet area.

Doppler quantification, and Doppler hemody-namic signs of elevated pressures (short aortic regurgitation half-time, pulmonary venous systolic flow reversal, and truncation of MR velocities) may provide the only echocardiographic clues to the true severity of acute MR.

DIASTOLIC FILLING/FILLING PRESSURES

Diastole encompasses the period of the cardiac cycle from closure of the aortic valve to closure of the mitral valve. During isovolumic relaxation, the LV untwists and de-stiffens. The rate of de-stiffening or relaxation normally is rapid and is characterized by τ or negative dP/dt. The rate of LV filling after mitral valve opening is determined by the instantaneous pressure gradient between LA and LV and the LV compliance (dV/dP). Impaired LV relaxation or reduced LV compliance are fundamental causes of abnormal diastolic filling that can be assessed accurately by echocar-diography. Diastolic function also is influenced by a number of other factors, including atrial transport function, ventricular interaction, pericardial constraint, ventricular–vascular coupling (vascular stiffening), and MR.

The severity of diastolic function relates inversely to prognosis in HF (both with preserved and with reduced EF) and directly to symptom severity and B-type natriuretic peptide (BNP) levels.[19–21] A single index of diastolic function analogous to EF remains elusive because of the complex physiology of diastole. Qualitative and quantitative Doppler techniques form the basis of contemporary echocardiographic assessment of ventricular filling pressures and diastolic filling.

Left Atrial Pressure

Estimation of LV and left atrial (LA) diastolic pres-sures from the pulmonary capillary wedge pres-sure (PCWP) at right heart catheterization is important in guiding management of the patient who has HF. An insensitive but specific sign of elevated LV end-diastolic pressure (LVEDP) is a "B bump" in the mitral valve M-mode (**Fig. 8**). Using the Bernoulli equation, a quantitative and noninvasive estimate of LAP can be derived from the peak V_{MR}. This jet velocity is determined by the systolic pressure gradient between LV and LA:

$$\Delta P = LV \text{ systolic pressure} - LA \text{ systolic pressure} = 4(V_{MR})^2.$$

Brachial artery systolic pressure (SBP) measured by sphygmomanometry is used to esti-mate LV systolic pressure. Therefore LAP equals SBP − $4(V_{MR})^2$. Applying this method, Gorscan

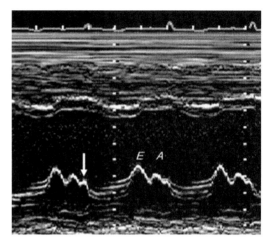

Fig. 8. M-mode cardiography through the mitral leaf-lets demonstrates a "B hump" (*arrow*) after the *A* excursion, indicating elevated LVEDP.

and colleagues[22] studied the correlation between the noninvasive measurement of LAP and simulta-neous mean PCWP in 35 stable inpatients who had HF and either primary or secondary chronic MR. This study found a strong correlation between echocardiographic and catheter measurements of LAP, even in the small subgroup (12 patients) who had phasic v waves 10 mm Hg above the mean wedge pressure ($r = 0.87$ versus $r = 0.88$).

Left Atrial Volume

With chronic elevations in LV diastolic pressure, the LAP must rise to maintain filling. In response to this increased wall stress, the LA enlarges and remodels. LAV has been shown to be an indepen-dent predictor of atrial fibrillation, stroke, HF, and cardiovascular death and has been proposed to be a marker of chronic diastolic dysfunction.[23] In support of this view, community-based studies have found LA size to be independently predictive of incident HFpEF.[17,24] An LAV of 32 mL/m² or greater was associated with increased incidence of congestive HF, independent of age, myocardial infarction, diabetes mellitus, hypertension, LV hypertrophy, and mitral inflow velocities (HR 1.97, 95% CI 1.4 to 2.7).[24] The prognostic signifi-cance of LA size in systolic HF is less clear, espe-cially because diastolic dysfunction is ubiquitous in this population. LAV, rather than linear dimen-sion, is the preferred method of quantification and is computed from the biplane area and length: LAV = (0.85) × (A_1) × (A_2)/L, where A_1 is the LA area from the four-chamber view, A_2 is LA area from the two-chamber view, and L is the LA length measured from mitral annulus mid-plane to supe-rior LA (**Fig. 9**).

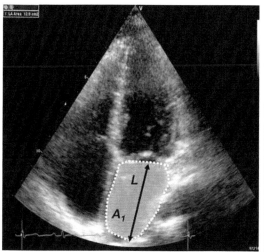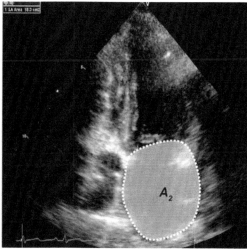

Fig. 9. Area—length method of computing LAV. The length *L* is chosen as the shorter LA length measured from apical two- or four-chamber. See text for details.

EARLY DIASTOLIC FLOW VELOCITY/LATE DIASTOLIC FLOW VELOCITY

Mitral inflow velocity curves reflect the instantaneous pressure gradient between the LA and LV during diastole. Pulse-wave Doppler at the mitral valve leaflet tips records an early diastolic flow velocity (E-wave velocity) followed by a late diastolic flow velocity (A-wave velocity) generated by atrial contraction. In the normal heart, approximately 85% of LV filling occurs during early diastole; therefore, E-wave velocity typically is greater than A-wave velocity. The time interval for the E-wave velocity to decelerate to the zero baseline is the deceleration time (DT) and reflects LV compliance.

Mitral inflow velocities follow a pattern of progression with increasing severity of diastolic abnormalitioo (**Fig. 10; Table 2**). With mild diastolic dysfunction, LV relaxation is impaired, resulting in reduced E-wave velocity and greater dependence on atrial contraction (higher A-wave velocity) for LV filling, that is, a ratio of E-wave velocity to A-wave velocity (E/A) less than 1. With moderate degrees of diastolic impairment caused by reduced LV compliance, pressures in the LA become elevated. The LA–LV gradient consequently is higher in early diastole, resulting in higher E-wave velocity and a "pseudo-normal" E/A ratio of 1 to 1.5. As LAP increases even further with severe diastolic dysfunction ("restrictive" pattern), the LV fills rapidly and equilibrates with the LA. The E-wave velocity, and therefore the E/A ratio, decreases with age, so that by age 50 years an E/A ratio of less than 1 may be normal. Maneuvers that lower LAP (pre-load), such as Valsalva's maneuvers, or the use of nitroglycerin, reduce E-wave velocity and thus can convert a restrictive pattern to a pseudo-normal pattern.

In patients who have dilated cardiomyopathy, the presence of a restrictive pattern is associated with poor prognosis, and the inability to convert a restrictive pattern to a pseudo-normal pattern with a Valsalva maneuver portends an even worse outcome.[25] The DT and E/A ratio also can be useful in semiquantitative estimation of LV filling pressures. In a study of patients who had ischemic cardiomyopathy, Giannuzi and colleagues[26] found that a DT of less than120 milliseconds has a high sensitivity and specificity for predicting a PCWP above 20 mm Hg, whereas an E/A ratio greater than 2 had a high specificity (99%) but low sensitivity (43%) for elevated PCWP.

SEMI-QUANTITATIVE ESTIMATION OF FILLING PRESSURES

The mitral E-wave velocity is related directly to LAP and inversely to LV relaxation. In patients who have systolic HF, increased filling pressure (high LAP) and reduced LV relaxation co-exist, so that E-wave velocity alone correlates poorly with mean LAP. Correcting E-wave velocity for abnormal LV relaxation enables accurate estimation of LAP or mean PCWP. The mitral annular velocity (E_m) and the flow propagation velocity (V_p) on color M-mode cardiography have been validated as measures of LV relaxation and have been combined with E-wave velocity to estimate PCWP.

Early diastolic motion of the mitral annulus is influenced by the motion of longitudinally oriented myocardial fibers. The lengthening of these fibers

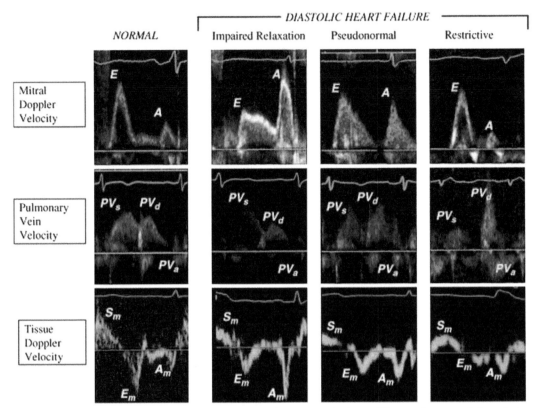

Fig. 10. Changes in Doppler echocardiographic profiles of patients who have different degrees of diastolic heart failure. As diastolic dysfunction worsens, the E/A ratio initially declines; then the stage of pseudo-normalization occurs. As filling pressures continue to rise, a restrictive filling pattern is seen. (*From* Fowler S, Narula J, Gurudevan S. Review of noninvasive imaging for hypertrophic cardiomyopathy syndromes and restrictive physiology. Heart Fail Clin 2006;2(2):218; with permission.)

in diastole results in mitral annular descent toward a relatively fixed apex. The velocity of early mitral annular (E_m) descent reflects LV relaxation and is independent of LAP. Using instrumented dogs, Nagueh and colleagues[27] confirmed that

E_m is relatively insensitive to acute alterations in pre-load compared with E-wave velocity. Because E-wave velocity is determined primarily by LAP and LV relaxation, correcting the E-wave velocity for LV relaxation (ie, the E/E_m ratio) allowed

Table 2
Grading of diastolic dysfunction

Pathophysiology	Normal	Grade I ↓ Relaxation	Grade II ↓ Relaxation ↑ LVEDP	Grade III (Reversible) ↓ Relaxation ↓ Compliance ↑ LVEDP	Grade III (Irreversible) ↓ Relaxation ↓↓ Compliance ↑↑ LVEDP
E/A	0.75–1.5	<0.75	0.75–1.5	>1.5	>1.5
DT (ms)	150–200	>200	>200	150–200	<150
IRT (ms)	50–100	>100	50–100	↓	↓
PV_s/PV_d	>1	$PV_s > PV_d$	$PV_s > PV_d$	$PV_s < PV_d$	$PV_s < PV_d$
PV_a (m/s)	<0.35	<0.35	≥0.35	≥0.35	≥0.35
a_{dur}-A_{dur}	<20	<20	≥20	≥20	≥20
E/E_m	<10	<10	≥10	≥10	≥10

accurate assessment of LAP or mean PCWP. An
E/E$_m$ ratio (measured at the lateral mitral annulus)
greater than 10 detected a PCWP higher than 15
mm Hg with a sensitivity of 97% and specificity
of 78%.[27] Similar findings were made using the
velocity measured at the septal mitral annulus,
with an E/E$_m$ ratio greater than 12 predicting
a PCWP greater than 15 mm Hg (**Fig. 11**).[27] The
septal annulus now is the preferred site for tissue
Doppler imaging, because this location is less
influenced by the pericardium.

Ommen and colleagues[28] compared the E/E$_m$
ratio with direct measurement of LVEDP in
patients referred for left heart catheterization. An
E/E$_m$ ratio less than 8 accurately predicted normal
LVEDP, and an E/E$_m$ ratio greater than 15 predicted an elevated LVEDP regardless of EF. E/E$_m$
values between 8 and 15 correlated with a wide
range of values of LVEDP, however. Thus, the E/
E$_m$ ratio alone is useful in dichotomizing patients
as having normal or high LVEDP but cannot clas-
sify intermediate values accurately or provide
quantitative measurement.

Several caveats are important when the E/E$_m$
ratio is used to estimate filling pressures. First,
the E/E$_m$ ratio is insensitive to preload changes in
patients who have impaired relaxation but not in
patients who have normal relaxation.[29] Moreover,
the E/E$_m$ ratio varies with changes in afterload.
Borlaug and colleagues[30] demonstrated in humans that E$_m$ is related inversely to arterial load,
particularly the late-systolic component caused
by arterial wave reflection. The E-wave velocity
was not influenced by arterial loading, so the
E/E$_m$ ratio varied directly with afterload. These
results may explain in part the observation that
the E/E$_m$ ratio increases with increasing age.[31]
Additionally, the E/E$_m$ ratio does not correlate
with PCWP in the setting of severe MR, probably
because the regurgitant lesion serves effectively
as afterload reduction.[32] A second limitation is
that E$_m$ measured at a single point in the heart is
assumed to represent global diastolic properties
of the heart. Wang and colleagues[33] used two-
dimensional speckle tracking to derive a global
measure of diastolic strain rate during isovolumic
relaxation (SR$_{ivr}$). Although impractical for routine
clinical use, the E/SR$_{ivr}$ ratio accurately predicted
PCWP when the E/E$_m$ ratio was indeterminate
(ie, in the range from 8–15) and had better accuracy than the E/E$_m$ ratio in patients who had
regional wall motion but preserved EF. Finally, in
constrictive pericarditis (CP), the E/E$_m$ ratio correlates inversely with PCWP ("annulus paradoxus,"
as discussed later). Pericardial constriction limits
the lateral expansion of the heart during diastole
and thereby must increase longitudinal myocardial

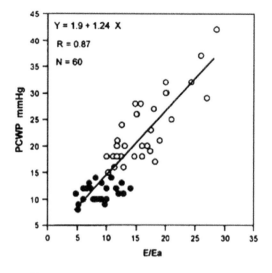

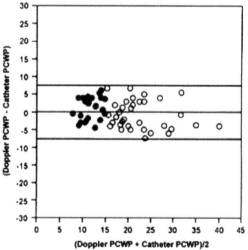

Fig. 11. The upper panel shows the relationship
between wedge pressure and E/Ea ratio in 60 patients
who had cardiac disease. Ea was measured at the
lateral side of the mitral annulus. The lower panel
shows the difference between the Doppler estimated
and invasively measured mean wedge pressure versus
the average of both observations. Solid circles indicate patients who had an impaired relaxation mitral
inflow pattern; open circles indicate patients who
had pseudo-normal or restrictive LV filling. (*From
Nagueh SF, Middleton KJ, Kopelen HA, et al. Doppler
tissue imaging: a noninvasive technique for evaluation of left ventricular relaxation and estimation of
filling pressures. J Am Coll Cardiol 1997;30:1531;
with permission.*)

motion. Because E$_m$ velocity increases in proportion to the severity of constriction, the E/E$_m$ ratio
is low despite the increase in LV filling pressure.[34]

Both the E/E$_m$ ratio and BNP levels correlate
with LV filling pressures. In patients admitted to
an ICU, the E/E$_m$ ratio demonstrated better

correlation with PCWP than BNP (r = 0.69 versus r = 0.32) with the optimal cut-off value for the E/E_m ratio greater than 15 predicting a PCWP greater than 15 mm Hg in patients who had reduced EF and an E/E_m ratio greater than 11 predicting a PCWP greater than 15 mm Hg in patients who had normal EF. The E/E_m ratio followed directional changes in PCWP accurately. Importantly, in patients who had cardiac disease, the E/E_m ratio was more sensitive and specific than a BNP level greater 400 pg/mL for a PCWP higher than 15 mm Hg, whereas the opposite was true in patients who did not have cardiac disease.[35]

Like E_m, the color M-mode propagation velocity, V_p, is an index of relaxation, so the E/V_p ratio also tracks with PCWP. V_p is obtained by placing the color M-mode cursor in the direction of mitral inflow as seen by color Doppler. The slope of the line along the edge of the first aliasing velocity in early diastole is the propagation velocity (normal > 50 cm/s) (**Fig. 12**). Garcia and colleagues[36] studied a heterogeneous patient group in a cardiac ICU and related PCWP to the E/V_p ratio. They found that a E/V_p ratio greater than 2 correlated with a PCWP greater than 15 mm Hg. In contemporary practice, E_m is used more commonly because it generally is easier to obtain and interpret than V_p. In addition, V_p can be artificially elevated when the LV cavity is small, as in hypertrophic or restrictive cardiomyopathy.

Pulmonary Venous Inflow

LA filling from the pulmonary veins provides additional insight into LV filling pressures. The normal pulmonary venous inflow velocity curve is characterized by inflow biphasic peaks in systole (PV_s) and diastole (PV_d) followed by a small atrial flow reversal (PV_a) whose duration is a_{dur} (see **Fig. 10**). The two systolic peaks can be resolved only by transesophageal echocardiography and correspond to LA relaxation and mitral annular descent toward the apex. PV_d, the velocity of diastolic flow into the LA, reflects the transmitral filling pressure gradient. With mitral valve opening, the LA and LV operate effectively as a single receiving chamber for pulmonary venous inflow, and therefore PV_d is influenced by the same determinants as E-wave velocity. Atrial contraction results in blood flow across the mitral valve as well as backward into the pulmonary veins. PV_a is determined by the interplay between compliance properties of the LA and LV and by atrial contractile function. In the normal heart with low LAP (ie, $PV_s/PV_d \geq 1$), PV_a is low (< 0.35 m/s), and a_{dur} is short. With increasing LAP pressure and reduced LV compliance, systolic flow into

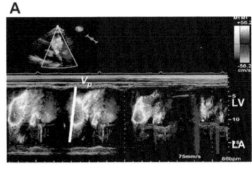

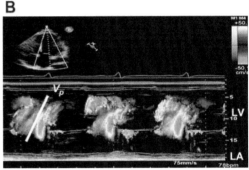

Fig. 12. V_p (*A*) in a normal subject and (*B*) in a patient who has cardiomyopathy. V_p is measured as the slope of the line along the first aliasing velocity, as indicated.

the LA decreases, PV_d exceeds PV_s and PV_a is greater than 0.35 m/s. In addition, a_{dur} is prolonged because of the increased flow reversal into the pulmonary veins. An a_{dur} 20 milliseconds greater than the duration of the mitral A wave (A_{dur}) was found to predict an LVEDP greater than 15 mm Hg with moderate sensitivity and specificity.[37]

Interrogation of pulmonary venous inflow is challenging in actual practice. From a transthoracic apical view, a sample volume is placed 1 to 2 cm inside the right superior pulmonary vein. At this depth, signal strength is limited, and it can be difficult to place the sample volume accurately.

PULMONARY CIRCULATION AND RIGHT HEART FUNCTION

RV dysfunction and secondary PH are critical determinants of functional capacity and survival in HF. Although PH in HF is caused primarily by pulmonary venous hypertension, there is little relationship between the degree of LV dysfunction and pulmonary artery pressure (PAP) because of the variable degree of diastolic impairment, MR, and LA size and compliance. Echocardiographic predictors of PH are a restrictive mitral inflow pattern and the severity of MR.[38]

RV function is an independent and additive prognosticator in PH complicating HF. The importance of RV function was illustrated by Ghio and colleagues,[39] who found that patients who had RV dysfunction and normal PAP had a prognosis similar to those who had normal RV function and PH, whereas those who had RV dysfunction and PH had considerably worse outcomes.

The complex geometry of the RV and suboptimal endocardial border definition preclude a reliable tomographic assessment of ventricular volumes and function. Because of the orientation of muscle fibers in the RV, contraction occurs predominantly along the longitudinal plane. Consequently, displacement of the tricuspid annulus toward the RV apex (tricuspid annular plane systolic excursion, TAPSE) is a reliable, easily measured surrogate for RV EF. In a population of patients who had advanced HF, Ghio and colleagues[40] showed that a TAPSE greater than 14 mm provided incremental prognostic information to functional class, LV function, and diastolic function and was measured more reliably than RV fractional area change or RV axis shortening. TAPSE is obtained by placing the M-mode cursor through the lateral tricuspid annulus and measuring the systolic motion of the annulus (Fig. 13).

Measures of RV diastolic function are analogous to those of the LV and are useful in characterizing various hemodynamic states. Unlike mitral inflow velocities, early and late tricuspid inflow peak velocities vary with respiration, increasing with inspiration because of increased systemic venous return and decreasing with expiration. Both superior vena cava and hepatic venous inflow patterns reflect the mechanics of RA filling and are characterized by systolic forward flow, diastolic forward flow, systolic flow reversal, and diastolic flow reversal (Fig. 14). These patterns of RA filling correlate with the jugular venous pressure curve. In normal subjects, the systolic forward flow is greater than the diastolic forward flow, and the systolic flow reversal and the diastolic flow reversal are low. With increasing RA pressure, the systolic forward flow decreases, and the diastolic forward flow increases, so that the diastolic forward flow is greater than the systolic forward flow; with severely increased RA pressure, the systolic flow reversal and the diastolic flow reversal become prominent. In patients who have cardiomyopathy both systolic flow reversal and diastolic flow reversal increase with inspiration. Tricuspid regurgitation (TR) results in a prominent S velocity.

Right ventricular systolic pressure (RVSP), which equals pulmonary artery systolic pressure (PASP) in the absence of RV outflow tract (RVOT) obstruction, is calculated reliably using the simplified Bernoulli equation from the velocity of the TR jet (V_{TR}) and RA pressure (RAP) (Fig. 15): RVSP = PASP = $4(V_{TR})^2$ + RAP. The RAP is estimated from bedside examination of the jugular venous pressure or is inferred from the inferior vena cava (IVC) dimension and the response to the "sniff" test (Table 3).[41] The normal IVC measures 15 to 25 mm and decreases by more than 50% with quiet inspiration. The absence of inspiratory IVC narrowing by more than 50% of the expiratory dimension suggests a RAP greater than 10 mm Hg, and distension of the IVC by more than 25 mm with lack of respiratory variation indicates an RAP of 20 mm Hg. These correlations are not accurate in ventilated patients because of positive-pressure ventilation, but a small IVC that collapses with respiration effectively excludes an

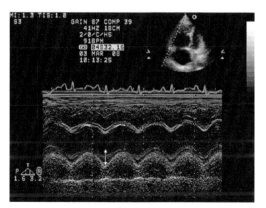

Fig. 13. Measurement of TAPSE in a patient who has pulmonary arterial hypertension. The M-mode cursor is placed through the lateral tricuspid annulus.

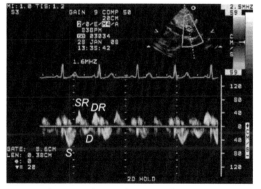

Fig. 14. Pulse Doppler evaluation of the hepatic veins demonstrates systolic (S) and diastolic (D) forward-filling velocities and flow reversal in systole (SR) and diastole (DR).

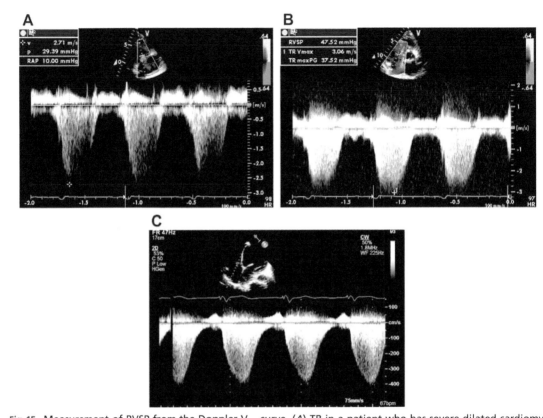

Fig. 15. Measurement of RVSP from the Doppler V_{TR} curve. (*A*) TR in a patient who has severe dilated cardiomy-opathy. Note the signal drop-out in the second half of systole. Peak V_{TR} is 2.7 m/s, and RVSP is 30 mm Hg. (*B*) Doppler interrogation from the basal short-axis view in the same patient. The TR signal intensity is much stronger because of better alignment of the Doppler beam with the regurgitant jet. The peak V_{TR} is 3.0 m/s, and RVSP is 38 mm Hg. (*C*) TR Doppler curve from another patient who has heart failure. The V_{TR} is 4 m/s, and RVSP is 75 mm Hg.

elevated RAP. Other two-dimensional echocardi-ography findings that correlate with elevated RAP include leftward bowing of the interatrial septum, dilatation of the coronary sinus, right-to-left shunting through a patent foramen ovale, and enlargement of the RA.

To avoid underestimation of RVSP, it is impor-tant to measure the peak V_{TR} using continuous-wave Doppler from a parallel intercept angle, usually from an apical four-chamber or RV inflow view. Agitated saline can be used to improve suboptimal Doppler signals. Overestimation will occur if the MR jet is confused for the TR jet, because V_{MR} usually is high, because of the greater pressure gradient between LV and LA. PH is diagnosed when the RVSP exceeds 35 mm Hg. In a large number of normal subjects RVSP has been found to increase with age and obesity, indicating that the normal range of RVSP may be as high as 40 mm Hg.[42] Applying a similar approach enables estimation of the pulmonary artery diastolic pressure (PADP) from the

pulmonary regurgitant jet velocity (V_{PR}): PADP = $4(V_{PR})^2$ + RAP.

The PAP is a surrogate for pulmonary vascular resistance (PVR). An abnormal PAP, whether derived from echocardiography or invasive measurement, is not synonymous with pulmonary vascular disease, however. The PAP may be elevated despite normal pulmonary vasculature because of increased flow through the pulmonary circulation, as occurs with left-to-right shunts, or passively elevated because of pulmonary venous hypertension. PVR accounts for both PCWP and CO and therefore is used in determining candidacy for heart transplantation and in assessing response to vasodilator therapy in HF. The PVR is calculated from catheter measurements: PVR = mean PAP − PCWP/CO. Abbas and colleagues[43] used echocardiography to assess the PVR noninvasively. These authors found good correlation (r = 0.93) between the V_{TR}/RVOT VTI ratio and catheter-based PVR using the equation PVR = 10 × (V_{TR}/RVOT VTI) + 0.16.

Table 3
Estimation of right atrial pressure

IVC Diameter (cm)	Respiratory Variation	Estimated RAP (mm Hg)
Small (<1.5)	Collapse	0–5
Normal (1.5–2.5)	Decrease by >50%	5–10
Normal	Decrease by <50%	10–15
Dilated (>2.5)	Decrease by <50%	15–20
Dilated	No change	>20

At a cut-off value of 0.2, the V_{TR}/RVOT VTI ratio had a sensitivity of 70% and specificity of 94% for determining a PVR greater than 2 Woods units.

Qualitative evidence of chronic RV pressure or volume overload includes RV chamber dilatation and hypertrophy. Acute RV dilatation and hypo-contractility can occur with acute pressure overload caused by major pulmonary embolism and may be distinguished from chronic RV disease by preserved RV apical contractility ("McConnell's sign") and the absence of RV hypertrophy.[44] The pattern of septal motion also provides insight into the hemodynamic state of the RV (**Fig. 16**). In RV volume overload, the leftward bowing of the interventricular septum occurs in diastole with normal systolic curvature, whereas pressure overload causes septal flattening in both systole and early diastole.[45]

CONSTRICTION VERSUS RESTRICTION

CP and restrictive cardiomyopathy (RCM) must be considered in any patient who has symptoms and signs of HF and normal systolic function. The clinical distinction between these two entities can be difficult, but in most cases echocardiography can aid in the diagnosis. Two-dimensional echocardiography findings characteristic of infiltrative restrictive cardiomyopathy include significant TR and MR, marked bi-atrial enlargement, and normal systolic function. A myocardium that is thickened and has a "sparkling" appearance on echocardiogram suggests amyloidosis, although the absence of these findings does not exclude amyloid or other infiltrative cardiomyopathy. Atrial enlargement typically is less prominent in CP. M-mode and two-dimensional findings suggestive of CP include a thickened pericardium, exaggerated septal motion, dilated IVC, and diastolic flattening of the LV posterior wall (**Fig. 17**). None of these findings are sensitive or specific.

The utility of echocardiography in distinguishing CP from RCM therefore rests primarily on its ability to demonstrate noninvasively the hallmark mechanisms of CP: (1) the dissociation of intracardiac and intrathoracic pressures and (2) exaggerated ventricular interdependence in diastolic filling. Because the rigid pericardium does not effectively transmit respiratory changes in intrathoracic pressure to the heart, the transmitral filling gradient

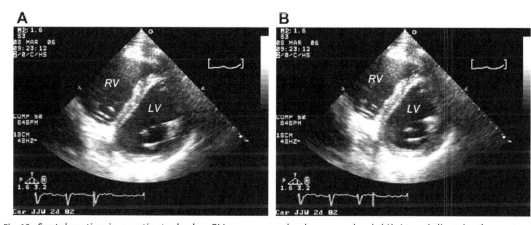

Fig. 16. Septal motion in a patient who has RV pressure and volume overload. (*A*) At end-diastole, the septum is mid-line, and the LV has a D-shape. (*B*) At end-systole, the septum remains mid-line because RV and LV pressures are equal.

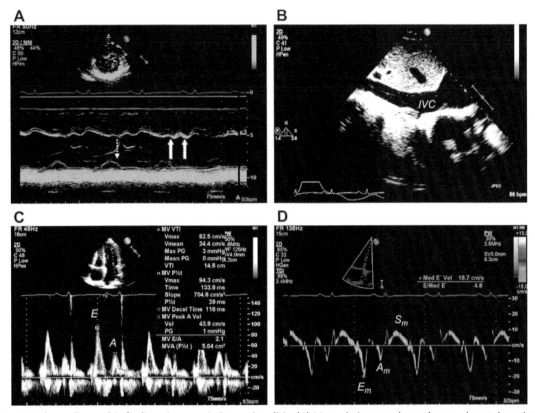

Fig. 17. Echocardiographic findings in constrictive pericarditis. (*A*) M-mode images show abnormal septal motion (*solid arrows*) and flattening of the posterior (*dashed arrow*) during early diastole. (*B*) The dilated IVC indicates elevated right atrial pressure. (*C*) Restrictive mitral inflow pattern with rapid deceleration time (116 ms). (*D*) Myocardial velocity at the basal medial septum is very high (E_m= 19.7 cm/s). The E/E_m is low (4.9) despite elevated filling pressures (annulus paradoxus). At subsequent right heart catheterization, the pulmonary capillary wedge pressure was 24 mm Hg.

(PCWP–LVP) tracks respiratory changes in the PCWP, decreasing with inspiration and increasing with expiration. Reciprocal respiratory changes occur in the RV filling gradient. Consequently, inspiration decreases the mitral E-wave and increases the tricuspid E-wave and hepatic vein diastolic velocity, whereas expiration produces opposite changes and increases diastolic flow reversal in the hepatic veins. Traditionally, a 25% variation in the peak E-wave velocity is used as the threshold value. An important caveat is that marked elevations in LAP blunt the effects of respiration on the LV filling gradient. Therefore, the absence of respiratory variation in E-wave velocity should not exclude the diagnosis of CP, especially when other features of CP are present.

Tissue Doppler of the mitral annulus is useful in differentiating CP from RCM. In myocardial disease, E_m is reduced (< 7 cm/s) because of abnormal myocardial relaxation, whereas in CP, E_m is normal or elevated. Pericardial constraint limits the lateral expansion of the heart, and longitudinal lengthening becomes exaggerated. As

filling pressure increases in CP, E_m increases linearly, exactly the opposite of its behavior in myocardial disease. Consequently, the E/E_m ratio is normal or reduced despite high filling pressures in CP (annulus paradoxus) but is low in myocardial disease (see **Fig. 17**).

SUMMARY

Qualitative and quantitative hemodynamic data can be obtained through echocardiography, making it a valuable noninvasive tool in the routine assessment of the patient who has HF. In addition to providing a hemodynamic profile, echocardiography provides unique and powerful prognostic data that cannot be obtained by catheterization. Thus, echocardiography is the diagnostic test of choice in the initial hemodynamic evaluation of HF.

REFERENCES

1. Stevenson LW. Are hemodynamic goals viable in tailoring heart failure therapy? Hemodynamic goals

are relevant. Circulation 2006;113(7):1020–7 [discussion 1033].

2. Hunt SA. ACC/AHA 2005 guideline update for the diagnosis and management of chronic heart failure in the adult: a report of the American College of Cardiology/American Heart Association Task Force on Practice Guidelines (Writing Committee to Update the 2001 Guidelines for the Evaluation and Management of Heart Failure). J Am Coll Cardiol 2005;46(6):e1–82.

3. Kass DA, Maughan WL, Guo ZM, et al. Comparative influence of load versus inotropic states on indexes of ventricular contractility: experimental and theoretical analysis based on pressure-volume relationships. Circulation 1987;76(6):1422–36.

4. Nishimura RA, Callahan MJ, Schaff HV, et al. Noninvasive measurement of cardiac output by continuous-wave Doppler echocardiography: initial experience and review of the literature. Mayo Clin Proc 1984;59(7):484–9.

5. Goldman JH, Schiller NB, Lim DC, et al. Usefulness of stroke distance by echocardiography as a surrogate marker of cardiac output that is independent of gender and size in a normal population. Am J Cardiol 2001;87(4):499–502, A8.

6. Lapu-Bula R, Robert A, De Kock M, et al. Relation of exercise capacity to left ventricular systolic function and diastolic filling in idiopathic or ischemic dilated cardiomyopathy. Am J Cardiol 1999;83(5):728–34.

7. Lang RM, Bierig M, Devereux RB, et al. Recommendations for chamber quantification: a report from the American Society of Echocardiography's Guidelines and Standards Committee and the Chamber Quantification Writing Group, developed in conjunction with the European Association of Echocardiography, a branch of the European Society of Cardiology. J Am Soc Echocardiogr 2005;18(12):1440–63.

8. Bargiggia GS, Bertucci C, Recusani F, et al. A new method for estimating left ventricular dP/dt by continuous wave Doppler echocardiography. Validation studies at cardiac catheterization. Circulation 1989;80(5):1287–92.

9. Tei C, Nishimura RA, Seward JB, et al. Noninvasive Doppler-derived myocardial performance index: correlation with simultaneous measurements of cardiac catheterization measurements. J Am Soc Echocardiogr 1997;10(2):169–78.

10. Cheung MM, Smallhorn JF, Redington AN, et al. The effects of changes in loading conditions and modulation of inotropic state on the myocardial performance index: comparison with conductance catheter measurements. Eur Heart J 2004;25(24):2238–42.

11. Peltier M, Slama M, Garbi S, et al. Prognostic value of Doppler-derived myocardial performance index in patients with left ventricular systolic dysfunction. Am J Cardiol 2002;90(11):1261–3.

12. Yamada H, Oki T, Tabata T, et al. Assessment of left ventricular systolic wall motion velocity with pulsed tissue Doppler imaging: comparison with peak dP/dt of the left ventricular pressure curve. J Am Soc Echocardiogr 1998;11(5):442–9.

13. Greenberg NL, Firstenberg MS, Castro PL, et al. Doppler-derived myocardial systolic strain rate is a strong index of left ventricular contractility. Circulation 2002;105(1):99–105.

14. Koyama J, Ray-Sequin PA, Falk RH. Longitudinal myocardial function assessed by tissue velocity, strain, and strain rate tissue Doppler echocardiography in patients with AL (primary) cardiac amyloidosis. Circulation 2003;107(19):2446–52.

15. Grayburn PA, Appleton CP, DeMaria AN, et al. Echocardiographic predictors of morbidity and mortality in patients with advanced heart failure: the Beta-blocker Evaluation of Survival Trial (BEST). J Am Coll Cardiol 2005;45(7):1064–71.

16. Levine TB, Levine AB, Bolenbaugh J, et al. Impact of left ventricular size on pharmacologic reverse remodeling in heart failure. Clin Cardiol 2000;23(5):355–8.

17. Melenovsky V, Borlaug BA, Rosen B, et al. Cardiovascular features of heart failure with preserved ejection fraction versus nonfailing hypertensive left ventricular hypertrophy in the urban Baltimore community: the role of atrial remodeling/dysfunction. J Am Coll Cardiol 2007;49(2):198–207.

18. Trichon BH, Felker GM, Shaw LK, et al. Relation of frequency and severity of mitral regurgitation to survival among patients with left ventricular systolic dysfunction and heart failure. Am J Cardiol 2003;91(5):538–43.

19. Bursi F, Weston SA, Redfield MM, et al. Systolic and diastolic heart failure in the community. JAMA 2006;296(18):2209–16.

20. Packer M. Abnormalities of diastolic function as a potential cause of exercise intolerance in chronic heart failure. Circulation 1990;81(2 Suppl):III78–86.

21. Persson H, Lonn E, Edner M, et al. Diastolic dysfunction in heart failure with preserved systolic function: need for objective evidence: results from the CHARM Echocardiographic Substudy-CHARMES. J Am Coll Cardiol 2007;49(6):687–94.

22. Gorcsan Jr, Snow FR, Paulsen W, et al. Noninvasive estimation of left atrial pressure in patients with congestive heart failure and mitral regurgitation by Doppler echocardiography. Am Heart J 1991;121(3 Pt 1):858–63.

23. Abhayaratna WP, Seward JB, Appleton CP, et al. Left atrial size: physiologic determinants and clinical applications. J Am Coll Cardiol 2006;47(12):2357–63.

24. Takemoto Y, Barnes ME, Seward JB, et al. Usefulness of left atrial volume in predicting first congestive heart failure in patients > or = 65 years of age with well-preserved left ventricular systolic function. Am J Cardiol 2005;96(6):832–6.

25. Pinamonti B, Di Lenarda A, Sinagra G, et al. Restrictive left ventricular filling pattern in dilated cardiomyopathy assessed by Doppler echocardiography: clinical, echocardiographic and hemodynamic correlations and prognostic implications. Heart Muscle Disease Study Group. J Am Coll Cardiol 1993;22(3):808–15.

26. Giannuzzi P, Imparato A, Temporelli PL, et al. Doppler-derived mitral deceleration time of early filling as a strong predictor of pulmonary capillary wedge pressure in postinfarction patients with left ventricular systolic dysfunction. J Am Coll Cardiol 1994;23(7):1630–7.

27. Nagueh SF, Sun H, Kopelen HA, et al. Hemodynamic determinants of the mitral annulus diastolic velocities by tissue Doppler. J Am Coll Cardiol 2001;37(1):278–85.

28. Ommen SR, Nishimura RA, Appleton CP, et al. Clinical utility of Doppler echocardiography and tissue Doppler imaging in the estimation of left ventricular filling pressures: a comparative simultaneous Doppler-catheterization study. Circulation 2000; 102(15):1788–94.

29. Firstenberg MS, Levine BD, Garcia MJ, et al. Relationship of echocardiographic indices to pulmonary capillary wedge pressures in healthy volunteers. J Am Coll Cardiol 2000;36(5):1664–9.

30. Borlaug BA, Melenovsky V, Redfield MM, et al. Impact of arterial load and loading sequence on left ventricular tissue velocities in humans. J Am Coll Cardiol 2007;50(16):1570–7.

31. De Sutter J, De Backer J, Van de Veire N, et al. Effects of age, gender, and left ventricular mass on septal mitral annulus velocity (E') and the ratio of transmitral early peak velocity to E' (E/E'). Am J Cardiol 2005;95(8):1020–3.

32. Olson JJ, Costa SP, Young CE, et al. Early mitral filling/diastolic mitral annular velocity ratio is not a reliable predictor of left ventricular filling pressure in the setting of severe mitral regurgitation. J Am Soc Echocardiogr 2006;19(1):83–7.

33. Wang J, Khoury DS, Thohan V, et al. Global diastolic strain rate for the assessment of left ventricular relaxation and filling pressures. Circulation 2007; 115(11):1376–83.

34. Ha JW, Oh JK, Ling LH, et al. Annulus paradoxus: transmitral flow velocity to mitral annular velocity ratio is inversely proportional to pulmonary capillary wedge pressure in patients with constrictive pericarditis. Circulation 2001;104(9):976–8.

35. Dokainish H, Zoghbi WA, Lakkis NM, et al. Optimal noninvasive assessment of left ventricular filling pressures: a comparison of tissue Doppler echocardiography and B-type natriuretic peptide in patients with pulmonary artery catheters. Circulation 2004; 109(20):2432–9.

36. Garcia MJ, Ares MA, Asher C, et al. An index of early left ventricular filling that combined with pulsed Doppler peak E velocity may estimate capillary wedge pressure. J Am Coll Cardiol 1997;29(2):448–54.

37. Rossvoll O, Hatle LK. Pulmonary venous flow velocities recorded by transthoracic Doppler ultrasound: relation to left ventricular diastolic pressures. J Am Coll Cardiol 1993;21(7):1687–96.

38. Enriquez-Sarano M, Rossi A, Seward JB, et al. Determinants of pulmonary hypertension in left ventricular dysfunction. J Am Coll Cardiol 1997;29(1):153–9.

39. Ghio S, Gavazzi A, Campana C, et al. Independent and additive prognostic value of right ventricular systolic function and pulmonary artery pressure in patients with chronic heart failure. J Am Coll Cardiol 2001;37(1):183–8.

40. Ghio S, Recusani F, Klersy C, et al. Prognostic usefulness of the tricuspid annular plane systolic excursion in patients with congestive heart failure secondary to idiopathic or ischemic dilated cardiomyopathy. Am J Cardiol 2000;85(7):837–42.

41. Kircher BJ, Himelman RB, Schiller NB. Noninvasive estimation of right atrial pressure from the inspiratory collapse of the inferior vena cava. Am J Cardiol 1990;66(4):493–6.

42. McQuillan BM, Picard MH, Leavitt M, et al. Clinical correlates and reference intervals for pulmonary artery systolic pressure among echocardiographically normal subjects. Circulation 2001;104(23): 2797–802.

43. Abbas AE, Fortuin FD, Schiller NB, et al. A simple method for noninvasive estimation of pulmonary vascular resistance. J Am Coll Cardiol 2003;41(6): 1021–7.

44. McConnell MV, Solomon SD, Rayan ME, et al. Regional right ventricular dysfunction detected by echocardiography in acute pulmonary embolism. Am J Cardiol 1996;78(4):469–73.

45. Louie EK, Rich S, Levitsky S, et al. Doppler echocardiographic demonstration of the differential effects of right ventricular pressure and volume overload on left ventricular geometry and filling. J Am Coll Cardiol 1992;19(1):84–90.

46. Nagueh SF, Middleton KJ, Kopelen HA, et al. Doppler tissue imaging: a noninvasive technique for evaluation of left ventricular relaxation and estimation of filling pressures. J Am Coll Cardiol 1997; 30(6):1527–33.

Assessment of Left Ventricular Systolic Function by Echocardiography

Martin G. St. John Sutton, MBBS, FRCP*, Ted Plappert, CVT,
Hind Rahmouni, MD

KEYWORDS

- Echocardiography • Remodeling • Heart failure
- Systolic function

Echocardiography serves an extremely important role in the diagnosis and management of patients with heart failure (HF). The various stages of structural and functional changes that constitute progressive left ventricle (LV) remodeling have all been characterized by two-dimensional echocardiography. In addition, echocardiography has defined the transition from compensated hypertrophy to LV dilatation and progression to end-stage HF. Echocardiography has also played an important role in clinical HF trials of β-adrenergic blocking agents and angiotensin-converting enzyme inhibitors and angiotensin receptor blockers and demonstrated their efficacy in HF. Echocardiography has been regarded as the single most useful diagnostic tool in the overall management of patients with HF.

EPIDEMIOLOGY OF HEART FAILURE

There is an estimated 25 to 30 million subjects with HF worldwide, and with an additional half a million new cases diagnosed each year in the United States alone. HF increases with age, and by the year 2035 there will be more than 75 million subjects over 75 years old in the United States so that as longevity increases, HF will increase to epidemic proportions. Already HF constitutes the most prevalent ICD coding for hospital discharge diagnosis in patients older than 65 years. The current prevalence of HF, its impact on employment status, combined with the poor quality of life, the adverse long-term prognosis, and the prohibitive health costs have resulted in HF becoming a high-priority health care initiative worldwide.

SYSTOLIC VERSUS DIASTOLIC HEART FAILURE

Approximately 35% to 50% of patients presenting with typical symptoms of dyspnea caused by pulmonary congestion and clinical signs of HF for the first time have preserved LV ejection fraction, and this has been variously called diastolic HF or HF with preserved LV function (ejection fraction >50%).[1,2] Clinical examination of the cardiovascular system does not reliably distinguish between systolic and diastolic HF (ejection fraction <50%), although chronic systemic hypertension and female gender are more commonly associated with diastolic than with systolic HF.[3] There are several reasons why diastolic HF took so long to be recognized as a discrete entity, not least of which was the notion that diastolic HF was regarded as relatively benign, difficult to define, and for which there was no specific therapy. Diastolic HF has subsequently been shown to have a significant morbidity and mortality, albeit lower than that associated with systolic HF.[4] The etiology in more than two thirds of systolic HF

This article originally appeared in *Heart Failure Clinics* 2009;5(2):177–190

University of Pennsylvania Medical Center, Philadelphia, PA, USA

* Corresponding author. Division of Cardiology, Department of Medicine, University of Pennsylvania Medical Center, 3400 Spruce Street, Philadelphia, PA 19104.

E-mail address: suttonm@mail.med.upenn.edu (M.G. St. John Sutton).

Ultrasound Clin 4 (2009) 167–180

doi:10.1016/j.cult.2009.04.005

patients (left ventricular ejection fraction [LVEF] <50%) is chronic ischemic heart disease caused by epicardial coronary stenoses or occlusions. The etiology in the remaining patients with systolic HF includes primary-idiopathic cardiomyopathy, hypertension, valvular heart disease, and myocarditis.

This article describes the various echocardiographic techniques that are both universally available and currently used routinely in the diagnosis and management of systolic HF. Echocardiography can be used to triage patients with systolic HF to optimize individual therapy to devices, surgery, or pharmacologic interventions. Brief mention is made of some clinical trials in HF that have used echocardiographic parameters as end points and of some novel technologies that include three-dimensional echocardiographic imaging and endocardial tracking algorithms that provide insight into global and regional myocardial strain, strain rate, and function.

LEFT VENTRICLE INTERNAL DIMENSIONS

M-mode echocardiography was the original noninvasive method for assessing LV size, LV mass, and contractile function (**Fig. 1**). Combined either with continuous LV pressure or cuff-systolic blood pressure measurements, M-mode echocardiographic estimates of LV dimensions and wall thicknesses enabled exploration of wall stress and strain as determinants of LV architecture and contractile function, myocardial relaxation, and mural and cavity mechanics in HF.[5,6] Moreover, M-mode echo measurements of LV dimensions

and wall thicknesses have been used extensively to assess LV mass in large, randomized-controlled clinical trials of hypertensive populations.[7–9] These studies have provided normative data; demonstrated the close relationship between LV size, mass, and body height; and aided in elucidating the different patterns of LV hypertrophy during eccentric versus concentric remodeling (**Fig. 2**).[8,9] M-mode echo continues to be used extensively in randomized clinical trials to quantify regression of LV hypertrophy following interventions to assess the efficacy of a variety of new pharmacologic antihypertensive agents and treatment regimens.

The major advantage of M-mode echocardiography is the high temporal resolution caused by the sampling frequency of 1000 cycles per second. The disadvantages of M-mode are that it assumes that the LV contracts concentrically and there are no regional LV wall motion abnormalities, that the LV wall thickness is uniform, and that contraction of the LV minor axis dimension sampled with two-dimensional echo guidance is truly representative of the whole ventricle. Furthermore, estimation of LV volumes from M-mode assumes fixed LV geometry and a fixed cavity short-to-long axis ratio that results in spuriously high ejection fractions. In systolic HF, the LV is almost invariably enlarged and this is associated with change in shape, and deviation from the normal axis ratio may confound quantification of LV volume and mass even in serial echoes over time.

LEFT VENTRICULAR VOLUMES

A number of different algorithms and geometric models have been used to assess LV end-diastolic and end-systolic volumes from a variety of imaging modalities including two-dimensional echocardiographic images. These echo volumes have been validated against volumes of casts of the LV, postmortem hearts, or MRI.

The LV is bullet-shaped and the recommendations of the American Society of Echocardiology for quantification of LV chamber volumes is Simpson's method of discs,[10] which requires manual digitization of the endocardial boundaries ideally from paired biplane images of the near-orthogonal apical four-chamber and the apical two-chamber views (**Fig. 3**). Accurate and reproducible estimates of LV volumes can be obtained, however, from single plane images of either the apical four-chamber or two-chamber views. Both of these correlate closely with biplane volumes, but are numerically different and cannot be used interchangeably with biplane volumes during serial

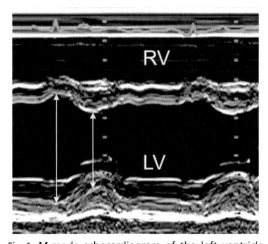

Fig. 1. M-mode echocardiogram of the left ventricle (LV) showing the septum and posterior wall. The arrows represent measurements of internal dimensions at end-diastole (*left arrow*) and at end-systole (*right arrow*).

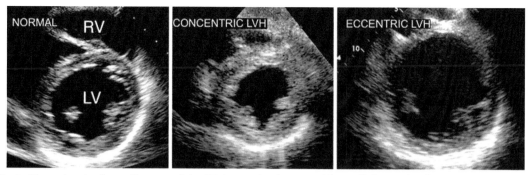

Fig. 2. Dimensional echocardiogram of the LV short axis of a normal heart (*left panel*), of an LV with concentric remodeling *(center panel)*, and an LV with eccentric remodeling (*right panel*).

follow-up.[11] Reproducibility of LV volumes varies because it depends on the quality of the echocardiographic images, identification of the endocardial boundaries, and the accuracy of manual digitization of the images (**Fig. 4**). All three of these factors vary from laboratory to laboratory from approximately 5% in busy experienced echo core laboratories to 10% and above in small laboratories where quantitative echocardiography is the exception rather than the rule.

Echocardiographic LV volumes are frequently used in HF trials as "clinical end points" that usually require the services of an experienced quantitative core laboratory because the expected change in LV volume from an intervention may be so small that it may be lost in the signal-to-noise ratio in a routine busy clinical laboratory.[12]

Recently, speckle-tracking technologies have been developed (AutoEF) using artificial intelligence and pattern recognition to facilitate endocardial recognition and provide continuous LV volumes almost instantaneously (**Fig. 5**).[13] Although the AutoEF system software in its current form functions well in normal hearts, it fares less well in the presence of mechanical valve prostheses or in large hearts with abnormal shape that typify HF.[14] The reproducibility of the automated LV volume estimates was superior to manual digitization as compared with the reproducibility typically obtained in a busy echo core laboratory using two-dimensional quantitative imaging.[14] In the authors' experience, however, automated volume computation systematically underestimated LV volumes calculated both by MRI and by manual digitization because of consistent failure to recognize the endocardium of the lateral wall.[14] Recently engineered software upgrades may improve the accuracy of automated volume quantification in hearts of varying sizes and shapes.

Commercially available software for three-dimensional echo full-volume quantitative analysis

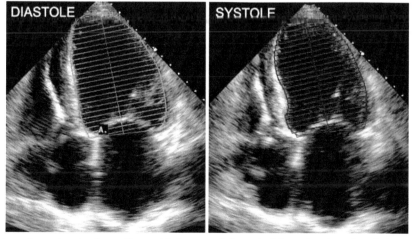

Fig. 3. Paired two-dimensional echocardiographic images of the apical four-chamber view (*left panel*) and apical two-chamber view (*right panel*) showing digitized endocardial boundaries for LV volume computations using Simpson's method.

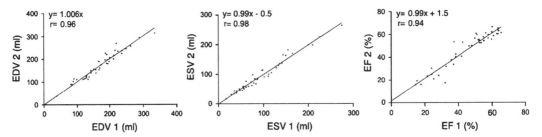

Fig. 4. Interobserver reproducibility of manually digitized LV end-diastolic volumes (EDV), end-systolic volumes (ESV), and ejection fraction (EF).

of LV volumes has demonstrated closer agreement and less variability than with assessment by two-dimensional when compared with volumes estimated by MRI, which is regarded as the gold standard for LV volume computation.[15] Independent of the three-dimensional method used for quantification of LV volumes, there are no assumptions regarding LV shape or plane positioning errors with three-dimensional echo, and volumes exhibit less scatter and less interobserver variability (**Fig. 6**). A number of studies have clearly demonstrated that three-dimensional echocardiography is superior to two-dimensional echocardiography for accurate and reproducible estimation of LV volumes.[15] Although three-dimensional echocardiography is being used with increasing frequency nationwide and is acknowledged to be superior to two-dimensional echo for volume

quantification, quantitative three-dimensional echocardiography has not yet been used in any randomized interventional clinical HF trials.

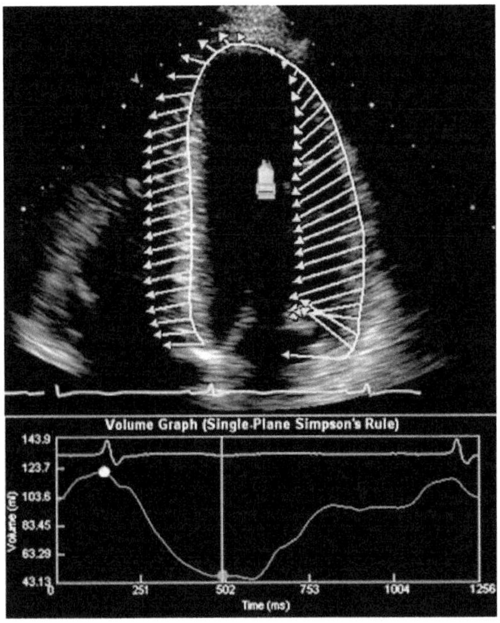

The importance of LV volumes resides in the fact that they provide powerful prognostic information pertaining to clinical outcome including mortality, recurrent HF requiring hospital admission, and recurrent myocardial function in patients with LV systolic dysfunction and HF. In a number of post–myocardial infarction and HF trials of patients with LV dysfunction and clinical HF (LVEF <40%), LV end-systolic volume has emerged as the single most important predictor of mortality and new-onset HF necessitating hospital admission.[16] Furthermore, the risk of a serious adverse cardiovascular event, including death, HF, or recurrent myocardial infarction, increases in direct proportion to increase in LV systolic volume (**Fig. 7**).[17] In addition, there is a striking direct relationship between LV volumes and incidence of ventricular arrhythmias[18] in survivors of myocardial infarction with residual LV dysfunction. The strong correlations between LV end-systolic volume and ventricular ectopy and between LV end-systolic volume and potentially life-threatening ventricular tachycardia persisted for at least 2 years postinfarction (**Fig. 8**).[18]

LEFT VENTRICLE SHAPE

The bullet-shape or prolate ellipsoidal shape of the normal human LV is conserved from infancy to old age. In systolic HF, however, the LV enlarges and as it does so the cavity shape becomes progressively distorted by the disproportionately greater increase in short axis than in long axis (**Fig. 9**), and this LV distortion is predictive of adverse clinical outcome.[19] Change in LV shape has been estimated echocardiographically and is usually expressed as an index of sphericity defined as the ratio of the LV short-axis diameter/LV long-axis length. Cavity shape becomes more spherical as the LV enlarges, because a sphere accommodates the greatest volume per unit perimeter of

Fig. 5. Velocity vector imaging uses speckle tracking to provide automated endocardial definition and LV volume computation.

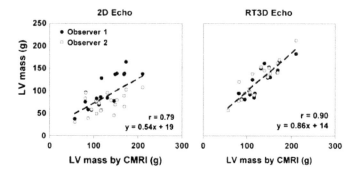

Fig. 6. Agreement between LV mass calculated from two-dimensional echocardiography and cardiac MRI (CMRI) that has become the gold standard (*left panel*), and agreement between LV mass by real-time three-dimensional echocardiography (RT3D) (*right panel*) and CMRI. Three-dimensional RT echo has a greater correlation coefficient with CMRI than two-dimensional echo and with less variability. (*From* Mor-Avi V, Sugeng L, Weinert L, et al. Fast measurement of left ventricular mass with real-time three-dimensional echocardiography: comparison with magnetic resonance imaging. Circulation 2004;110:1814–8; with permission.)

any geometric configuration. An alternative echo-cardiographic method for estimating LV cavity shape at end-diastole and end-systole is by indexing cavity volume to the volume of a sphere with a diameter equal to LV cavity length measured in the apical four-chamber view.[20] As LV volume increases, the shape-sphericity index increases toward unity, which would represent a perfect sphere. Change in cavity shape to a more spherical configuration is associated with poor outcome that persists even after adjusting for LV volumes.

LEFT VENTRICLE GLOBAL FUNCTION
Ejection Fraction

The most frequent assessment of LV function is ejection fraction, which can be derived as the difference between end-diastolic and end-systolic

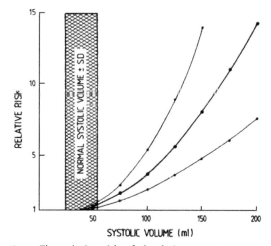

Fig. 7. The relative risk of death increases exponentially with increasing LV end-systolic volume. This relationship demonstrates the importance of end-systolic volume for early risk stratification. (*From* White HD, Norris RM, Brown MA, et al. Left ventricular end-systolic volume as the major determinant of survival after recovery from myocardial infarction. Circulation 1987;76:44–51; with permission.)

volumes, which represents stroke volume, expressed as a percentage of end-diastolic volume:

$$EDV - ESV = SV(\text{stroke volume})$$

$$LVEF = SV/EDV \times 100\%$$

LVEF describes global left ventricular cavity function, and normal values independent of age or gender are greater than 55%. Although LVEF is dimensionless and exquisitely sensitive to perturbations in loading conditions, it has been shown to be a powerful predictor of clinical outcome in patients with and without HF from valvular heart disease and ischemic and idiopathic LV dysfunction. LVEF has been used to define inclusion and exclusion criteria for multiple randomized clinical trials assessing the efficacy of angiotensin-converting enzyme inhibitors, angiotensin receptor blockers, vasodilators and β-adrenergic receptor blockers, and resynchronization devices in patients with HF.[21–24] LVEF is used to stratify risk and appropriateness of HF patients for adjuvant device therapies that include epicardial constraint, biventricular pacing, mitral valve replacement, ventricular-assist devices, cardiac transplantation, internal cardiac defibrillators, and novel pharmacologic interventions.[21–25]

Although LVEF should be calculated from end-diastolic and end-systolic volumes obtained from digitized paired biplane orthogonal apical images, visual estimates of LVEF by experienced level three trained echocardiologists correlate very closely with those obtained from digitized images and are used extensively in clinical practice for risk stratification, clinical decision making, and interventional therapies.

Left Ventricle Fractional Shortening

Linear measurements of the LV short-axis dimensions at end-diastole and end-systole by two-dimensional directed M-mode echo can be

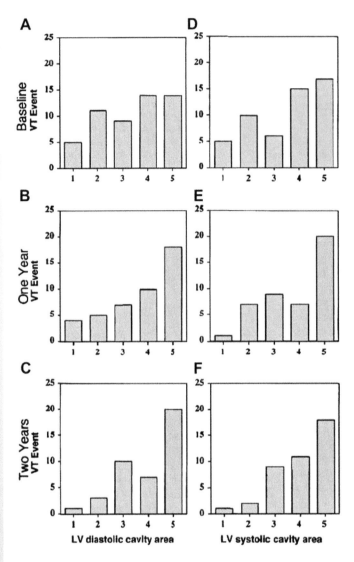

Fig. 8. The relationships between ventricular tachycardia and LV end-diastolic (A–C) cavity area and size and LV end-systolic (D–F) cavity size at baseline, at 1 year, and at 2 years indicating that the incidence of life-threatening ventricular tachycardia increases in direct proportion to LV size. (*From* St. John Sutton M, Lee D, Rouleau JL, et al. Left ventricular remodeling and ventricular arrhythmias after myocardial infarction. Circulation 2003;107:2577–82; with permission.)

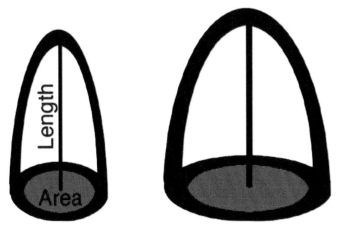

Fig. 9. Schematic showing that the LV enlarges more by increasing the short axis than the long axis and in so doing, the LV becomes more spherical, transitioning from a prolate ellipse at left to an ellipse with a disproportionately greater area at the base.

used to estimate fractional systolic LV shortening as an index of contractile function as:

$$\%\Delta LVD = (LVED - LVES/LVED) \times 100\%$$

The percent change in M-mode measurements of LV minor axis dimensions, although providing some information about LV function, is often confounded when regional variation in function or abnormal septal motion are present. Although the same caution is required when interpreting mid-wall fractional shortening, which requires measurement of LV wall thickness, mid-wall fractional shortening is useful in detecting LV systolic dysfunction in patients with LV hypertrophy.[26]

Regional Left Ventricle Function

Detection of regional variation in myocardial function at rest can be demonstrated as decreased regional myocardial thickening, and reduced endocardial-wall motion during systole provides insight into the etiology of HF. Regional variation in LV function not apparent at rest can be unveiled by stress testing with treadmill exercise, dobutamine, or Persantine in HF patients in conjunction with echocardiographic imaging using currently available conventional protocols. The LV is divided into 17 myocardial segments, similar to the prior 16-segment model except for the apical cap (segment 17), which represents the most distal apical myocardium that extends beyond the LV cavity (**Fig. 10**). The rationale of the stress test in patients with HF is to establish an ischemic etiology, which relies on the fact that coronary flow may be of normal magnitude and distribution

at rest with proximal coronary stenosis of 85% to 90%. During exercise stress, a proximal 50% stenosis at the same location may be flow limiting and result in diminished regional myocardial perfusion and blunted contraction. Echocardiographic imaging is obtained at rest and at peak tolerated stress during which time each of the 17 myocardial segments is analyzed for the extent of systolic thickening and endocardial motion. Normal regional wall thickening is graded 1, hypokinesis is graded 2, akinesis is graded 3, and dyskinesis is graded 4. A wall motion score index is determined as the sum of all scores divided by the number of analyzable segments.[10] This echocardiographic wall motion score index provides information about the location, size, and transmurality of the infarction and how extensive is the region of border zone myocardium at risk.[10]

Left Ventricle Mass

Calculation of left ventricular mass is most frequently obtained using M-mode echocardiography for which measurement of LV cavity diameter, LV posterior wall, and septal thicknesses are required at end-diastole. The algorithm used to calculate LV mass is modeled on prolate ellipsoidal geometry and uniform wall thickness in both short and long axes. This allows calculation of the volume of two ellipses, one with the total volume based on the epicardial surface and the second ellipse (cavity volume) based on the endocardial surface of the LV. Subtraction of end-diastolic cavity volume from the total volume of the epicardial ellipse and multiplying this by the

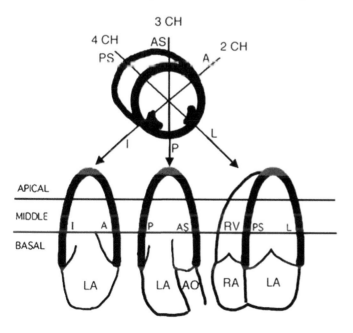

Fig. 10. Schema of the 17-segment model of the LV with the apical cap representing the seventeenth segment. This is the schematic used for assessing regional LV function in which each segment is graded 1 through 4, and a total score is derived by summation of all available scores and by dividing the total by the number of scores evaluated.

density of muscle (1.04) provides an approximation of LV muscle mass. Limitations of LV mass estimations include errors in measurements of wall thickness that are amplified by a cube function in calculating LV mass. Determinations of LV mass may be confounded in severely dilated hearts with altered cavity geometry and regional wall variation in wall thickness or wall motion.

Relative Wall Thickness and Mass/Volume Ratio

Relative wall thickness (RWT) is defined as:

$$RWT = 2 \times PWTd/LVDd$$

RWT is virtually unchanged throughout life in structurally normal hearts exposed to the normal range of systolic blood pressure (>0.42). Development of systolic HF from systemic hypertension is characterized by concentric remodeling and an increase in RWT, whereas systolic HF caused by chronic severe volume overload from aortic or mitral regurgitation (MR) is associated with eccentric hypertrophic remodeling and reduction in RWT.

In spite of the technical limitations inherent in LV mass calculations from M-mode, two-dimensional and three-dimensional echo, knowledge of LV mass especially as it relates to mass/volume ratio is important, because this ratio remains constant throughout life unless eccentric or concentric remodeling are induced similar to RWT. When the stimulus for remodeling is counterbalanced by therapeutic intervention, the mass/volume ratio reverts toward normal. LV mass in HF patients varies widely from patients who develop severe LV hypertrophy as in nonischemic idiopathic cardiomyopathy to those with ischemic dilated cardiomyopathy who exhibit a limited or inadequate hypertrophic response because of myocytes loss or malfunction and are without the capacity to elaborate contractile proteins.

Wall Stress and Stress-Shortening

Systolic HF is characterized by LV dilatation that initially increases systolic wall stress at the LV endocardium and at the LV mid-wall proportional to the increase in LV size. Meridional end-systolic wall stress (MWS-σ) can be calculated from M-mode echo measurements of LV cavity radius (r), LV wall thickness (h), and cavity length (circumferential stress) with simultaneous direct or indirect (cuff systolic blood pressure) measurement of LV systolic pressure (P).

$$MWS(\sigma) = P \times r/2h(1+h/2r)$$

Circumferential wall stress (CWS-σ) correlates more closely with cavity emptying but requires two-dimensional echocardiography measurement of cavity length.

$$CWS(\sigma) = P \times b/h(1 - h/2b)(1 - hb/2a)$$

Where "a" and "b" are the major and minor LV cavity axes.

Wall stress is a major determinant of LV cavity architecture, LV hypertrophy, and contractile function. In compensated congestive HF, initial LV dilatation increases wall stress that is transduced by stretch-activated mechanoreceptors that trigger a hypertrophic response by the angiotensin-1 receptor. Hypertrophy results in an increase in LV wall thickness that normalizes wall stress and preserves and stabilizes LV contractile function. There is a strong inverse relationship between systolic wall stress and ejection phase indices including ejection fraction, fractional shortening of the LV internal dimensions, and velocity of circumferential fiber shortening (**Fig. 11**). As systolic wall stress increases, so ejection fraction decreases. This is important from a therapeutic perspective because reducing wall stress is accompanied by improvement in ejection fraction. This is the fundamental principle underlying the use of vasodilator therapy in patients with HF before the onset of irreversible myocardial

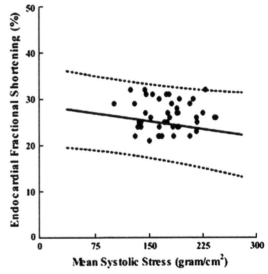

Fig. 11. Inverse relationship between LV function (percent of endocardial fractional shortening) and mean systolic stress in normal subjects showing that as systolic stress increases, LV function deteriorates. Reducing LV loading (systolic wall stress) conditions with vasodilators in patients with heart failure invokes this mechanical principle. (*From* Aurigemma GP, Zile MR, Gaasch WH. Contractile behavior of the left ventricle in diastolic heart failure: with emphasis on regional systolic function. Circulation 2006;113: 296–304; with permission.)

damage occurs at which point they fall off the normal stress-shortening relationship, leftward and downward. The effects of therapeutic interventions aimed at altering LV loading conditions and contractile function can be readily assessed echocardiographically.

The natural history of systolic HF is a progressive deterioration in pump function with the inability to elaborate sufficient hypertrophy to normalize wall stress and prevent the escalation to HF. Assessment of wall stress can be achieved easily by M-mode or two-dimensional measurements of LV cavity radius (diameter/2), wall thickness, and for circumferential wall stress cavity length. In individual patients the slope of the relationship between changes in end-systolic wall stress and end-systolic diameter over a series of perturbations in LV loading conditions provides an index of contractile function that is independent of load.[6] The limitation of calculating wall stress in HF is that the currently used stress equations make the assumption that the material properties of the myocardium are homogeneous and that there are no regional wall motion abnormalities. These conditions are not met in patients with HF of ischemic etiology, who comprise approximately two thirds of all HF patients.

Although estimation of regional and global wall stress assumes that myocardial material properties are homogeneous throughout the LV and calculations become uninterpretable, myocardial strain or deformation can be measured and used as a surrogate for wall stress. Strain is defined in physical terms as the change in myocardial length over resting length:

Strain, $(\epsilon) = \Delta L/L_0$

$\Delta L = (L_t - L_0)$
L_n – resting length
L_t = length at a specific time "t"

Measurements of myocardial strain can be obtained from tissue Doppler imaging using echocardiography with high temporal and spatial accuracy[27–29] and ideally should be related to the long axis of the myocardial fibers. Echo measurements of myocardial strain correlate closely with strain measurements derived from sonomicrometry crystals and from MRI using myocardial tagging techniques.[30] Tissue Doppler imaging measures myocardial velocity at two locations, whereas sonomicrometry and MRI measure movement between two points. Acquisition of strain measurements from echocardiography is relatively simple, but highly dependent on image and signal quality and consistency. Furthermore,

measurement of strain with tissue Doppler imaging is angle dependent and limited to apical echocardiographic images so that only longitudinal strain can be quantified.

An alternative echocardiographic method for assessing myocardial strain that also correlates with LVEF uses speckle tracking technology. This is based on the interference from back-scattered ultrasound waves from neighboring structures that create a speckled pattern that remains stable throughout the cardiac cycle (**Fig. 12**).[31,32] This technique, unlike tissue Doppler imaging, is not angle dependent and enables assessment of radial and circumferential strain in addition to longitudinal strain (**Fig. 13**).[31,32] Strain rate is the rate of change of strain over unit time:

Strain rate = $d\epsilon/dt$

Multidimensional strain and strain rate analyses are attractive because they are based on fundamental physiologic principles of myocardial mechanics, obtainable noninvasively and as such provide insight into the mechanisms of HF, and also serve as a clinical tool for long-term follow-up.

Left Ventricular Pressure-Volume Relations, Left Ventricular Elastance

Further insight into LV chamber function in systolic HF can be obtained by integrating echocardiographic images with pressure or displacement to construct pressure volume loops or pressure-LV short axis area loops with acoustic quantification. From these constructs, single beat estimates of end-systolic pressure-volume relations, stroke work, LV elastance, preload-adjusted maximal power index, and recruitable work can be quantified using two-dimensional echocardiography.[33] Although such studies do clarify current understanding of LV global function in HF, the need for continuous LV or central aortic pressure makes them user-unfriendly methodologies and impractical for widespread use in randomized clinical HF trials, and the same can be said for calculation of systolic wall stress.

Mitral Regurgitation

MR is almost ubiquitous in patients with severe systolic HF regardless of its etiology and the more severe the HF, the greater the likelihood of hemodynamically significant MR. There are different pathoetiologic mechanisms that are distinguishable echocardiographically, although the mitral valve leaflets may be intrinsically normal. The two major causes of MR in HF are ischemic MR that is associated with regional LV wall motion

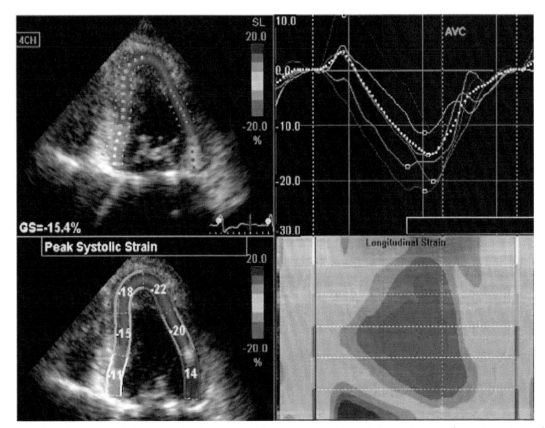

Fig. 12. Peak longitudinal strain obtained using speckle tracking during systolic contraction from six regions of interest that are angle independent and occur almost simultaneously in this normal subject.

abnormalities and nonischemic cardiomyopathy. Both ischemic and nonischemic HF exhibit progressive LV remodeling and cavity dilatation.

Ischemic MR is associated with a poor prognosis and usually results from ischemia of the papillary muscles or subjacent LV wall, and the severity of MR worsens with the increased demands for exercise stress. Ischemic MR is important to diagnose because it can often be rectified by myocardial revascularization alone, or

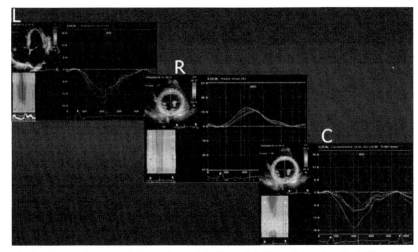

Fig. 13. Schematic showing a plot out of circumferential (C), radial (R), and longitudinal (L) strains from a normal subject in whom there is the usual regional temporal coordination of contraction.

by revascularization combined with surgical repair of the mitral valve. The diagnosis of ischemic MR can readily be made with transthoracic two-dimensional echo Doppler used in conjunction with exercise or pharmacologic stress that exacerbates the degree of MR.

Recognition of MR and assessment of its severity is important because if MR is left untreated it leads to progressive LV dilatation from volume overload that increases wall stress, reduces ejection fraction, and escalates the downward course to HF.[34] MR begets LV dilatation and LV dilatation begets further MR and initiates the remodeling process of progressive deterioration in contractile function that if detected early can be rectified. The severity of MR can often be ameliorated unless irreversible LV dysfunction has supervened. Improvement in MR can be achieved either by reducing LV loading conditions with vasodilators; by surgical repair of the mitral valve; by epicardial restraint devices; or by resynchronization therapy provided that LV dyssynchrony and a prolonged QRS (>120 milliseconds) duration are present.

Color flow Doppler is exquisitely sensitive to MR, allowing detection of even the most trivial MR signal. There are numerous methods for semi-quantification of MR by visual estimation of the color flow Doppler jet area and grading severity from 1+ (mild) through 4+ (severe), and true quantification of MR using proximal isovelocity surface area to assess regurgitant volume and effective mitral regurgitant orifice area.

Development of MR in HF of nonischemic etiology is directly related to progressive LV dilatation with disproportionately greater increase in the short axis diameter than in cavity length resulting in a more spherical LV. This change in LV cavity shape separates the two papillary muscles in space with no change in chordal length thereby disrupting normal mitral leaflet area of coaptation causing leaflet tenting and changing the angles that the papillary muscles subtend to the center of the plane of the mitral valve annulus. This distortion of LV that disrupts the normal mitral valve and subvalve apparatus is also accompanied by dilatation of the mitral annulus that facilitates MR. The diagnosis of secondary MR in dilated nonischemic cardiomyopathy is easily established by transthoracic Doppler echocardiography and should be detected early in the course of the remodeling process so that appropriate remedial therapy can

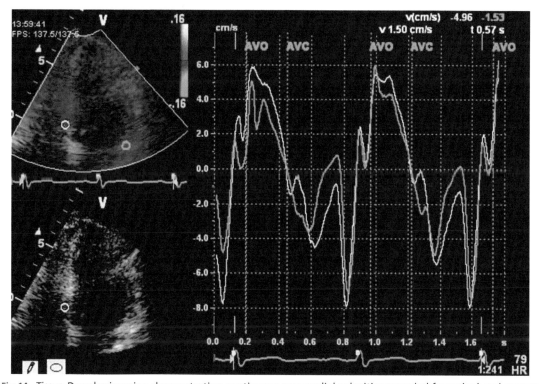

Fig. 14. Tissue Doppler imaging demonstrating continuous myocardial velocities recorded from the basal septum (*yellow*) and basal lateral wall (*green*) from a normal subject. Peak velocities from both regions occur almost simultaneously during LV ejection, indicated by the period between aortic valve opening (AVO) and aortic valve closure (AVC) showing the high degree of temporal coordination of contraction.

be instituted before MR escalates the onset of irreversible LV dysfunction.

Left Ventricle Dyssynchrony

Approximately one third of patients presenting with the symptoms and clinical stigmata of congestive HF have prolonged QRS duration on ECG. QRS duration has been used to establish the presence of LV dyssynchrony. Recent serial echocardiographic studies have demonstrated that cardiac resynchronization therapy (CRT) in patients with advanced HF (New York Heart Association symptom class III/IV) attenuates and more frequently reverses LV remodeling in two thirds of patients.[35–38] The reason postulated for the 30% of nonresponders is a combination of technical problems with the coronary sinus having unfavorable anatomy, or that in spite of the QRS greater than 120 milliseconds there is little evidence for LV dyssynchrony being present. The search for a reliable echocardiographic predictor for LV dyssynchrony and an optimal response to CRT has proved elusive. Initial use of Doppler parameters as predictors of clinical outcome in the PROSPECT randomized trial involved measuring the time interval from the beginning of QRS to both the peak and the onset of peak systolic myocardial velocity (see **Fig. 14**) in the basal two or six myocardial segments to determine the differences in the duration of this time interval between segments.[39] Although this enabled detection of LV dyssynchrony there was no single echo parameter that reliably or consistently predicted response to CRT.[39] The use of Doppler echocardiography and CRT in HF patients is discussed elsewhere in this issue and is not discussed here, other than to mention that echocardiography has characterized the short- and long-term effects of CRT, defined the concept of reversed LV remodeling, and is partly responsible for the role of CRT in patients with symptomatic HF.

SUMMARY

Echocardiography serves an extremely important role in the diagnosis and management of patients with HF. The various stages of structural and functional changes that constitute progressive LV remodeling including changes in loading conditions, hypertrophy, dilatation, cavity shape, mitral annulus, and subvalve apparatus and development of MR are associated with worsening symptoms and quality of life and have all been characterized by two-dimensional echocardiography. In addition, echocardiography has defined the transition from compensated hypertrophy to LV dilatation and progression to end-stage (New York Heart Association class III/IV) HF.

Echocardiography has also played an important role in clinical HF trials of β-adrenergic blocking agents and angiotensin-converting enzyme inhibitor and angiotensin receptor blocker and demonstrated their efficacy in HF. These agents have become standard of care the treatment of HF. It is not surprising that echocardiography has been regarded as the single most useful diagnostic tool in the overall management of patients with HF.

REFERENCES

1. Vasan RS, Levy D. Defining diastolic HF: a call for standardized diagnostic criteria. Circulation 2000; 101:2118–21.
2. Zile MR, Gaasch WH, Carroll JD, et al. Heart failure with a normal ejection fraction: is measurement of diastolic function necessary to make the diagnosis of diastolic HF? Circulation 2001;104:779–82.
3. Kitzman DW, Gardin JM, Gottdiener JS, et al. Importance of HF with preserved systolic function in patients >65 years of age. Am J Cardiol 2001;87: 413–9.
4. Smith GL, Masoudi FA, Vaccarino V, et al. Outcomes in HF patients with preserved ejection fraction: mortality, readmission, and functional decline. J Am Coll Cardiol 2003;41:1510–8.
5. Grossman W, Jones D, McLaurin LP. Wall stress and patterns of hypertrophy in the human left ventricle. J Clin Invest 1975;56:14–23.
6. Reichek N, Wilson JR, St. John Sutton M, et al. Noninvasive determination of left ventricular end-systolic stress: validation of the method and initial application. Circulation 1982;65:99–108.
7. Gerdts E, Zabalgoitia M, Bjornstad H, et al. Gender differences in systolic left ventricular function in hypertensive patients with electrocardiographic left ventricular hypertrophy (the LIFE study). Am J Cardiol 2001;87:980–3.
8. Devereux RB, Roman MJ, de Simone G, et al. Relations of left ventricular mass to demographic and hemodynamic variables in American Indians: the Strong Heart Study. Circulation 1997;96:1416–23.
9. Devereux RB, Bella JN, Palmieri V, et al. Left ventricular systolic dysfunction in a biracial sample of hypertensive adults: The Hypertension Genetic Epidemiology Network (Hyper GEN) Study. Hypertension 2001;38:417–23.
10. Lang RM, Bierig M, Devereux RB, et al. A report from the American Society of Echocardiography's Nomenclature and Standards Committee and the Task Force on Chamber Quantification, developed in conjunction with the American College of Cardiology Echocardiography Committee, the American Heart Association, and the European Association

of Echocardiography, a branch of the European Society of Cardiology. J Am Soc Echocardiogr 2005;18:1440–63.

11. St. John Sutton M, Otterstat JE, Plappert T, et al. Quantitaion of Left Ventricular Volumes and Ejection Fraction in Post-infarction Patients from Biplane and Single Plane Two Dimensional Echocardiograms. A Prospective Longitudinal Study of 1113 Echocardiograms. Eur Heart J 1998;19:808–16.

12. St. John Sutton M, Plappert T. Core lab, no core lab or automated LVEF? Eur J Echocardiogr 2007;8: 239–40.

13. Cannesson M, Tanabe M, Suffoletto MS, et al. A novel two-dimensional echocardiographic image analysis system using artificial intelligence-learned pattern recognition for rapid automated ejection fraction. J Am Coll Cardiol 2007;49:217–26.

14. Rahmouni HW, Ky B, Plappert T, et al. Clinical utility of automated assessment of left ventricular ejection fraction using artificial intelligence-assisted border detection. Am Heart J 2008;155:562–70.

15. Mor-Avi V, Sugeng L, Weinert L, et al. Fast measurement of left ventricular mass with real-time three-dimensional echocardiography: comparison with magnetic resonance imaging. Circulation 2004; 110:1814–8.

16. St. John Sutton M, Pfeffer MA, Plappert T, et al. Quantitative two dimensional echocardiographic measurements are major predictors of adverse cardiovascular events following acute myocardial infarction: the protective effects of captopril. Circulation 1994;89:68–75.

17. White HD, Norris RM, Brown MA, et al. Left ventricular end-systolic volume as the major determinant of survival after recovery from myocardial infarction. Circulation 1987;76:44–51.

18. St. John Sutton M, Lee D, Rouleau JL, et al. Left ventricular remodeling and ventricular arrhythmias after myocardial infarction. Circulation 2003;107: 2677 82.

19. St. John Sutton M, Pfeffer MA, Moye LA, et al. Cardiovascular death and left ventricular remodeling two years after myocardial infarction: baseline predictors and impact of long-term use of captopril. Information from the Survival and Ventricular Enlargement (SAVE) trial. Circulation 1997;96: 3294–300.

20. Lamas GA, Vaughan DE, Parisi AF, et al. Effects of left ventricular shape and captopril therapy on exercise capacity after anterior wall acute myocardial infarction. Am J Cardiol 1989;63:1167–73.

21. Pfeffer MA, Braunwald E, Moyé LA, et al. Effect of captopril on mortality and morbidity in patients with left ventricular dysfunction after myocardial infarction. Results of the survival and ventricular enlargement trial. The SAVE Investigators. N Engl J Med 1992;327:669–77.

22. The SOLVD Investigators. Effect of enalapril on mortality and the development of HF in asymptomatic patients with reduced left ventricular ejection fractions. N Engl J Med 1992;327:685–91.

23. Bristow MR, Krause-Steinrauf H, Nuzzo R, et al. Effect of baseline or changes in adrenergic activity on clinical outcomes in the beta-blocker evaluation of survival trial. Circulation 2004;110:1437–42.

24. Abraham WT, Fisher WG, Smith AL, et al. Cardiac resynchronization in chronic HF. N Engl J Med 2002; 346:1845–53.

25. Mann DL, Acker MA, Jessup M, Acorn Trial Principal Investigators and Study Coordinators. Clinical evaluation of the CorCap Cardiac Support Device in patients with dilated cardiomyopathy. Ann Thorac Surg 2007;84(4):1226–35.

26. Aurigemma GP, Zile MR, Gaasch WH. Contractile behavior of the left ventricle in diastolic heart failure: with emphasis on regional systolic function. Circulation 2006;113:296–304.

27. Sutherland GR, Stewart MJ, Groundstroem KW, et al. Color Doppler myocardial imaging: a new technique for the assessment of myocardial function. J Am Soc Echocardiogr 1994;7:441–58.

28. Edvardsen T, Skulstad H, Urheim S, et al. Regional myocardial function during acute myocardial ischemia assessed by strain Doppler echocardiography. J Am Coll Cardiol 2001;37:726–30.

29. Abraham TP, Nishimura RA. Myocardial strain: can we finally measure contractility? J Am Coll Cardiol 2001;37:731–4.

30. Gotte MJW, van Rossum AC, Twisk JWR, et al. Quantication of regional contractile function after infarction: strain analysis superior to wall thickening analysis in discriminating infarct from remote myocardium. J Am Coll Cardiol 2001;37:808–17.

31. Korineck J, Wang J, Sengupta PP, et al. Two-dimensional strain-A Doppler independent ultrasound method for quantitation of regional deformation: validation in vitro and in vivo. J Am Soc Echocardiogr 2005;18:1247–53.

32. Artis NJ, Oxborough DL, Williams G, et al. Two-dimensional strain imaging: a new echocardiographic advance with research and clinical applications. Int J Cardiol 2008;123:240–8.

33. Senzaki H, Chen C-H, Kass DA. Singe beat estimation of end-systolic pressure-volume relation in humans: a new method with the potential for non-invasive application. Circulation 1996;94:2497–506.

34. Grigioni F, Enriquez-Sarano M, Zehr KJ, et al. Regurgitation: long-term outcome and prognostic implications with quantitative Doppler assessment. Circulation 2001;103:1759–64.

35. St. John Sutton MG, Plappert T, Abraham WT, et al. Effect of cardiac resynchronization therapy on left ventricular size and function in chronic HF. Circulation 2003;107:1985–90.

36. Linde C, Gold MR, Abraham WT, et al. Randomized trial of cardiac resynchronization in mildly symptomatic HF patients and in asymptomatic patients with left ventricular dysfunction and previous HF symptoms. J Am Coll Cardiol 2008; in press.

37. Cleland JG, Daubert JC, Erdmann E, et al. The effect of cardiac resynchronization on morbidity and mortality in HF. N Engl J Med 2005;352:1539–49.

38. Yu C, Chau E, Sanderson JE, et al. Tissue Doppler echocardiographic evidence of reverse remodeling and improved synchronicity by simultaneously delaying regional contraction after biventricular pacing therapy in HF. Circulation 2002;105:438–45.

39. Chung ES, Leon AR, Tavazzi L, et al. Results of the predictors of response to CRT (PROSPECT) trial. Circulation 2008;117:2608–16.

Upper Extremity Venous Doppler Ultrasound

Therese M. Weber, MD*, Mark E. Lockhart, MD, MPH,
Michelle L. Robbin, MD

KEYWORDS

- Hemodialysis arteriovenous fistula • Venous system
- Venous thrombosis • Fistula • Arterial anatomy

Sonography plays a major role in evaluating the upper extremity venous system. The most widely used applications include evaluation for thrombus and vessel patency, localization during venous access procedures, preoperative venous mapping for hemodialysis arteriovenous fistula (AVF) and graft placement, and postoperative hemodialysis AVF and graft assessment. Knowledge of anatomy, scanning technique, and attention to detail are important to the success of demonstrating abnormalities in the upper extremity venous system. Sonographic evaluation of the upper extremity venous system is more challenging than evaluation of the lower extremity venous system.

This article presents methods that allow easy identification of the sometimes complex anatomy and the avoidance of pitfalls that can lead to common and uncommon errors.

NORMAL ANATOMY

The venous anatomy of the neck and arm is illustrated in **Fig. 1**.

Deep Venous System

The more clinically important aspect of the venous system of the upper extremity is the deep system, especially the proximal aspect of the venous system including the internal jugular vein, the subclavian vein, and the brachiocephalic vein. One easy way to tell if a vein is superficial or deep is to assess whether it has an artery running with it. In the upper extremity only deep veins have arteries running with them. The radial and ulnar veins in the forearm, which usually are paired, unite caudal to the level of the elbow to form the brachial veins. The brachial veins in the upper arm join with the basilic vein at a variable location, typically at the level of the teres major muscle. The confluence of the brachial and basilic veins continues as the axillary vein, which passes through the axilla from the teres major muscle to the first rib. As the axillary vein crosses the first rib, it becomes the lateral portion of the subclavian vein. The medial portion of the subclavian vein receives the smaller external jugular vein and the larger internal jugular vein to form the brachiocephalic (innominate) vein. Bilateral brachiocephalic veins join to form the superior vena cava.

The authors define the central veins as the brachiocephalic veins and superior vena cava, which usually cannot be demonstrated sonographically. Some angiographers include the subclavian vein when they discuss central veins. Therefore, it is important to be very specific about the vein segment examined in describing sonographic findings. The presence or absence of significant central stenosis or thrombosis needs to be inferred by evaluating the transmitted cardiac pulsatility and respiratory phasicity in the medial subclavian vein and caudal internal jugular vein, as discussed later.

Superficial Venous System

The superficial venous system of the upper extremity comprises the cephalic vein located more laterally and the basilic vein located more medially. The basilic and cephalic veins typically

This article originally appeared in *Radiologic Clinics of North America* 2007;45(3):513–524
Department of Radiology, University of Alabama at Birmingham, 619 19th Street, South, JT N312, Birmingham, AL 35249-6830, USA
* Corresponding author.
E-mail address: tweber@uabmc.edu (T.M. Weber).

Ultrasound Clin 4 (2009) 181–192
doi:10.1016/j.cult.2009.04.010

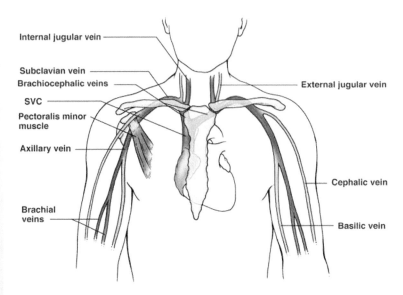

Internal jugular vein

Subclavian vein
Brachiocephalic veins

SVC

Pectoralis minor
muscle

Axillary vein

Brachial
veins

External jugular vein

Cephalic vein

Basilic vein

Fig. 1. Normal venous anatomy. The deep veins of the arm (*dark blue*) include the brachial vein and axillary vein. The brachiocephalic vein is formed by the internal jugular and subclavian veins. The two brachiocephalic veins join to become the superior vena cava. Superficial veins (*light blue*) include the cephalic vein, basilic vein, and external jugular vein.

have a variably larger vein connecting them caudally near the elbow, the median antecubital vein.

Normal Arterial Anatomy

The brachial artery begins in the upper arm at the lower margin of the teres major muscle tendon and usually ends about 1 cm below the elbow where is divides into the radial and ulnar arteries. Anatomic variants of the radial artery include a high take-off or high bifurcating radial artery. In some cases, the radial artery may take off from the cranial aspect of the brachial artery in the upper arm. One way to distinguish a high take-off of the radial artery from a large elbow branch artery is to follow it into the forearm down to the radial artery region at the wrist. A large arterial branch to the elbow traverses toward the elbow and does not extend into the forearm. Rarely, the ulnar artery may be absent.

SONOGRAPHIC EXAMINATION TECHNIQUE

Sonographic evaluation of the upper extremity venous system is more technically challenging than evaluation of the lower extremity venous system. These technical challenges include the inability to compress the subclavian vein because of the overlying clavicle and the need to differentiate large venous collaterals from normal veins in cases of venous obstruction.

The patient is scanned in a supine position with the examined arm abducted from the chest and with the patient's head turned slightly away from the examined arm. Real-time B-mode imaging

with spectral and color flow analysis is performed using the highest frequency linear transducer that still gives adequate penetration. Typically the examination is best performed using a 5- to 10-MHz linear-array transducer moving to a higher frequency in the upper arm and forearm if possible. A curved-array transducer or sector transducer may be useful in larger individuals, especially in the axillary area, because of the increased depth of penetration and larger field of view.

All veins are examined with compression every 1 to 2 cm in the transverse plane. Gray-scale transverse images with and without compression or cine clips during compression are obtained from the cranial aspect of the internal jugular vein in the neck near the mandible to the thoracic inlet caudally. Longitudinal color and spectral images are performed also. The subclavian vein is evaluated from its medial to lateral aspect with longitudinal color and spectral images, demonstrating transmitted respiratory variability, cardiac pulsatility, and color fill-in. An inferiorly angled, supraclavicular approach with color Doppler is necessary to demonstrate the superior brachiocephalic vein and the medial portion of the subclavian vein. Use of a small-footprint sector probe in or near the suprasternal notch may facilitate visualization of the brachiocephalic veins and the cranial aspect of the superior vena cava. The midportion of the subclavian vein, located deep to the clavicle, frequently is imaged incompletely. An infraclavicular, superiorly angled approach is used to demonstrate the lateral aspect of the subclavian vein. Frequently, the subclavian vein can be compressed.

Spectral waveform evaluation is critical to upper extremity venous evaluation. Documentation of normal flow features in the medial subclavian vein is extremely important, because it confirms patency of the brachiocephalic vein and superior vena cava, which cannot be examined directly. Each spectral image is evaluated for spontaneous, phasic, and nonpulsatile flow. These samples are obtained in the longitudinal plane of the vessel with angle of insonation maintained at less than 60° (**Fig. 2**). Spectral analysis of the caudal internal jugular vein and medial subclavian vein is mandatory to evaluate for the presence of transmitted cardiac pulsatility and respiratory phasicity. Loss of this pulsatility may be caused by a more central venous stenosis or obstruction (**Fig. 3**).[1] A normal spectral tracing should return to baseline.

Spectral tracings from the medial subclavian vein should be compared with tracings from the lateral subclavian vein. A change between the two tracings suggests subclavian vein stenosis in the midportion of the subclavian vein. Response to a brisk inspiratory sniff or Valsalva's maneuver may assist in evaluating venous patency. With a sniff, the internal jugular vein or subclavian vein normally decreases in diameter or collapses completely. Patients who have significant stenosis or obstruction of the central brachiocephalic vein or superior vena cava lose this response.[1]

Peripheral Deep Venous System

The remainder of the examination includes compression every 1 to 2 cm of the axillary vein, the cranial, midportion, and caudal aspect of the brachial veins, and the basilic and cephalic veins

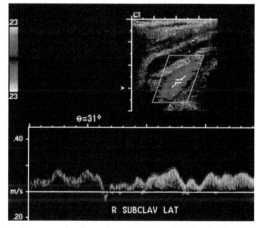

Fig. 2. Normal subclavian vein. Longitudinal color and spectral Doppler of the subclavian vein shows normal filling of the vessel with color. There is normal transmitted respiratory phasicity and cardiac pulsatility with transient reversal of flow below baseline.

in the upper arm. Evaluation of the axilla may be limited by body habitus with subsequent limitation in seeing the vessels sonographically. Typically, the upper extremity is imaged to the antecubital fossa. If the patient has focal pain or swelling or a palpable mass in the forearm, the symptomatic area is assessed sonographically. Vessels in the forearm usually are assessed only as part of a focused evaluation of a painful or swollen area or a palpable cord.

Potential Pitfalls

Pitfalls to avoid include[2–4]

1. Axillary versus cephalic vein: The axillary vein can be traced through its anatomic course into the subclavian vein. In addition, the cephalic vein, a superficial vein, does not have an adjacent artery running along its course. It may be necessary to abduct the arm further, bend the elbow, and place the hand near the patient's head to access the axilla adequately. Excessive abduction, however, can cause alteration in the venous waveform that falsely suggests a more proximal venous stenosis or occlusion. This alteration resolves with a change in position.
2. Caudal occlusion of the internal jugular vein: It is imperative to follow the caudal aspect of the internal jugular vein into the junction with the medial subclavian vein as it forms the brachiocephalic vein. The internal jugular vein usually is in close proximity to the carotid artery. A vein located further away probably represents a collateral vessel. An additional pitfall is that normal respiratory phasicity may be seen in well-developed collaterals. The collaterals usually follow the course of the occluded vein. Collaterals frequently are multiple, somewhat serpiginous veins, rather than the normal single vein following the associated artery.
3. Mirror-image artifact: Because of reflection from the lung apex or clavicle, mirror-image artifact may give the appearance of two subclavian veins in the supraclavicular region

IMAGING PROTOCOL

Training, skill, and experience are extremely important in performing all vascular ultrasound examinations, including upper extremity venous Doppler ultrasound. Participation in one of the vascular accreditation programs, such as the American College of Radiology or the Intersocietal Commission for the Accreditation of Vascular Laboratories, is strongly recommended.

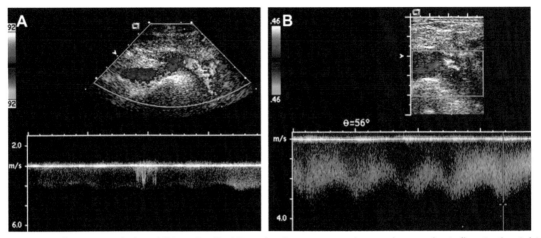

Fig. 3. Central venous occlusion. (*A*) Longitudinal Doppler demonstrates abnormal monophasic flow in the right brachiocephalic vein (Doppler gate). (*B*) Extremely high-velocity flow (329 cm/s) in the vein suggests high-grade stenosis at this level.

The upper extremity venous imaging protocol includes the following images for each deep venous segment:

1. Transverse gray-scale image at rest and with compression or a cine clip of the compression maneuver
2. Longitudinal color Doppler with spectral waveform demonstrating transmitted cardiac and respiratory variability
   A. Internal jugular vein—cranial and caudal portions
   B. Subclavian vein—mid, medial, lateral
   C. Axillary vein
   D. Brachial vein—cranial, mid, caudal
   E. Basilic vein—upper arm
   F. Cephalic vein—upper arm

CLINICAL DIAGNOSIS

Undiagnosed and untreated deep venous thrombosis (DVT) can result in the fatal outcome of pulmonary embolism. In 12% to 16% of pulmonary embolism cases, the source of thrombus is the upper extremities.[5,6] Fatal pulmonary embolism caused by DVT of the upper extremity has been reported.[7]

Wells and colleagues[8] previously demonstrated that the use of a clinical model allows the physician to determine accurately the probability that a patient has DVT before diagnostic tests are performed. Clinical factors associated with increased probability of DVT include active cancer, immobility, localized tenderness along the distribution of the deep venous system, swollen entire extremity, pitting edema confined to the symptomatic extremity, collateral superficial veins, and

previously documented DVT. The D-dimer assay has a high negative predictive value, and D-dimer is a sensitive but nonspecific marker for DVT.[9–11] Wells and colleagues[12] concluded that DVT can be ruled out in a patient who is judged clinically unlikely to have DVT and who has a negative D-dimer test and that ultrasound evaluation can be omitted safely in these patients. A problem may arise when a D-dimer is obtained without first evaluating the clinical model. D-dimer may be positive in patients who have had recent surgery or trauma, infection, atherosclerosis, congestive heart failure, or disseminated intravascular coagulation and in pregnant, puerperal, or elderly individuals. This work addressed lower extremity DVT and did not address central lines, a frequent cause of upper extremity DVT (UEDVT).

UPPER EXTREMITY VENOUS THROMBOSIS

The most common indication for venous Doppler ultrasound of the upper extremity is to identify DVT. Indications for upper extremity venous Doppler ultrasound, as listed in the 2006 American College of Radiology practice guideline for the performance of peripheral venous ultrasound examination, include but are not limited to[13]

1. Evaluation of possible venous obstruction or thrombus in symptomatic or high-risk asymptomatic individuals
2. Assessment of dialysis access grafts
3. Venous mapping before harvest for arterial bypass or reconstructive surgery
4. Evaluation of veins before venous access
5. Evaluation for DVT in patients suspected of having pulmonary embolism

6. Follow-up for patients who have known venous thrombosis

Other causes include pain and or swelling at the site of prior phlebotomy or intravenous access site and, uncommonly, effort-related thrombosis. The pathogenesis of effort-related thrombosis is related to an anatomic constriction of the vein by the clavicle and first rib complex associated with repetitive trauma to the vein and resultant changes in the vein wall itself.[14] Radiation therapy, effort-induced thrombosis, and malignant obstructions from compression or direct venous invasion by adjacent tumor or metastatic nodal disease are more common causes of venous obstruction in the chest and arm than in the lower extremities.

Unlike the lower extremity, most cases of UEDVT are related to the presence of a central venous catheter or electrode leads from an implanted cardiac device. Thirty-five percent to 75% of patients who have upper extremity venous catheters develop thrombosis, approximately 75% of which are asymptomatic.[15–17] The complication rate varies greatly, depending on whether the catheter access site is the subclavian or the internal jugular vein. Examining only patients who had symptomatic UEDVT, Trerotola and colleagues[18] found a greater incidence of DVT in patients who had subclavian venous access than in those who had internal jugular access. Thirteen percent of the patients who had subclavian venous catheters had DVT, compared with only 3% of patients who had internal jugular vein catheters. Thus, the placement of large-bore catheters into the subclavian vein is to be discouraged, especially in patients who have end-stage renal disease for whom dialysis access is being considered. The development of subclavian vein stenosis or thrombosis would limit dialysis access possibilities for that upper extremity.

Only 12% to 16% of patients who have UEDVT develop pulmonary embolism.[6,19] Most acute pulmonary emboli in patients who have UEDVT occur in untreated patients.[5,20] The risk of pulmonary embolism is greater in catheter-related UEDVT than in UEDVT from other causes.[21] Associated complications such as venous stasis and insufficiency caused by venous thrombosis are less common and less severe in the upper extremity than in the leg. Physiologic factors that exist in the leg, such as exposure of the deep venous system to high hydrostatic pressure, do not exist in the arm. The tendency toward development of extensive collateral venous pathways in the arm and chest after venous thrombosis or obstruction contributes to these differences.

ACUTE DEEP VENOUS THROMBOSIS

Current literature shows the sensitivity of venous Doppler ultrasound for UEDVT to range from 78% to 100% and its specificity to range from 82% to 100%.[22–27] The acute deep vein thrombus is seen as an enlarged, tubular structure filled with thrombus showing variable echogenicity and absence of color Doppler flow (**Fig. 4**). Nonocclusive thrombus may show flow outlining the thrombus, with a variable appearance depending on whether the nonocclusive thrombus is acute or chronic. Nonocclusive thrombus usually does not result in enlargement of the vein (**Fig. 5**). When obstruction is incomplete, monophasic flow is demonstrated when the luminal narrowing is significant enough to affect the transmitted cardiac pulsatility and respiratory phasicity from the thorax. As with lower extremity venous Doppler ultrasound, attention to detail is important in areas of duplicated veins to avoid overlooking thrombus in one of the paired veins (**Fig. 6**).

Spectral analysis can assist in the evaluation of central thromboses. The presence of a nonpulsatile waveform (similar to portal venous flow) strongly suggests central venous disease such as thrombosis, stenosis, or extrinsic compression from an adjacent mass.[22] It is important to compare the suspicious waveform with the contralateral side to confirm its presence on only the symptomatic side. Patel and colleagues[28] found that absent or reduced cardiac pulsatility was a more sensitive parameter in patients who had unilateral venous thrombosis, even though respiratory phasicity often was asymmetric. In bilateral subclavian vein

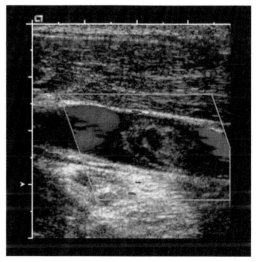

Fig. 4. Occlusive deep venous thrombosis. On longitudinal color Doppler of internal jugular vein, no flow is present around the heterogeneous clot.

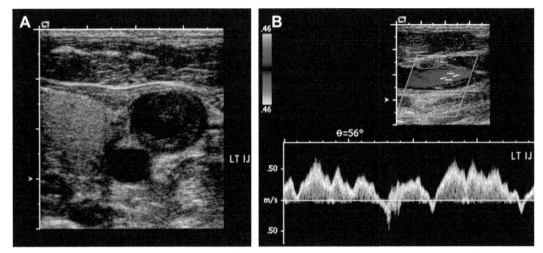

Fig. 5. Nonocclusive deep venous thrombosis. (*A*) Transverse gray-scale image shows hypoechoic thrombus that does not completely fill the internal jugular vein. (*B*) On longitudinal color and spectral Doppler, flow is present in the vein alongside the clot, and normal respiratory phasicity is present.

or superior vena cava occlusions the process is bilateral, and a high level of suspicion must be maintained to detect central thrombus or stenosis. Also, because of high-volume flow, there may be absence of phasicity without stenosis in the central veins if a hemodialysis graft is present in the upper arm (**Fig. 7**).

CHRONIC DEEP VENOUS THROMBOSIS

As in the lower extremity, diagnosis of chronic venous disease may be more difficult than the diagnosis of acute venous disease. Suggestive findings include frozen valve leaflets, synechia, recanalized veins with internal channels of flow, and small-caliber veins with noncompressible, thickened walls (**Fig. 8**).[22] In some cases of chronic venous thrombosis, the vein may be collapsed, fibrosed, and not visible sonographically in the expected anatomic location. For example, if only one brachial vein is demonstrated, chronic scarring from prior DVT of the other brachial vein should be suggested.

Flow direction and collateral pathways should be noted also. In rare cases of brachiocephalic thrombosis, drainage may occur in a retrograde fashion

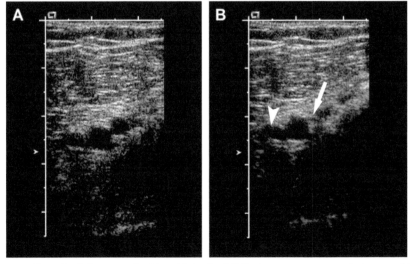

Fig. 6. Deep venous thrombosis in one paired brachial vein. (*A*) On transverse gray-scale image of brachial veins, paired veins are visible without compression. (*B*) A potential pitfall in detecting deep vein thrombosis is shown as one of the two paired brachial veins compresses normally (*arrow*). The other does not compress because of occlusive clot (*arrowhead*).

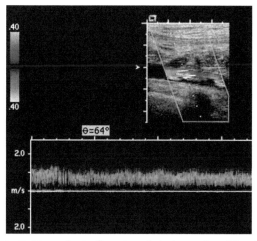

Fig. 7. Monophasic flow in subclavian vein without stenosis. Longitudinal color and spectral Doppler show monophasic waveforms due to high flow volumes from an upper arm hemodialysis graft. There was no central stenosis present on angiography.

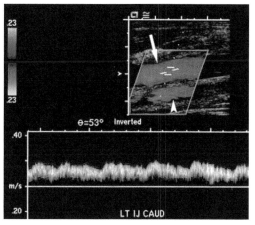

Fig. 9. Brachiocephalic vein occlusion. Reversal of flow is present on color Doppler of the internal jugular vein (*arrow*). Note the internal jugular vein and carotid artery (*arrowhead*) both demonstrate cranial flow.

through the internal jugular vein to collateral vessels (**Fig. 9**). In cases of occluded veins, the development of large venous collaterals may be mistaken for the thrombosed vessel. Collateral veins are tortuous venous structures that are not in the normal venous location, adjacent to the artery (**Fig. 10**). These collateral veins may show normal respiratory phasicity because they communicate with veins that are subject to changes in intrathoracic pressure.

The presence of a chronic thrombus in a symptomatic patient without evidence for new acute thrombus suggests postthrombotic syndrome.

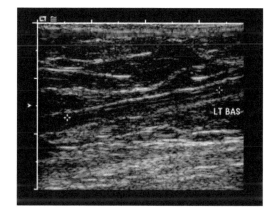

Fig. 8. Chronic superficial venous thrombosis. On longitudinal gray-scale image, thickening of the basilic vein (*cursors*) is present at site of previous catheter placement. The basilic vein is a superficial vein and usually does not require anticoagulation if a thrombus is present.

Postthrombotic syndrome is the most common late complication of DVT. Signs and symptoms include pain, edema, hyperpigmentation, and skin ulceration. Without the presence of acute thrombus, anticoagulant therapy is not indicated.[29] Therefore, it is important in patient management to differentiate acute from chronic changes whenever possible. Rubin and colleagues[30,31] demonstrated that sonographic elasticity imaging, a technique that measures tissue hardness, can discriminate between acute and chronic thrombi and can perform at least as well as thrombus echogenicity. Although this technique currently is not available commercially, it may play a future diagnostic role.

Areas of stenosis related to prior thrombosis or line placement can be demonstrated with gray-scale and color Doppler examination. A segment of vein may be narrowed significantly relative to the adjacent segments. Thickening or irregularity of the vein wall may be present. Turbulence with aliasing on color Doppler or high-velocity flow on spectral analysis may be demonstrated in these areas. Flow in the narrowed segment is not normal and may show increased pulsatility as compared with dampened, nonphasic flow in the more peripheral waveform (**Fig. 11**).[22]

Other vascular entities, such as a carotid artery to internal jugular fistula, may be associated with upper extremity swelling and mimic DVT (**Fig. 12**). Additional factors may alter venous hemodynamics. Pain and colleagues[32] demonstrated significant alteration of axillary venous

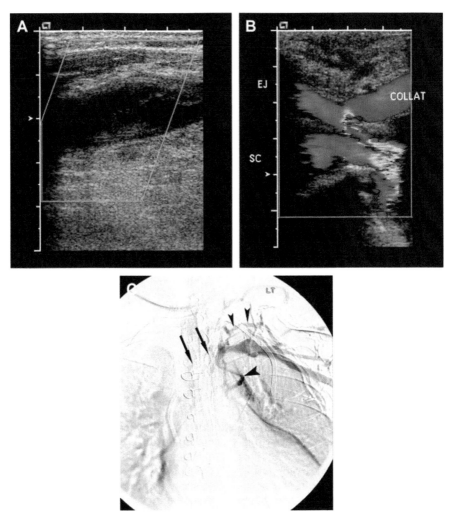

Fig. 10. Occlusive deep venous thrombosis with collaterals. (*A*) Color Doppler of internal jugular vein shows thrombus without visible flow. (*B*) A large collateral vessel is visible communicating with the external jugular vein as it bypasses the level of internal jugular vein obstruction, confirming the chronic component of the obstruction. (*C*) Catheter venogram in another patient shows absence of contrast in the left brachiocephalic vein (*arrows*) and presence of collateral vessels (*arrowheads*).

flow patterns in patients who had axillary lymph node dissection and breast cancer–related lymphedema. The etiology of breast cancer–related edema is multifactorial, and abnormalities of venous drainage are a contributory factor. Further investigation is needed.

When Doppler findings are indeterminate, especially regarding central thrombosis or stenosis, or when there is high clinical suspicion for UEDVT without confirmatory sonographic findings, correlation with MR venography or catheter venography may be needed. In the authors' experience, the most frequent indications for MR venography are suspected central thrombosis and stenosis with unilateral or bilateral abnormal respiratory phasicity in the medial subclavian vein and internal jugular vein.

VENOUS ACCESS PROCEDURES

In patients who need venous access or catheterization, upper extremity venous Doppler ultrasound can identify an appropriate vessel for access. This access vessel should be screened for the possibility of central stenosis or occlusion. Ultrasound also can demonstrate the target vessel during the procedure to improve the accuracy of venipuncture, decrease potential complications, and reduce procedure time. The variability in location of vascular structures relative to external

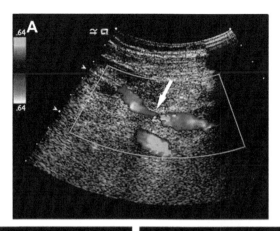

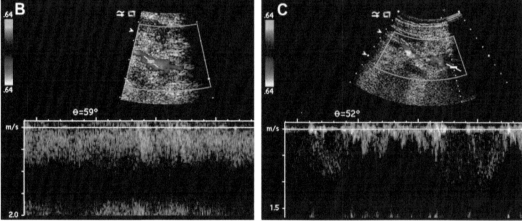

Fig. 11. Stenosis of cephalic vein. (A) Longitudinal color Doppler of the cephalic vein demonstrates focal narrowing (arrow) of the vessel with aliasing. (B) Spectral Doppler shows a waveform that is abnormally monophasic. (C) Medial to the area of stenosis, spectral Doppler shows normal venous phasicity.

landmarks is a strong reason to use ultrasound. Povoski and Zaman[33] recommend the use of preoperative ultrasound in patients who have had previous central venous access associated with deep venous thrombosis to assess for central stenosis or occlusion. In addition, they recommend intraprocedural venography when there is difficulty advancing the guidewire or catheter centrally or when preoperative ultrasound is negative despite previous central venous access with DVT. In an existent catheter that has been in place for a prolonged time, upper extremity ultrasound can demonstrate thrombus or fibrin sheath around a catheter (Fig. 13).

SONOGRAPHIC EVALUATION BEFORE AND AFTER PLACEMENT OF HEMODIALYSIS ACCESS
Preoperative Mapping

Ultrasound vascular mapping before hemodialysis access placement now is an established procedure. Robbin and colleagues[34] demonstrated

that preoperative sonographic mapping before placement of hemodialysis access can change surgical management, with an increased number of AVFs placed and an improved likelihood of selecting the most functional vessels. Superficial and deep veins of the forearm and upper arm, as well as arteries, are evaluated for their suitability for graft or fistula placement. Criteria such as the diameter of the vein and the depth of the superficial vein from the skin are used to determine whether a fistula or a graft is recommended.[35]

Arteriovenous Fistula Maturity Assessment

Ultrasound also has a role after access placement. Upper extremity venous Doppler ultrasound can play a key role in addressing the two primary goals of the Vascular Access Work Group of the National Kidney Foundation, to increase the prevalence and use of native AVFs and to detect access dysfunction before occlusion.[36] Ultrasound evaluation will play an increasingly important role in

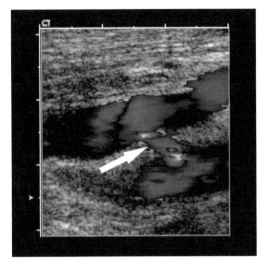

Fig. 12. Carotid-jugular fistula. Color Doppler shows direct communication (*arrow*) between the carotid artery and internal jugular vein. Arterialized flow was present in the internal jugular vein (not shown).

determining the maturity of a hemodialysis AVF.[37,38] Using color duplex ultrasound surveillance, Grogan and colleagues[38] found an unexpectedly high prevalence of critical stenoses in patent AVFs before initiation of hemodialysis and concluded that stenoses seem to develop rapidly after arterialization of the upper extremity superficial veins. They postulated that turbulent flow conditions in AVFs might play a role in inducing progressive vein wall and valve leaflet intimal thickening, although stenoses may be caused by

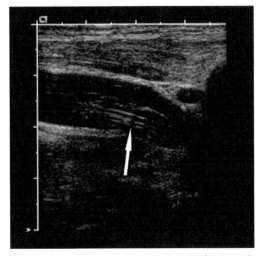

Fig. 13. Clot around catheter. Gray-scale Doppler shows occlusive clot surrounding an existing jugular venous catheter (*arrow*), a common complication of venous catheter placement.

venous abnormalities that predate AVF placement. Detection of stenosis, graft degeneration, or pseudoaneurysm formation may be important in triaging the patient toward appropriate care.[39] Ultrasound may prove useful in triaging patients toward the appropriate therapy for an immature AVF. When an AVF has low-volume flow, and one or more accessory or competing veins that may be sumping flow from the AVF are detected, ligation of accessory vein branches may be useful.[40]

Because of the large amounts of arterialized flow in the hemodialysis access, there may be changes in the spectral venous flow characteristics of the draining vein. Specifically, there may be loss of the normal respiratory phasicity in the absence of central stenosis or occlusion. This loss of phasicity occurs more commonly in patients who have upper extremity hemodialysis grafts than in those who have fistulas.

SUMMARY

It is important to understand thoroughly the normal anatomy and common variations of the upper extremity veins and arteries to avoid misdiagnosis. This understanding is particularly important because the incidence of upper extremity venous disease is increasing. The widespread use of central venous catheters, percutaneous interventional procedures performed with access through the upper extremity venous system, and implanted cardiac devices is increasing the number of patients who have upper extremity thrombosis. Ultrasound plays an important role in evaluating the upper extremity venous system and is the initial imaging modality of choice. When sonographic findings are equivocal or nondiagnostic, especially regarding central thrombosis, correlation using MR venography or catheter venography may be helpful. Ultrasound can provide an accurate, rapid, low-cost, portable, noninvasive method for screening, mapping, and surveillance of the upper extremity venous system.

ACKNOWLEDGMENTS

The authors thank Trish Thurman for her assistance in manuscript preparation.

REFERENCES

1. Gooding GA, Hightower DR, Moore EH, et al. Obstruction of the superior vena cava or subclavian veins: sonographic diagnosis. Radiology 1986; 159(3):663–5.
2. Kremkau FW, Taylor KJ. Artifacts in ultrasound imaging. J Ultrasound Med 1986;5(4):227–37.

3. Reading CC, Charboneau JW, Allison JW, et al. Color and spectral Doppler mirror-image artifact of the subclavian artery. Radiology 1990;174(1):41–2.
4. Pozniak MA, Zagzebski JA, Scanlan KA. Spectral and color Doppler artifacts. Radiographics 1992; 12(1):35–44.
5. Horattas MC, Wright DJ, Fenton AH, et al. Changing concepts of deep venous thrombosis of the upper extremity–report of a series and review of the literature. Surgery 1988;104(3):561–7.
6. Monreal M, Lafoz E, Ruiz J, et al. Upper-extremity deep venous thrombosis and pulmonary embolism–a prospective study. Chest 1991;99(2):280–3.
7. Campbell CB, Chandler JG, Tegtmeyer CJ, et al. Axillary, subclavian, brachiocephalic vein obstruction. Surgery 1977;82(6):816–26.
8. Wells PS, Anderson DR, Bormanis J, et al. Value of assessment of pretest probability of deep-vein thrombosis in clinical management. Lancet 1997; 350(9094):1795–8.
9. Wells PS, Brill-Edwards P, Stevens P, et al. A novel and rapid whole-blood assay for D-dimer in patients with clinically suspected deep vein thrombosis. Circulation 1995;91(8):2184–7.
10. Freyburger G, Trillaud H, Labrouche S, et al. D-dimer strategy in thrombosis exclusion–a gold standard study in 100 patients suspected of deep venous thrombosis or pulmonary embolism: 8 DD methods compared. Thromb Haemost 1998;79(1):32–7.
11. Brill-Edwards P, Lee A. D-dimer testing in the diagnosis of acute venous thromboembolism. Thromb Haemost 1999;82(2):688–94.
12. Wells PS, Anderson DR, Rodger M, et al. Evaluation of D-dimer in the diagnosis of suspected deep-vein thrombosis. N Engl J Med 2003;349(13):1227–35.
13. ACR practice guideline for the performance of peripheral venous ultrasound examination. In: Practical guidelines and technical standards. Reston (VA): American College of Radiology; 2006. p. 863–6.
14. Aziz S, Strachley OJ, Whelan TJ Jr. Effort-related axillosubclavian vein thrombosis. A new theory of pathogenesis and a plea for direct surgical intervention. Am J Surg 1986;152(1):57–61.
15. Bonnet F, Loriferne JF, Texier JP, et al. Evaluation of Doppler examination for diagnosis of catheter-related deep vein thrombosis. Intensive Care Med 1989;15(4):238–40.
16. McDonough JJ, Altemeier WA. Subclavian venous thrombosis secondary to indwelling catheters. Surg Gynecol Obstet 1971;133(3):397–400.
17. Luciani A, Clement O, Halimi P, et al. Catheter-related upper extremity deep venous thrombosis in cancer patients: a prospective study based on Doppler US. Radiology 2001;220(3):655–60.
18. Trerotola SO, Kuhn-Fulton J, Johnson MS, et al. Tunneled infusion catheters: increased incidence of symptomatic venous thrombosis after subclavian versus internal jugular venous access. Radiology 2000;217(1):89–93.
19. Becker DM, Philbrick JT, Walker FB IV. Axillary and subclavian venous thrombosis. Prognosis and treatment. Arch Intern Med 1991;151(10):1934–43.
20. Mustafa S, Stein PD, Patel KC, et al. Upper extremity deep venous thrombosis. Chest 2003;123(6): 1953–6.
21. Kooij JD, van der Zant FM, van Beek EJ, et al. Pulmonary embolism in deep venous thrombosis of the upper extremity: more often in catheter-related thrombosis. Neth J Med 1997;50(6):238–42.
22. Chin EE, Zimmerman PT, Grant EG. Sonographic evaluation of upper extremity deep venous thrombosis. J Ultrasound Med 2005;24(6):829–38.
23. Baarslag HJ, van Beek EJ, Koopman MM, et al. Prospective study of color duplex ultrasonography compared with contrast venography in patients suspected of having deep venous thrombosis of the upper extremities. Ann Intern Med 2002;136(12):865–72.
24. Knudson GJ, Wiedmeyer DA, Erickson SJ, et al. Color Doppler sonographic imaging in the assessment of upper-extremity deep venous thrombosis. Am J Roentgenol 1990;154(2):399–403.
25. Baxter GM, Kincaid W, Jeffrey RF, et al. Comparison of colour Doppler ultrasound with venography in the diagnosis of axillary and subclavian vein thrombosis. Br J Radiol 1991;64(765):777–81.
26. Bernardi E, Piccioli A, Marchiori A, et al. Upper extremity deep vein thrombosis: risk factors, diagnosis, and management. SeminVasc Med 2001; 1(1):105–10.
27. Fraser JD, Anderson DR. Venous protocols, techniques, and interpretations of the upper and lower extremities. Radiol Clin North Am 2004;42(2):279–96.
28. Patel MC, Berman LH, Moss HA, et al. Subclavian and internal jugular veins at Doppler US: abnormal cardiac pulsatility and respiratory phasicity as a predictor of complete central occlusion. Radiology 1999;211(2):579–83.
29. Buller HR, Agnelli G, Hull RD, et al. Antithrombotic therapy for venous thromboembolic disease: the Seventh ACCP Conference on Antithrombotic and Thrombolytic Therapy. Chest 2004;126(3 Suppl): 401S–28S.
30. Rubin JM, Xie H, Kim K, et al. Sonographic elasticity imaging of acute and chronic deep venous thrombosis in humans. J Ultrasound Med 2006;25(9): 1179–86.
31. Rubin JM, Aglyamov SR, Wakefield TW, et al. Clinical application of sonographic elasticity imaging for aging of deep venous thrombosis: preliminary findings. J Ultrasound Med 2003;22(5):443–8.
32. Pain SJ, Vowler S, Purushotham AD. Axillary vein abnormalities contribute to development of lymphoedema after surgery for breast cancer. Br J Surg 2005;92(3):311–5.

33. Povoski SP, Zaman SA. Selective use of preoperative venous duplex ultrasound and intraoperative venography for central venous access device placement in cancer patients. Ann Surg Oncol 2002;9(5):493–9.

34. Robbin ML, Gallichio MH, Deierhoi MH, et al. US vascular mapping before hemodialysis access placement. Radiology 2000;217(1):83–8.

35. Allon M, Lockhart ME, Lilly RZ, et al. Effect of preoperative sonographic mapping on vascular access outcomes in hemodialysis patients. Kidney Int 2001;60(5):2013–20.

36. National Kidney Foundation. K/DOQI clinical practice guidelines for vascular access, 2000. Am J Kidney Dis 2001;37(Suppl 1):S7–64.

37. Robbin ML, Chamberlain NE, Lockhart ME, et al. Hemodialysis arteriovenous fistula maturity: US evaluation. Radiology 2002;225(1):59–64.

38. Grogan J, Castilla M, Lozanski L, et al. Frequency of critical stenosis in primary arteriovenous fistulae before hemodialysis access: should duplex ultrasound surveillance be the standard of care? J Vasc Surg 2005;41(6):1000–6.

39. Lockhart ME, Robbin ML. Hemodialysis access ultrasound. Ultrasound Q 2001;17(3):157–67.

40. Beathard GA, Arnold P, Jackson J, et al. Physician operators forum of RMS lifeline. Aggressive treatment of early fistula failure. Kidney Int 2003;64(4):1487–94.

Ultrasound Evaluation of the Lower Extremity Veins

Ulrike M. Hamper, MD, MBA[a],[*],
M. Robert DeJong, RDMS, RVT, RCDS[a],
Leslie M. Scoutt, MD[b]

KEYWORDS

- Deep venous thrombosis • Sonographic anatomy
- Differential diagnosis • Venous insufficiency
- Pathophysiology

Over the past 2 decades venous ultrasonography (US) has become the standard primary imaging technique for the initial evaluation of patients for whom there is clinical suspicion of deep venous thrombosis (DVT) of the lower extremity veins. It has replaced the venogram and other diagnostic studies such as impedance plethysmography, various radionuclide studies, and conventional CT because of its noninvasive nature, the ease with which it can be performed in skilled hands, and its proven efficacy. Compression US first was described as a means of diagnosing DVT in 1986 by Raghavendra and colleagues[1] and was introduced into clinical practice in 1987 by Cronan and colleagues[2–7] from the United States and Appleman and colleagues[8] from the Netherlands. In the ensuing years multiple articles were published establishing venous US as the examination of choice for the diagnosis of venous thrombosis, further refining the US technique and diagnostic criteria with gray-scale imaging, and also Incorporating the newly developed technique of Doppler US.

This article addresses the role of duplex US and color Doppler US (CDUS) in today's clinical practice for the evaluation of patients suspected of harboring a thrombus in their lower extremity veins. Clinical presentation and differential diagnoses, technique, and diagnostic criteria for both acute and chronic DVT are reviewed. In addition, sonographic evaluation of venous insufficiency is addressed.

CLINICAL PRESENTATION AND DIFFERENTIAL DIAGNOSIS

Acute DVT is a significant health problem affecting approximately 2 million people in the United States per year. Pulmonary embolism (PE) is the most dreaded complication of an untreated DVT and is reported to occur in about 50% to 60% of untreated cases with a 25% to 30% mortality rate.[4,9–12] Predisposing factors for DVT include prolonged bed rest, congestive heart failure, prior DVT, pelvic and lower extremity surgery, coagulopathies, immobilization, trauma, pregnancy, malignancies, indwelling catheters, intravenous drug abuse, dehydration, travel (probably because of prolonged immobility), and endothelial injury. In addition, oral contraceptive use, obesity, and systemic diseases such as systemic lupus erythematosus, lupus anticoagulant, nephritic syndrome, Behçet's disease, nocturnal hemoglobinuria, polycythemia vera, and hyperviscosity syndromes may predispose a patient to thromboembolism formation.

The signs and symptoms of DVT often are nonspecific, and thus the clinical diagnostic accuracy is poor. Extremity swelling, pain, and edema place the patient at risk for DVT. Significant

This article originally appeared in *Radiologic Clinics of North America* 2007;45(3):525–547

[a] Department of Radiology and Radiological Science, Johns Hopkins University, School of Medicine, 600 N Wolfe Street, Baltimore, MD 21287, USA

[b] Yale University, School of Medicine, 20 York Street, 2-272WP New Haven, CT 06504, USA

[*] Corresponding author.

E-mail address: umhamper@jhu.edu (U.M. Hamper).

Ultrasound Clin 4 (2009) 193–216
doi:10.1016/j.cult.2009.04.003

thrombus can be present in asymptomatic patients, however. The clinical accuracy for the diagnosis of acute DVT has been reported to be about 50% in symptomatic patients.[13–16] Localized pain and calf tenderness are reported in approximately 50% of cases, but pain on forced dorsiflexion of the toes, the so-called "Homan's sign," is an unreliable diagnostic criterion and is present in only 8% to 30% of symptomatic patients harboring a DVT. Furthermore, the Homan's sign can be elicited in nearly 50% of symptomatic patients who do not have a DVT as a cause of their symptoms.[4,17] A palpable cord caused by a thrombosed superficial vessel can be present with or without involvement of the deep venous system.[4] US examination is highly sensitive and specific for the diagnosis of DVT: several series have reported sensitivities and specificities approaching 95% to 100% for the diagnosis of DVT in the proximal lower extremity. The most common causes for false-negative examinations are venous duplication, infrapopliteal thrombus, and nonocclusive focal or segmental DVT. Therefore, expeditious sonographic evaluation of patients suspected of having DVT may aid in rapid initiation of therapeutic measures to decrease the potential for developing complications such as PE or postthrombotic venous insufficiency. The limitations of US in accurately diagnosing calf vein thrombosis and DVT in obese patients is addressed later.

EXAMINATION TECHNIQUE AND NORMAL SONOGRAPHIC ANATOMY

The choice of transducer for evaluating the lower extremity veins depends on the patient's body habitus and the depth of the vessel to be studied. The examination is preferentially performed with a high-resolution 5- to 7.5-MHz linear array transducer. For very superficial veins (ie, the greater or small saphenous veins), a 10-MHz transducer may be optimal. For large patients a lower-frequency (2.5- or 3.5-MHz) curvilinear transducer may be necessary. In general, the transducer with the highest frequency allowing adequate penetration provides the best spatial resolution. Appropriate gain settings must be applied to ensure that the vessels are free of artifactual internal echoes and that thrombus is not mistaken for echoes caused by slow-flowing blood. In addition, CDUS imaging parameters must be optimized for sensitivity to slow, low-volume flow.

The lower extremity venous system consists of a superficial system, the saphenous veins and their tributaries, and a deep system. A more detailed description of the superficial venous plexus is presented later in the section discussing venous insufficiency. Briefly, the great saphenous vein (GSV) joins the common femoral vein (CFV) just superior to its bifurcation. It travels medially in the thigh and calf extending inferiorly to the level of the foot (**Fig. 1**A). It measures about 3 to 5 mm in

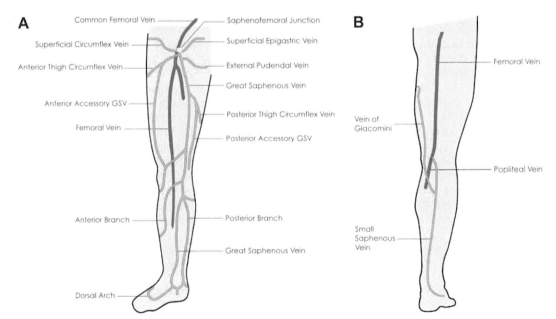

Fig. 1. (A) The great saphenous vein and its major tributaries. (B) The small saphenous vein. (*Adapted from* Weiss RA, Feied CF, Weiss MA. Vein diagnosis and treatment. New York: McGraw-Hill; 2001.)

diameter at the level of the saphenofemoral junction, tapering to about 1 to 3 mm in diameter at the level of the ankle (see **Fig. 1A**). Measurement of the GSV is important before harvesting for autologous vein grafting. The small saphenous vein (SSV) (formerly called the "lesser saphenous vein") extends from the ankle along the posterior aspect of the calf to insert at variable levels into the posterior proximal or mid popliteal vein (PV) (**Fig. 1B**). The diameter of the SSV tapers from 2 to 4 mm proximally to about 1 to 2 mm distally. Both the GSV and SSV may become enlarged and varicose in patients who have venous insufficiency or congestive heart failure. Thrombosis of these vessels may occur with ensuing superficial thrombophlebitis (**Fig. 2**).

The deep venous system includes the CFV, the deep femoral or profunda femoris vein, the femoral vein (FV) (previously called the "superficial femoral vein"), and the PV as well as the paired anterior and posterior tibial veins and the peroneal veins

(**Fig. 3**). The CFV is the continuation of the external iliac vein and extends from the level of the inguinal ligament to the level of the bifurcation into the FV and profunda femoris vein. The profunda femoris vein lies medial to the accompanying artery and can be evaluated only in its most proximal portion. The CFV lies medial to the accompanying artery. The FV travels medial to the femoral artery through the adductor canal in the distal thigh. To avoid confusion among clinicians, the term "femoral vein" (FV) should be used instead of the previously designated term "superficial femoral vein" to describe that part of the deep venous system caudal to the bifurcation of the CFV. (In a survey performed by Bundens and colleagues,[18] more than 70% of surveyed internists regarded the "superficial femoral vein" as part of the superficial and not the deep venous system and thus were under the assumption that superficial femoral vein thrombosis did not require treatment.) The PV is the continuation of the FV after its exit from

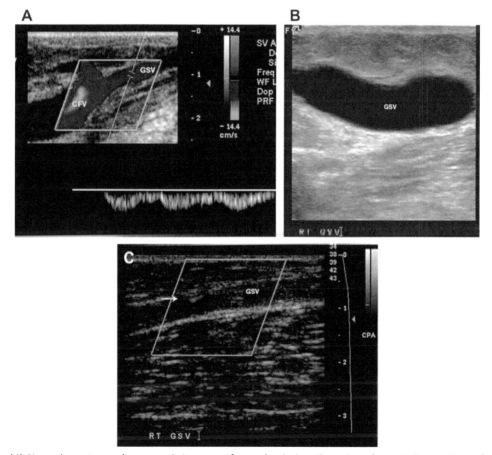

Fig. 2. (*A*) Normal greater saphenous vein/common femoral vein junction—Doppler gate in greater saphenous vein. (*B*) Large greater saphenous vein in a patient who has congestive heart failure. (*C*) Sagittal US of thrombosed greater saphenous vein with only a trickle of peripheral flow (*arrow*).

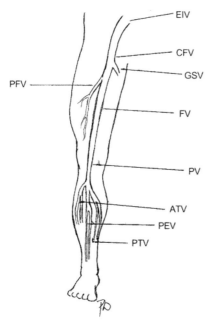

Fig. 3. The anatomy of the deep venous system. ATV, anterior tibial veins; CFV, common femoral vein; EIV, external iliac vein; FV, femoral vein; GSV, greater saphenous vein; PEV, peroneal veins; PFV, profunda femoris vein; PTV, posterior tibial veins; PV, popliteal veins.

the adductor canal in the posterior distal thigh. The PV is located anterior to its accompanying artery and courses through the popliteal space into the proximal calf. In general, the deep veins in the thigh are wider in diameter than the accompanying artery unless the veins are duplicated. Duplication of the FV or PV can be seen in 20% to 35% of patients. Duplication of the FV can be segmental. It is important to mention these anatomic variants so that thrombosis in one of the duplicated limbs is not missed (Fig. 4). The paired anterior tibial veins are accompanied by their corresponding artery and arise from the popliteal vein traversing the anterior calf compartment along the interosseous membrane to the dorsum of the foot. The tibioperoneal trunk originates from the PV slightly distal to the anterior tibial veins and bifurcates into the paired posterior tibial veins and peroneal veins, both of which are accompanied by their respective arteries. The peroneal veins course medial to the posterior aspect of the fibula, whereas the posterior tibial veins course through the posterior calf muscles posterior to the tibia and along the medial malleolus. In addition, the muscles of the calf are drained by gastrocnemius and soleus veins, which do not have accompanying arteries.

In a patient suspected of having DVT, the deep venous system should be evaluated from just

above the inguinal ligament to the trifurcation of the popliteal vein in the upper calf, every 2 to 3 cm, with compression. In addition, evaluation of the external iliac veins and calf veins, including anterior and posterior tibial veins and peroneal veins, can be performed. The iliac vein, CFV, and FV are best evaluated with the patient in a supine position (Fig. 5A). The popliteal veins can be studied with the patient supine and the leg flexed 20° to 30° and externally rotated or in a decubitus position with the study side up (Fig. 5B). The anterior tibial veins are best identified initially at the posterior medial ankle. When followed up the leg, the peroneal veins, which originate from the lateral ankle, are posterior to the anterior tibial veins. The anterior tibial veins run between the tibia and fibula anteriorly.

According to the American College of Radiology practice guidelines and technical standards, lower extremity Duplex sonography should include compression, color, and spectral Doppler sonography with assessment of phasicity and venous flow augmentation.[19] A complete examination includes evaluation of the full length of the CFV and saphenofemoral junction, the proximal portion of the deep femoral vein, the FV, and the PV. These veins are imaged in the transverse plane with and without compression with mild transducer pressure every 2 to 3 cm from the level of the CFV to the distal FV in the adductor canal and the PV to the popliteal trifurcation. In obese patients compression in the adductor canal may be difficult. Sometimes a two-hand technique, pushing the leg into the transducer with the free hand from behind, may help achieve adequate compression (Fig. 5C). A normal pulse of color flow Doppler signal in a suboptimally compressed or poorly visualized segment is reassuring of at least partial patency and excludes the possibility of occlusive thrombus. Compression of a normal vein completely collapses the venous lumen (Figs. 6 and 7), whereas the presence of DVT prevents coaptation of the vein walls (see Figs. 6 and 7). In the authors' laboratory, color flow Doppler US is used routinely because it speeds the identification of the vessels and facilitates identification of deeply located vessel segments. Color should fill the entire lumen of normal veins, but color flow is diminished or absent in partially or completely thrombosed veins (Fig. 8). Sometimes, particularly in veins with slow flow, squeezing the calf will augment venous flow, resulting in complete color filling of a vessel. Doppler spectral analysis is performed to assess phasicity and augmentation responses following squeezing of the calf or plantar flexion of the foot and is helpful as a secondary means of assessing patency of

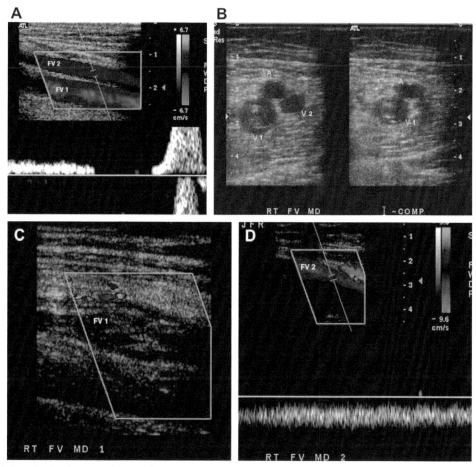

Fig. 4. (A) Sagittal color Doppler US of duplicated femoral vein (FV). (B) Transverse US of duplicated femoral vein demonstrating noncompressibility of thrombosed limb (V1). (C) Sagittal color Doppler US limb of a duplicated femoral vein (FV1). (D) Sagittal color Doppler US of normal flow in duplicated femoral vein (FV2).

the more proximal veins, particularly the iliac veins (see **Fig. 8**E, F). If a thrombus is identified in any segment of the veins, augmentation is not performed to avoid detaching the clot and thereby causing a PE. Because of the risk of superficial thrombophlebitis extending into the deep venous system, the authors also routinely study the GSV at its junction with the CFV (see **Fig. 8**F–H). Because of its increased sensitivity to low-velocity, low-volume flow, pwer Doppler US sometimes is useful in identifying early recanalization of thrombosed veins or in detecting minimal flow in nearly occluded venous segments, deep vessels, or the smaller calf veins. Power Doppler, however, does not indicate directionality of flow and is affected adversely by patient motion or calcifications.

The normal veins are easily compressible by slight transducer pressure (see **Figs. 6** and **7**). If one cannot compress the veins because of swelling or pain, one can attempt indirect evaluation using a Valsalva maneuver, observation of the presence or absence of respiratory phasicity, and augmentation techniques. Following a Valsalva maneuver, a normal vein expands to more than 50% of its diameter from baseline. The Valsalva maneuver has the most pronounced effect on the veins near the inguinal ligament. Proximal pelvic DVT or external compression of the pelvic veins blunts the normal dilatation of the CFV following a Valsalva maneuver. Evaluation of respiratory phasicity and augmentation also can provide indirect assessment of adjacent vein segments. Proximal (cephalic) obstruction caused by pelvic venous thrombosis or external compression of the pelvic veins by ascites, pelvic mass, or hematoma dampens respiratory phasicity in the CFV (**Fig. 9**). Distal (caudal) DVT blunts the normal augmentation of venous flow achieved by squeezing the leg inferior to the point of insonation. Valsalva maneuvers also can be used to evaluate venous insufficiency. With the patient supine, a temporary reversal of

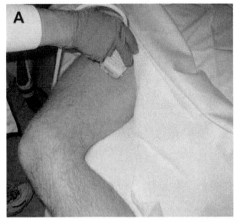
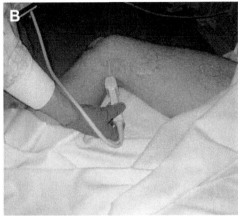
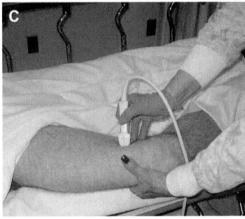

Fig. 5. (A) Transverse scan demonstrating the imaging technique of the femoral vein with the patient in a supine position. (B) Transverse scan demonstrating the imaging technique of the popliteal vein with the leg flexed and externally rotated. (C) "Two-hand technique" to visualize the femoral vein (FV) in the adductor canal.

flow occurs if the valves are incompetent. (This phenomenon is discussed in more detail at the end of the article). Likewise changes in the venous spectral tracing can indicate more proximal cardiovascular disease. For example, in patients who have elevated right atrial pressure caused by congestive heart failure or tricuspid insufficiency, the spectral venous waveform can be quite pulsatile, mimicking a waveform more typical of the hepatic veins or inferior vena cava (**Fig. 10**).[20]

CONTROVERSIAL ISSUES VIS-À-VIS THE EXAMINATION TECHNIQUE

US evaluation of the calf veins remains controversial because of its unproven clinical value and cost effectiveness, and the American College of Radiology practice guidelines do not require their evaluation. It has been shown that isolated calf vein thrombosis rarely causes significant pulmonary emboli and thus is assumed to be a benign, self-limiting disease.[21] Hence, patients who have isolated calf DVT rarely receive anticoagulation therapy in clinical practice because the risk of bleeding from the anticoagulation therapy is considered to be higher than the risk of PE even though several studies have shown that approximately 20% of calf DVTs ultimately extend into the more superior deep venous system in the thigh.[21] In addition, US evaluation of the calf veins is less accurate than evaluation of veins in the thigh because the veins in the calf are much smaller; therefore it is difficult to be certain that all of the calf vessels, some of which are duplicated, are free of thrombus. Other studies stress the clinical importance of calf vein thrombosis and argue that the 4% to 10% risk of potential bleeding with anticoagulation therapy is safer than the 20% to 30% risk of propagation and potential 5% risk for development of PE.[22,23] In a study by Badgett and colleagues,[24] a complete venous examination including calf veins altered clinical management in about 30% of patients. The practice in the authors' laboratory is to evaluate the calf veins only in

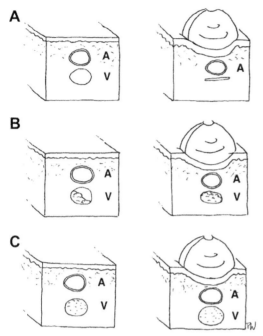

Fig. 6. Transverse compression of normal and thrombosed veins. (*A*) Compression of a normal vein completely collapses the venous lumen. (*B*) Compression of a nonocclusive, thrombosed vein partially collapses the venous lumen. (*C*) Compression of a completely thrombosed vein prevents venous coaptation.

patients who have focal, persistent, or worsening calf symptoms.

Another controversy in the radiologic and surgical literature centers around the necessity of routinely performing bilateral lower extremity venous US examinations versus the appropriateness of performing a unilateral examination if symptoms are limited to one leg. Some studies recommend routine performance of bilateral venous US studies of the lower extremities because thrombus can occur in either leg in up to 23% of patients who have bilateral symptoms.[25] A study by Cronan[3] concluded that the likelihood of finding DVT in patients who have bilateral lower extremity symptoms is related to their predisposing risk factors, and that bilateral lower extremity sonography is indicated only in patients who have a risk factor for DVT, not in those who are at risk only for cardiac disease.

Other studies suggest that examination of an asymptomatic leg is unnecessary because, although thrombosis may occur in the asymptomatic leg in up to 14% of patients, these patients typically have DVT in the symptomatic leg as well.[25–28]

An additional concern centers on the issue of performing limited examinations. Some authors have suggested a limited compression examination of the FV and PV because of the low rate of reported isolated FV thrombosis. Several studies, however, have shown that omitting the FV and evaluating only the CFVs and PVs would lead to a decrease in sensitivity because isolated thrombosis of the FV occurs in 4% to 6% of cases.[26,29] Another issue concerns the usefulness of performing augmentation in all patients being evaluated for DVT. A study by Lockhart and colleagues[30] questions the usefulness of performing venous flow augmentation maneuvers with duplex sonography because of its lack of clinical benefit and the added discomfort for the patient who has swollen and painful legs. The authors recommend using augmentation as an adjunct only in uncertain cases rather than as a routine diagnostic component of the lower extremity DVT examination.

Finally, the recent development of multislice and/or multidetector techniques in CT has led to a reconsideration of the role of CT in the diagnosis of DVT when included as part of a pulmonary angiography study. A study by Kim and colleagues[31] demonstrated that multislice helical CT detected DVT that had been missed by venous sonography in five patients, but US detected DVT that was missed by CT in one patient. On the other hand, Kim and colleagues reported[31] that indirect multidetector CT is as accurate as sonography in the detection of femoropopliteal DVT and has the advantage over sonography of being able to evaluate the pelvic veins and inferior vena cava. Particularly in a patient undergoing CT pulmonary angiography in the ICU, the use of indirect CT venography of the lower extremities may be a reasonable alternative to sonography.[32] One must, however, consider carefully the increased radiation dose from multidetector CT when considering the use of this imaging approach to diagnose DVT.

SONOGRAPHY OF ACUTE DEEP VENOUS THROMBOSIS

The hallmark gray-scale findings of acute DVT include noncompressibility of the vessel as well as direct visualization of the thrombus (see **Fig. 6**; **Figs. 11** and **12**). Thrombus may be anechoic or hypo- or hyperechoic. Anechoic or hypoechoic thrombi are thought to be more recent, although the distinction is not precise. Clot echogenicity alone cannot be used to assess the age of a clot.[33] In addition, very slowly flowing blood may be sufficiently echogenic to mimic the appearance of clot (**Fig. 13A**).[34] In this instance,

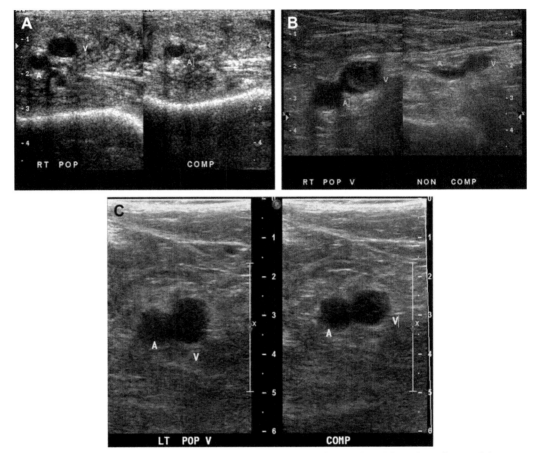

Fig. 7. Transverse sonograms demonstrating compression response of normal and thrombosed veins. (*A*) Compression of a normal popliteal vein completely collapses the venous lumen. Only the popliteal artery (A) remains on compression view. (*B*) Compression of a nonocclusive thrombosed popliteal vein partially collapses the venous lumen (V). (*C*) Compression of a completely thrombosed popliteal vein prevents venous coaptation.

however, the compression US is normal (**Fig. 13B**). Changes in vein caliber with respiration or Valsalva maneuver are lost also when thrombus is present. Thrombi may occlude the lumen completely or partially, and they may be adherent to the wall or free floating (**Fig. 14**). On CDUS a filling defect can be seen indicating nonocclusive thrombus, or there may be complete absence of flow (**Fig. 15**).

In a large, pooled series of DVT studies, the accuracy of compression US for DVT has been shown to reach 95% with 98% specificity.[4] In other series sensitivities and specificities range from 88% to 100% and from 92% to 100%, respectively. Additional studies report a sensitivity of 95%, specificity of 99%, and accuracy of 98% for color Doppler flow imaging.[35,36] Sensitivities for isolated calf vein thrombosis are lower, ranging from 60% to 80%.[4,37,38] Protocols and techniques for evaluation of the calf veins have not been established definitively.

PITFALLS AND LIMITATIONS OF DIAGNOSIS OF ACUTE DEEP VEIN THROMBOSIS

The classic clinical signs of DVT cannot be trusted because a variety of abnormalities can mimic the signs and symptoms of acute DVT. Cronan and colleagues[6] showed that in approximately 10% of patients studied for acute DVT, ancillary findings were diagnosed by sonography along with a normal deep venous examination. US can readily distinguish those entities from venous pathology.

A variety of conditions that may cause clinical signs and symptoms indistinguishable from DVT may be caused by other underlying pathology such as adenopathy (groin swelling), arterial aneurysms, or stenoses/occlusions (**Fig. 16**), soft tissue

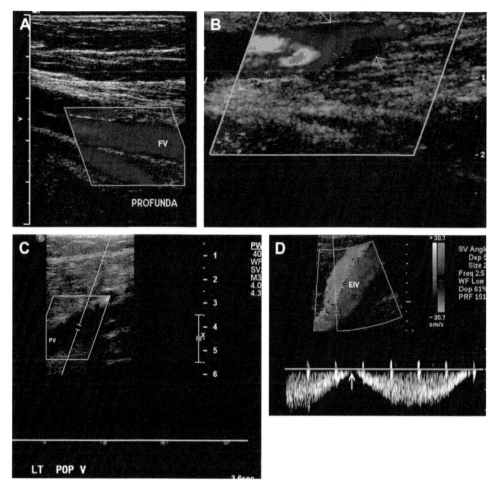

Fig. 8. (*A*) Normal veins demonstrating color flow filling the entire vessel lumen. FV, femoral vein. (*B*) Partial venous thrombosis demonstrating focal absence of color flow (*arrows*). (*C*) Occlusive venous thrombosis demonstrating complete absence of color flow in the popliteal vein. Also note absence of venous waveform on duplex spectrum. (*D*) Normal respiratory phasicity of the right iliac vein. Note return of flow to baseline during inspiration (*arrow*). (*E*) Augmentation maneuver demonstrates surge of flow in right popliteal vein when squeezing the calf (*arrow*). (*F*) Normal color flow Doppler appearance of the junction of the greater saphenous vein (GSV) and the common femoral vein (CFV). (*G*) Thrombosis of the left greater saphenou vein (GSV) near the junction with the common femoral vein (*arrow*). (*H*) Six days later the greater saphenous vein thrombosis has extended into the common femoral vein (V) as demonstrated on the transverse compression images.

tumors, hematomas or abscesses, muscle tears, and diffuse soft tissue edema (**Fig. 17**). Proximal obstruction by an extrinsic mass, such as adenopathy, pseudoaneurysm, or hematoma, may limit the compressibility of veins and produce the same clinical signs of DVT (see **Fig. 9**B; **Fig. 18**). Simple popliteal synovial cysts or cysts that communicate with the posterior bursa around the knee (Baker's cysts) can, when ruptured, cause mass effect and simulate the pain and swelling associated with popliteal DVT (**Fig. 19**). Popliteal artery aneurysm may cause calf pain and swelling (**Fig. 20**). Congestive heart failure or tricuspid insufficiency with secondary venous distension

and leg swelling and edema may cause a clinically false-positive result. Often in these patients a very pulsatile venous waveform is observed (see **Fig. 10**).[20] A patent SSV filled with thrombus may be mistaken for a thrombosed PV (**Fig. 21**). Acute or chronic clot may be difficult to differentiate, as discussed later.

False-negative US studies can occur in obese patients or in patients who have very edematous extremities. The FV in the adductor canal region may be difficult to evaluate. Small nonocclusive thrombi in the profunda femoris vein may be missed. Thrombosis of a duplicated FV (see **Fig. 4**B) may go undetected, and more proximal

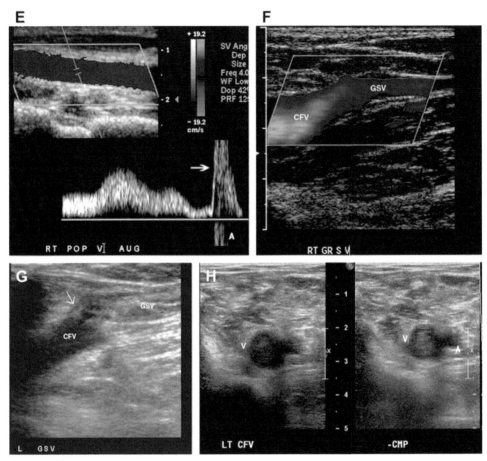

Fig. 8. (continued)

iliac vein thrombosis often is difficult to demonstrate. Loss of phasicity in the CFV or distal iliac vein should be noted as a secondary sign indicating a more proximal thrombosis or compression by masses or collections (see **Figs. 16** and **18**).

It is important to recognize these pitfalls and limitations to lessen the chance of potentially severe consequences of an erroneous or missed diagnosis of DVT. False-negative imaging results may deprive the patient of appropriate anticoagulation therapy and potentially result in clot propagation, PE, and death, whereas a false-positive result may result in unnecessary anticoagulation with the associated risk of bleeding.

SONOGRAPHY OF CHRONIC DEEP VENOUS THROMBOSIS

The differentiation of acute or chronic DVT by imaging methods and clinical parameters often is difficult. In about one fourth of patients, the DVT resolves completely after adequate treatment regimens. Serial studies, however, have shown persistent abnormal findings on compression US 6 to 24 months later in 54% of patients who had acute DVT.[4] Without an US evaluation showing resolution of the acute DVT, recurrent DVT may be indistinguishable from chronic disease. On compression US both acute and chronic DVT may show noncompressibility of the vessel. In chronic DVT, the vessel walls often are thickened with decreased compliance (**Fig. 22A**). Veins may recanalize to a certain extent after an acute DVT (**Fig. 22B**). Residual clot, however, may manifest as organized echogenic material along the vein walls and mimic the sonographic appearance of acute clot. Because noncompressibility of a vein is a sonographic sign of both chronic and acute DVT, care must be taken to differentiate the two entities so that patients do not receive unnecessary anticoagulation therapy for a chronic condition. Some US findings that may help distinguish acute from chronic DVT are atretic segments (inability to identify a normal vein next to the artery), echogenic weblike filling defects within

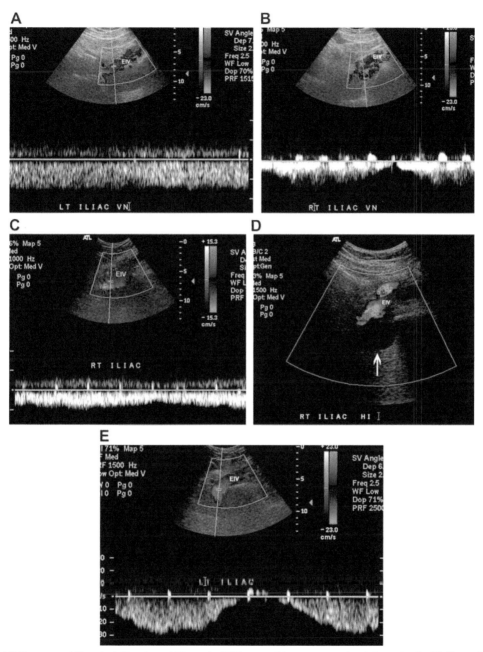

Fig. 9. (A) Dampened flow in left external iliac vein (EIV) caused by more proximal thrombosis. (B) Normal respiratory phasicity flow in right external iliac vein (EIV). (C) Dampened flow in right external iliac vein (EIV) caused by compression by fluid collection with loss of respiratory phasicity. (D) Right groin fluid collection (*arrow*). (E) Normal respiratory phasicity in left external iliac vein (EIV).

the vein (see **Fig. 22**B), collateral vessels (**Fig. 23**B), and valvular damage with reflux and resultant chronic deep venous insufficiency. Chronic thrombus usually is more echogenic and may calcify (**Fig. 23**A). Chronic thrombi may demonstrate thickened vein walls with a reduced venous diameter (see **Fig. 22**A). In addition, the size of the vein is helpful. In acute DVT the vein usually is enlarged, whereas in chronic DVT it is normal, small, or diminutive. Recent studies

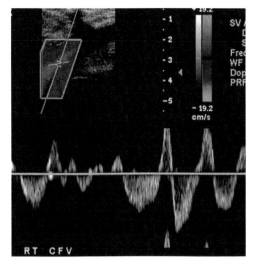

Fig. 10. Pulsatile spectral waveform in right common femoral vein (CFV) caused by tricuspid insufficiency.

demonstrating the contribution of in vitro US elasticity imaging to assess clot age may be promising for clinical use in the future.[39]

CHRONIC VENOUS INSUFFICIENCY

Venous insufficiency is a common but often undiagnosed condition with a prevalence estimated at 25% in women and 15% in men.[40–43] The clinical significance of varicose veins is not merely cosmetic, because chronic venous insufficiency may cause significant pain and swelling of the lower extremities and ultimately may result in debilitating skin changes ranging from discoloration and induration to cutaneous and soft tissue breakdown (ie, venous stasis ulcers). Treatment costs are estimated to be as high as 3 billion dollars per year in the United States[44] and to comprise up to 1% to 3% of the total health care budget in developed countries.[45–47] Recently developed minimally invasive catheter techniques have revolutionized treatment options for patients who have varicose veins. Hence, it is important that radiologists become familiar with the US technique for evaluation of venous reflux.

Early on, patients who have venous reflux may present with leg pain and swelling and may not have obvious visible varicosities. Such patients often are referred for lower extremity venous US examinations to rule out DVT, and both clinician and radiologist may overlook the diagnosis of venous insufficiency. Hence, venous insufficiency is a diagnosis that should be considered in the patient presenting with leg pain or swelling and a negative DVT US examination, particularly in someone who has persistent or recurrent symptoms. Patients who have venous reflux also may complain of leg soreness, burning, aching, throbbing, cramping, and/or muscle fatigue. Symptoms are typically exacerbated by standing or warm weather. The severity of a patient's symptoms is not necessarily related to the size or number of the varicosities or even to the amount of reflux, and significant symptoms may occur even before varicosities are clinically apparent. Over time, patients may develop chronic skin or soft tissue changes ranging from swelling and discoloration to inflammatory dermatitis and, ultimately, chronic, nonhealing leg ulcers.

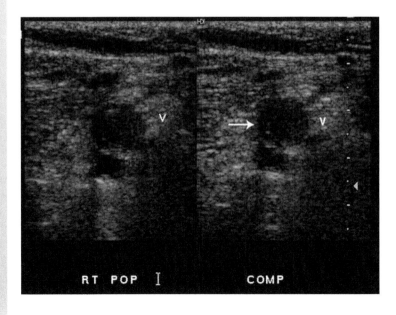

Fig. 11. Complete venous thrombosis. Transverse views of the right popliteal vein demonstrate noncompressible vein caused by acute thrombus (arrow).

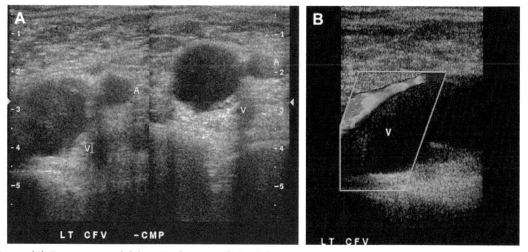

Fig. 12. (A) Transverse and (B) sagittal views of the left common femoral vein (V) demonstrate hypoechoic thrombus and expansion of the venous lumen.

Pathophysiology

Normally, venous blood flow is directed from the superficial venous system of the lower extremities through the GSV, SSV, and perforators toward the deep venous system and the heart by a series of competent, one-way valves as well as by contraction of the foot and calf muscles.[48] Valve failure is the primary cause of venous insufficiency. An incompetent valve results in retrograde flow of blood and venous pooling, which in turn dilates the more caudal veins, resulting in a cascading effect of sequential failure of more and more valves. The precise pattern of varicosities that develop depends on exactly which valves fail.

Because the tributaries of the GSV and SSV are not protected by a fascial layer, they are more prone to dilate. Primary pump failure of the calf muscles, venous obstruction from DVT, and extrinsic venous compression are much less common causes of venous insufficiency.

Risk factors for the development of venous insufficiency include any condition that distorts and/or weakens the venous valves or results in venous dilation or volume overload or increases hydrostatic pressure. Hence, risk factors include genetic predisposition, prior DVT, pregnancy, age, obesity, and occupations or activities that require prolonged standing, running, or lifting.[49] The incidence of varicose veins is nearly twice as

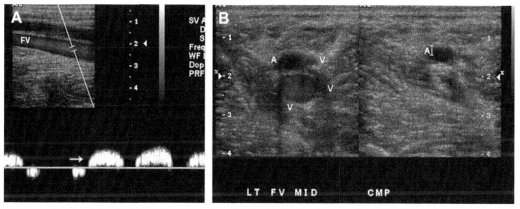

Fig. 13. Slow-flowing blood mimicking acute thrombosis. (A) Sagittal view of the left femoral vein demonstrates echogenic material in the venous lumen. Note venous waveform on duplex spectrum, however. (B) With transverse compression the venous lumen (V) collapses completely.

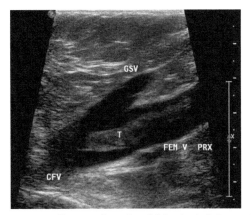

Fig. 14. Free-floating thrombus (T) in the left femoral vein (FV) extending into the common femoral vein (CFV).

high in women as in men,[50] probably because of multiple factors including cyclic hormonal changes. Venous insufficiency also is more common in industrialized Western countries; the increased incidence is postulated to be largely secondary to either genetic predisposition and/or diet.[51]

Venous Anatomy of the Superficial Veins of the Lower Extremity

The anatomy of the deep venous system in the lower extremity has been described earlier in this article. One should note here, however, several features that help discriminate the deep venous system from the superficial venous system. The veins of the deep venous system in the thigh and calf are surrounded by muscles and a deep fascial layer that help propel blood back toward the heart by means of the primary muscle pump and also help prevent reflux by limiting dilatation of the deep veins. The deep veins also always accompany an artery. The superficial veins, on the other hand, are found in the subcutaneous tissues and do not accompany an artery. A thin superficial fascial layer surrounds the saphenous trunks but not their tributaries. Thus, major branches of the saphenous system are more prone to dilate and develop reflux.

There are three major subdivisions of the superficial venous system in the lower extremity: the GSV, the SSV, and the lateral subdermic venous systems. There is substantial variability in the anatomy of the superficial venous system and in the distribution of the communicating veins (perforators) between the deep and superficial venous system.

As mentioned previously, the GSV originates medially on the foot, courses anteromedially around the medial malleolus at the ankle, and ascends anteromedially up the calf and thigh in a relatively straight line, joining the CFV medially near the groin (see **Fig. 1**A). There always is a terminal valve at the saphenofemoral junction and usually one or two subterminal valves within 1 to 2 cm of the terminal valve. The GSV is typically 3 to 4 mm in diameter in the upper thigh and is contained in an oval fascial envelope resulting in a characteristic appearance in cross-section that

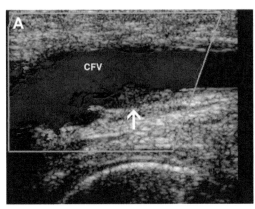
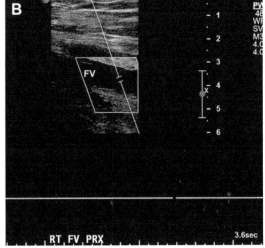

Fig. 15. (A) Color Doppler filling defect in the common femoral vein (CFV) caused by mural thrombus (arrow). (B) Absence of color flow and spectral waveform in completely thrombosed right femoral vein. Note color flow in adjacent femoral artery.

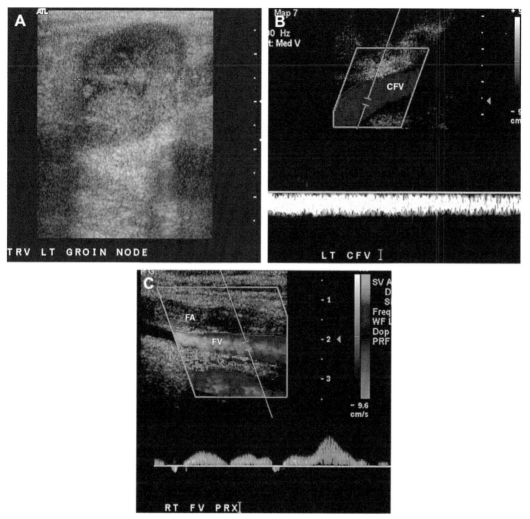

Fig. 16. False-positive clinical findings mimicking DVT. (*A*) Groin adenopathy (*between calipers*) causing leg swelling and pain. (*B*) Dampening of flow in adjacent patent left common femoral vein (CFV). (*C*) Right femoral artery thrombosis (FA) causing pain. Note normal flow in adjacent femoral vein (FV).

has been compared with an "Egyptian eye" (**Fig. 24**).[52] The most important branches of the GSV in the thigh are the posteromedial and anteromedial thigh veins, which arise in the upper to mid thigh. The lateral and medial cutaneous femoral branches, the external circumflex iliac vein, the superficial epigastric vein, and the external pudendal vein are all found near the saphenofemoral junction and terminal valves; the later three branches course superiorly (see **Figs. 1A** and **24**). These branches, although they may be large, are contained by the oval echogenic fascial envelope. It is estimated that 60% of patients who have varicosities have reflux in the GSV system.

The SSV originates laterally on the dorsum of the foot, passes posterior to the lateral malleolus at the ankle, and ascends the calf posteriorly, like the seam in an old-fashioned stocking (see **Fig. 1B**). The exact point of termination of the SSV into the deep system is quite variable. In most people, the SSV terminates directly into the PV near the popliteal crease, but the SSV may join the GSV in the lower thigh through the vein of Giacomini or even may empty directly into the FV in the thigh. The SSV also is surrounded by a fascial layer in the upper calf and typically is not wider than 3 mm in diameter. The SSV runs close to the tibial and sural nerves, which may explain the pain associated with varicosities arising from the SSV.

The lateral subdermic venous system consists of a group of small veins found laterally above

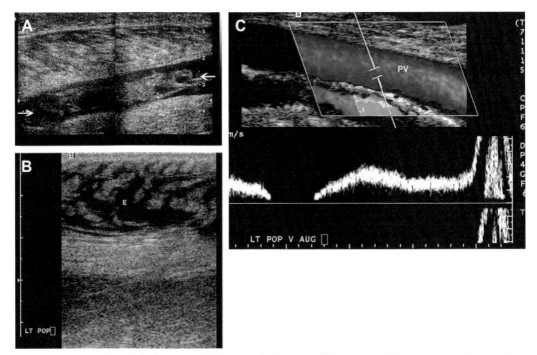

Fig. 17. False-positive clinical findings mimicking DVT. (*A*) Large calf hematoma (*between arrows*) secondary to a muscular tear. (*B*) Diffuse soft tissue edema (E) of the lower extremity. (*C*) The underlying popliteal vein (PV) was patent.

and below the knee. These veins have variable communications with the deep system. Reflux in the lateral subdermic venous system typically results in a fine telangiectasic web of superficial varicosities posterolaterally above or below the knee. Such spider-vein varicosities often occur in younger women (probably resulting from a genetic predisposition) and typically are not associated with truncal varicosities or significant pain and swelling.

Numerous short, perforating veins direct flow from the superficial to the deep system. The exact number and location of these perforators is quite variable. In general these veins are short, straight, and run perpendicular or at a slight angle from the GSV or SSV toward the deep venous system. The most common named groups are the Hunterian perforators (near the medial aspect of the upper adductor canal); Dodd's perforators (in the lower medial thigh); Boyd's perforators (in the mid calf);

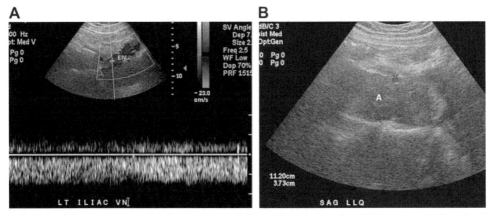

Fig. 18. Clinically false-positive results for DVT caused by groin adenopathy. (*A*) Dampened flow in the left external iliac vein (EIV) caused by (*B*) large groin adenopathy (A) from prostate cancer (between calipers).

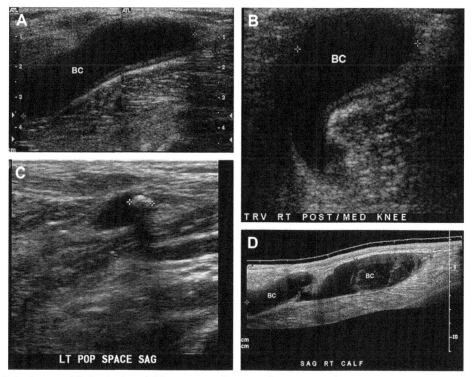

Fig. 19. Baker's cysts. (*A*) Sagittal and (*B*) transverse images of a simple Baker's cyst (BC). (*C*) Sagittal view of a complex Baker's cyst (BC) with calcifications (between calipers). (*D*) Sagittal view of a ruptured Baker's cyst (BC) extending into the lower calf (between calipers).

and Crockett's perforators (in the lower postero-medial calf) (**Fig. 25**). When incompetent, these perforators dilate focally and may cause "blow outs," point tenderness, or even ulceration where they join the superficial system.

Method of Examination

Designing a treatment plan for a patient who has varicose veins requires identification of the highest as well as the lowest point of reflux. In addition, the source of reflux must be identified for every

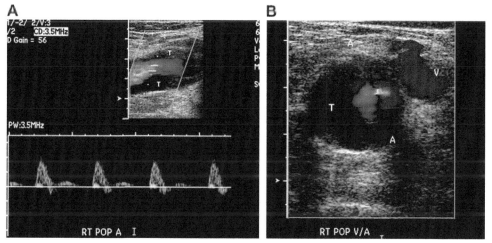

Fig. 20. Popliteal artery aneurysm. (*A*) Sagittal and (*B*) transverse color Doppler US of a partially thrombosed popliteal artery aneurysm (A) causing pain and calf swelling. Note absence of flow in the thrombosed portion (T).

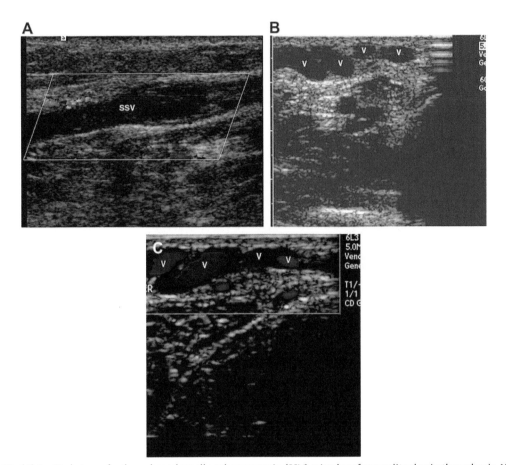

Fig. 21. (*A*) Sagittal view of a thrombosed small saphenous vein (SSV) mistaken for popliteal vein thrombosis. Note the very superficial location of the small saphenous vein and absence of an accompany artery. (*B*) Gray-scale image and (*C*) color Doppler US of superficial varicosities (V) causing pain and swelling, thus clinically mimicking DVT.

varicosity. This identification is accomplished by a combination of visual inspection and Doppler US. US examination can be quite lengthy in a patient who has numerous varicosities because patterns of reflux are highly variable and often are quite complex, with multiple sources of reflux.

The Doppler US examination for reflux begins with a standard US examination of the deep system performed with the patient in the supine position to exclude DVT. The patient then stands, and the legs are inspected visually to identify all varicose veins, because the examination should be tailored to address all varicosities in question. In general, reflux in the GSV tends to involve the medial (inner) thigh, whereas reflux in the SSV causes varicosities in the posterior calf. Telangiectastic varices developing laterally around the knee typically are secondary to reflux in the lateral

subdermic venous system. Because not all symptomatic varicosities are visible, the examiner should remember to ask the patient where it hurts.

Doppler assessment of reflux always should be performed with the patient in the standing position. Because the examination can be time consuming, it may be helpful to have a walker, table, or counter to help support the patient as well as a stool for the examiner. Either color or pulse Doppler can be used, and three different maneuvers can be attempted to elicit reflux:

1. Augmentation: The leg is squeezed from below, directing flow toward the heart. If blood flows back toward the feet for more than 0.5 seconds following augmentation, the examination is positive for reflux (**Fig. 26**), although some examiners require a full second of reflux before considering

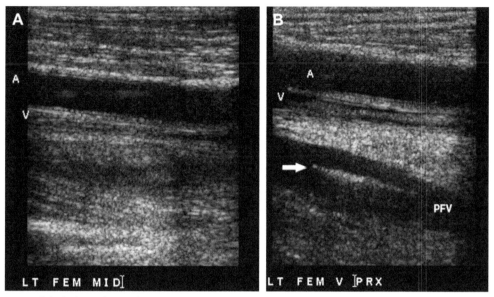

Fig. 22. DVT. (*A*) Thickened irregular vessel walls in a patient who has chronic DVT (V). (*B*) Linear fibrin strand in left profunda femoris vein (PFV), a sequela from prior DVT (*arrow*).

the examination to be positive. Transient retrograde flow is normal and serves to push back the valve leaflets, causing them to close.

2. Valsalva maneuver: Reflux can be assessed in the thigh after the Valsalva maneuver because the resultant increased intra-abdominal pressure causes retrograde flow through incompetent valves (**Fig. 27**). Although this technique is sensitive, it works well only in the upper thigh. If the terminal and/or subterminal valves in the

GSV are competent, the Valsalva maneuver will not detect more distal points of reflux.

3. Direct or retrograde compression: Direct compression above the point of Doppler interrogation propels blood toward the feet in the setting of an incompetent valve. Although it is easiest to assess for reflux in the longitudinal plane using color or pulse Doppler interrogation, with experience the examination can be performed more efficiently in the transverse

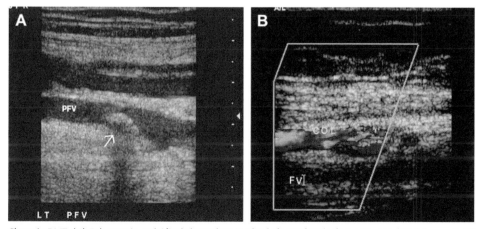

Fig. 23. Chronic DVT. (*A*) Echogenic, calcified thrombus in the left profunda femoris vein (PFV) (*arrow*). (*B*) Collateral vessels (COL) in a patient who has chronic thrombosis of the right femoral vein (FV).

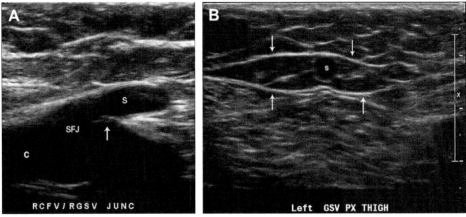

Fig. 24. Normal greater saphenous vein. (A) Longitudinal image at the saphenofemoral junction (SFJ). Note the junction of the more superficial and smaller greater saphenous vein (S) with the deeper and larger common femoral vein (C). The greater saphenous vein runs medial to the femoral vessels and joins the common femoral vein in the groin. Arrow indicates terminal valve. (B) Transverse image of the greater saphenous vein (S) within its surrounding echogenic elliptical fascial sheath creating an appearance similar to a stylized "Egyptian eye" (arrows). Tributaries of the greater saphenous vein pierce this fascial envelope and run more superficially in the subdermal fat and connective tissue.

plane with color Doppler while angling the transducer toward the head or feet (**Fig. 28**).

In addition to Doppler interrogation, gray-scale imaging can be helpful. Often the valves themselves can be visualized directly in the GSV. If the valve leaflets are scarred, thickened, or retracted and do not meet in the midline, reflux is likely. Similarly, if the GSV measures more than 6 mm in diameter, reflux is also likely.

The standard or minimum US examination should assess for reflux in the deep venous system at the levels of the CFV (above and below the saphenofemoral junction), FV (upper, mid, and low), and PV as well as in the GSV, from the saphenofemoral junction to the knee including the origin of the major tributaries and the PV-SSV junction. Full examination of the SSV and GSV below the knee need not be performed unless varicosities are noted in the calf. All varicosities should be traced back to the origin of reflux. In this way, reflux in major branches of the GSV or SSV or reflux originating from incompetent perforators may be identified even in the absence of truncal reflux in the GSV and SSV.

SUMMARY

DVT of the lower extremities is a common clinical entity and, if left untreated, may result in chronic disability producing the postphlebitic syndrome

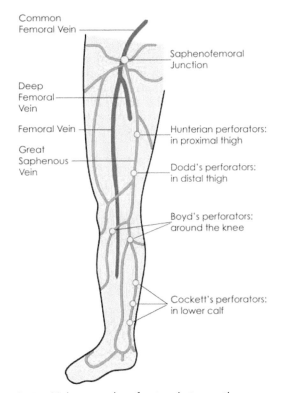

Fig. 25. Major named perforators between the superficial and deep venous system in the lower extremity. (Adapted from Weiss RA, Feied CF, Weiss MA. Vein diagnosis and treatment. New York: McGraw-Hill; 2001.)

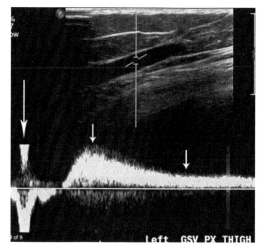

Fig. 26. Reflux in the greater saphenous vein following augmentation. Note sharp, short increase in volume and velocity of blood flow directed toward the head when the leg is squeezed from below (*long arrow*). Subsequently, there is prolonged reversed flow of blood toward the feet lasting well over several seconds (*short arrows*).

or potentially life-threatening and devastating outcomes such as PE. Compression US now is recognized as the most appropriate primary initial imaging modality for evaluating patients at risk for a peripheral DVT, and its accuracy in diagnosing acute or chronic DVT is well established in patients who have lower extremity symptoms. The CFV,

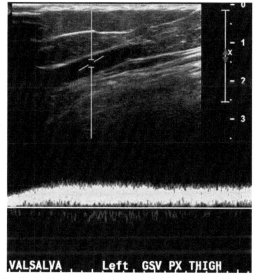

Fig. 27. Reflux in the greater saphenous vein following a Valsalva maneuver. Prolonged reflux (ie, reversed flow in the greater saphenous vein), is noted when the patient increases intra-abdominal pressure by performing a Valsalva maneuver.

FV, and PV are examined routinely. The need for evaluation of the calf veins remains controversial, however. US also is helpful in evaluating patients who have chronic venous changes such as the postphlebitic syndrome and venous insufficiency.

The advantages of US include the noninvasiveness of the examination, lack of ionizing radiation, lack of need for intravenous nephrotoxic contrast media, relatively low cost, and portability so that even the most critically ill patients in the ICU can be examined. A thorough knowledge of regional vascular anatomy, equipment sensitivity, and scanning techniques is required. Despite its limitations in less well-visualized areas such as the iliac and calf veins, US is the most appropriate initial study to perform in patients suspected of harboring a lower extremity DVT. If US studies are nondiagnostic or equivocal, further evaluation with multidetector CT or MR venography may occasionally be necessary.

The signs and symptoms of venous insufficiency overlap with those of DVT. Hence, in a patient presenting with leg pain and swelling, the possibility of venous insufficiency may be overlooked by both clinician and the radiologist because of the overriding and more immediate concern of excluding DVT, a more serious and potentially life-threatening problem. Thus, in the acute setting, Doppler US examination of the lower extremities typically is performed solely to assess for DVT. The clinician and radiologist, however, should remember that venous insufficiency is a common cause of false-negative US examination of the lower extremities and should consider this diagnosis in patients who have leg pain and/or swelling and a negative Doppler US, particularly if symptoms are recurrent or if varicosities are visible. Consideration then should be given to referral for a more extensive Doppler evaluation of the lower extremities to evaluate for reflux.

Although more than 60% of varicosities are caused by reflux in the GSV and its major branches, other tributaries and perforators should be examined based on the patient's symptoms, visual inspection, and physical examination (focal tenderness, bulging, ulcers). If the point of origin of reflux cannot be identified by following the GSV or SSV distally, the examiner should begin at the varicosity and follow it proximally, being careful to identify the highest point of reflux. The examiner should remember that there can be complex patterns of reflux and multiple sites of origin involving tributaries and perforators with or without truncal reflux. It is important to make the diagnosis of chronic venous insufficiency, both to diagnose the cause of the patient's symptoms and because new, minimally invasive

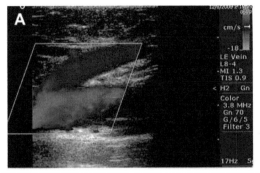

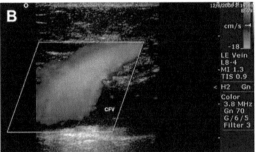 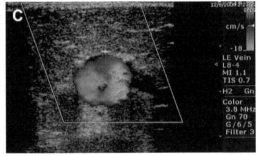

Fig. 28. (*A*) Color baseline examination reveals blood in the common femoral vein and greater saphenous vein heading away from the transducer toward the head (and therefore is color-coded *blue*). (*B*) Color reflux following augmentation (or the Valsalva maneuver): blood flow in the greater saphenous vein is toward the feet and away from the transducer (and therefore is color-coded *red*). Note no blood flow is noted in the deeper common femoral vein (CFV) because competent valves in the common femoral vein prevent reflux of blood toward the feet. (*C*) Imaging in the transverse plane with the transducer angled toward the feet demonstrates blood flowing away from the transducer (ie, refluxing toward the feet and therefore color-coded *red*).

percutaneous techniques such as ambulatory phlebectomy, sclerotherapy, and endovascular thermal ablation have revolutionized treatment of this common, debilitating problem.

REFERENCES

1. Raghavendra BN, Horii SC, Hilton S, et al. Deep venous thrombosis: detection by probe compression of veins. J Ultrasound Med 1986;5:89–95.
2. Cronan JJ. History of venous ultrasound. J Ultrasound Med 2003;22:1143–6.
3. Cronan JJ. Deep venous thrombosis: one leg or both legs? Radiology 1996;200:429–31.
4. Cronan JJ. Venous thromboembolic disease: the role of ultrasound. Radiology 1993;186:619–50.
5. Cronan JJ, Leen V. Recurrent deep venous thrombosis: limitations of US. Radiology 1989;170:739–42.
6. Cronan JJ, Dorfman GS, Grusmark J. Lower-extremity deep venous thrombosis: further experience with and refinements of US assessment. Radiology 1988;168:101–7.
7. Cronan JJ, Dorfman GS, Scola FH, et al. Deep venous thrombosis: US assessment using vein compression. Radiology 1987;162:191–4.
8. Appelman PT, DeJong TE, Lampmann LE. Deep venous thrombosis of the leg: US findings. Radiology 1987;163:743–6.
9. Huisman MV, Buller HR, ten Cate JW, et al. Unexpected high prevalence of silent pulmonary embolism in patients with deep venous thrombosis. Chest 1989;95:498–502.
10. Monreal M, Ruiz J, Olazabal A, et al. Deep venous thrombosis and the risk of pulmonary embolism. A systematic study. Chest 1992;102:677–81.
11. Moser KM, Fedullo PF, LitteJohn JK, et al. Frequent asymptomatic pulmonary embolism in patients with deep venous thrombosis. JAMA 1994;271:223–5.
12. Perone N, Bounameaux H, Perrier A. Comparison of four strategies for diagnosing deep vein thrombosis: a cost-effectiveness analysis. Am J Med 2001;110:33–40.
13. Barnes RW, Wu KK, Hoak JC. Fallibility of the clinical diagnosis of venous thrombosis. JAMA 1975;234(6):605–7.

14. Haeger K. Problems of acute deep venous thrombosis. I. The interpretation of signs and symptoms. Angiology 1969;20:219–23.

15. Salzman EW. Venous thrombosis made easy. [editorial]. N Engl J Med 1986;314:847–8.

16. Rosen MP, Weintraub J, Donohoe K, et al. Role of lower extremity US in patients with clinically suspected pulmonary embolism. J Vasc Interv Radiol 1995;6:439–41.

17. Browse NR. Deep vein thrombosis. BMJ 1969;4:676–8.

18. Bundens WP, Bergan JJ, Halasz NA, et al. The femoral vein. A potentially lethal misnomer. JAMA 1995;274:1296–8.

19. American College of Radiology. Practical guidelines and standards for performance of the peripheral venous ultrasound examination. Reston (VA): American College of Cardiology; 2006.

20. Abu-Yousef MM, Kakish ME, Mufid M. Pulsatile venous Doppler flow in lower limbs: highly indicative of elevated right atrium pressure. AJR Am J Roentgenol 1996;167:977–80.

21. Gottlieb RH, Widjaja J, Mehra S, et al. Clinically important pulmonary emboli: does calf vein US alter outcomes? Radiology 1999;211:25–9.

22. Lohr JM, Kerr TM, Lutter KS, et al. Lower extremity calf thrombosis: to treat or not to treat? J Vasc Surg 1991;14:618–23.

23. Coon WW. Anticoagulant therapy. Am J Surg 1985;150:45–9.

24. Badgett DK, Comerota MC, Khan MC, et al. Duplex venous imaging: role for a comprehensive lower extremity examination. Ann Vasc Surg 2000;14:73–6.

25. Naidich JB, Torre JR, Pellerito JS, et al. Suspected deep venous thrombosis: is US of both legs necessary? Radiology 1996;200:429–31.

26. Fard MN, Mostaan M, Zahed Pour Anaraki M. Utility of lower-extremity duplex sonography in patients with venous thromboembolism. J Clin Ultrasound 2001;29:92–8.

27. Sheiman RG, McArdle CR. Bilateral lower extremity US in the patient with unilateral symptoms of deep venous thrombosis: assessment of need. Radiology 1995;194:171–3.

28. Nix ML. Should bilateral venous duplex imaging be performed in a patient with unilateral leg symptoms? J Vasc Technol 1994;18:211–2.

29. Frederick MG, Hertzberg BS, Kliewer MA, et al. Can the US examination for lower extremity deep venous thrombosis be abbreviated? A prospective study of 755 examinations. Radiology 1996;199:45–7.

30. Lockhart ME, Sheldon HI, Robbin ML. Augmentation in lower extremity sonography for the detection of deep venous thrombosis. AJR Am J Roentgenol 2005;184:419–22.

31. Kim T, Murakami T, Hori M, et al. Efficacy of multislice helical CT venography for the diagnosis of deep venous thrombosis: comparison with venous sonography. Radiat Med 2004;22:77–81.

32. Taffoni MJ, Ravenel JG, Ackerman SJ. Prospective comparison of indirect CT venography versus venous sonography in ICU patients. AJR Am J Roentgenol 2005;185:457–62.

33. Murphy TP, Cronan JJ. Evolution of deep venous thrombosis: a prospective evaluation with US. Radiology 1990;177:543–8.

34. Maki DD, Kumar N, Nguyen B, et al. Distribution of thrombi in acute lower extremity deep venous thrombosis: implications for sonography and CT and MR venography. AJR Am J Roentgenol 2000;175:1299–301.

35. Cornuz J, Pearson SD, Polak JF. Deep venous thrombosis: complete lower extremity venous US evaluation in patients without known risk factors—outcome study. Radiology 1999;211:637–41.

36. Heijboer H, Buller HP, Lensing AWA, et al. A comparison of real-time compression ultrasonography with impedance plethysmography for the diagnosis of DVT in symptomatic outpatients. N Engl J Med 1993;329:1365–9.

37. Yucel EK, Fisher JS, Egglin TK, et al. Isolated calf venous thrombosis: diagnosis with compression US. Radiology 1991;179:443–6.

38. Rose SC, Zwiebel WJ, Nelson BD, et al. Symptomatic lower extremity deep venous thrombosis: accuracy, limitations, and role of color duplex flow imaging in diagnosis. Radiology 1990;175:639–44.

39. Rubin JM, Xie H, Kim K, et al. Sonographic elasticity imaging of acute and chronic deep venous thrombosis in humans. J Ultrasound Med 2006;9:1179–86.

40. Callam MJ. Epidemiology of varicose veins. Br J Surg 1994;81:167–73.

41. Brand FN, Dannenburg AL, Abbott RD, et al. The epidemiology of varicose veins: the Framingham Study. Am J Prev Med 1988;4:96–101.

42. Beaglehole R. Epidemiology of varicose veins. World J Surg 1986;10:898–902.

43. Evans CJ, Allan PL, Lee AJ, et al. Prevalence of venous reflux in the general population on DUS scanning: the Edinburgh vein study. J Vasc Surg 1998;28:767–76.

44. McGuckin M, Waterman R, Brooks J, et al. Validation of venous leg ulcer guidelines in the United States and United Kingdom. Am J Surg 2002;183:132–7.

45. Kurz X, Kahn SR, Abenhaim L, et al. Chronic venous disorders of the leg: epidemiology, outcomes, diagnosis and management. Summary of an evidence-based report of the VEINES task force. Int Angiol 1999;18:83–102.

46. Ruckley CV. Socioeconomic impact of chronic venous insufficiency and leg ulcers. Angiology 1997;48:67–9.

47. Van den Oever R, Hepp B, Debbaut B, et al. Socio-economic impact of chronic venous insufficiency: an underestimated public health problem. Int Angiol 1998;17:161–7.

48. Caggiati A, Bergan JJ, Gloviczki P, et al. Nomenclature of the veins of the lower limbs: an international interdisciplinary consensus statement. J Vasc Surg 2002;36(3):416–22.

49. Weiss RA, Feied CF, Weiss MA. Vein diagnosis and treatment. A comprehensive approach. New York: McGraw Hill Publishing; 2001. p. 4.

50. Coon WW, Willis PW, Keller JB. Venous thromboembolism and other venous disease in the Tecumseh community health study. Circulation 1973;48:839–46.

51. Alexander CJ. The epidemiology of varicose veins. Med J Aust 1972;1:215–8.

52. Caggiati A. Fascial relationships of the long saphenous vein. Circulation 1999;100:2547–9.

Musculoskeletal Ultrasound Intervention: Principles and Advances

Luck J. Louis, MD, FRCPC

KEYWORDS

- Ultrasound • Musculoskeletal intervention
- Prolotherapy • Barbotage • Ganglion cysts • Ganglia

The use of ultrasonography in interventional musculoskeletal radiology is well established[1–3] and is used primarily to guide needle placement for injections, aspirations, and biopsies. The chief advantage of ultrasound imaging is its ability to perform real-time, multiplanar imaging without ionizing radiation. It is relatively inexpensive, is widely available, and permits comparison with the asymptomatic side. Conversely, the modality is operator dependent and requires detailed knowledge of the relevant anatomy, often resulting in a long learning curve. As well, physically deep and osseous lesions may not be visualized readily.

An exhaustive review of ultrasound-guided musculoskeletal intervention is beyond the scope of this section. The foremost goals of this chapter, then, are to present core principles and practical information that can be applied to most procedures. This includes a discussion of guidelines and precautions regarding the use of corticosteroids, a medication that is commonly injected under ultrasound guidance into soft tissues and joints. After this, various aspects of intra-articular intervention will be presented, including suggested routes of access for several major joints. Intratendinous calcium aspiration and intratendinous prolotherapy performed under ultrasound guidance are relatively new variations on old concepts. Both have shown great potential in the treatment of refractory chronic tendon disorders and will be described in detail. Finally, intervention of bursae and ganglion cysts will be reviewed.

GENERAL PRINCIPLES

The choice of ultrasound probe is critical. High-frequency (7–12 MHz), linear array transducers should be used routinely. To visualize deep structures such as the hip in larger patients, lower frequency curvilinear probes may be required. However, such probes should be avoided when possible because they are prone to anisotropic artifact. Anisotropy is a phenomenon in which the appearance of a structure varies depending on the angle from which it is being examined. Anisotropic artifact is common when imaging acoustically reflective, highly organized structures such as ligaments, tendons, muscles, and nerves. When the insonating sound beam is not perpendicular to the structure of interest, the sound reflects off of the structure and away from the transducer, resulting in a hypoechoic "drop off" (Fig. 1).

Regardless of the transducer selected, a complete sonographic examination (including color Doppler) of the area to be punctured is required to define the relationship of adjacent critical structures to be avoided such as nerves and vessels. Only then can a needle trajectory be planned safely. Areas of superficial infection should also be avoided when selecting a needle

This article originally appeared in *Radiologic Clinics of North America* 2008;46(3):515–533

Sections of Musculoskeletal and Emergency Trauma Radiology, Department of Radiology, Vancouver General Hospital, University of British Columbia, 899 W.12th Ave., Vancouver, BC V5Z 1M9, Canada

E-mail address: luck.louis@vch.ca

Ultrasound Clin 4 (2009) 217–236
doi:10.1016/j.cult.2009.04.009

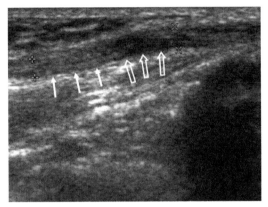

Fig. 1. Anisotropic artifact. Longitudinal sonogram of the ulnar nerve (*solid arrows*) at the level of the wrist using a linear, high-frequency transducer. As the nerve curves toward the transducer face, the insonating sound beams are no longer perpendicular to the nerve. As a result, the nerve appears hypoechoic (*open arrows*), simulating disease. Curvilinear transducers often exacerbate anisotropy because the insonating beams from the ends of the transducer face tend not to be perpendicular to the structure being examined.

path to prevent deeper spread. These include areas of cellulitis, septic bursitis, and abscess. In cases of aspiration or biopsy of suspected malignancy, magnetic resonance (MR) imaging should be performed before the procedure, and the proposed needle route should be discussed with an orthopedic oncologic surgeon to avert unnecessary transgression of anatomic compartments that may complicate surgical management.[4]

One common localization technique is to perform the puncture without direct ultrasound guidance.[5] In this "safe injection" technique, the lesion is first scanned transversely, and its

maximum width is determined. Two dots are marked on the skin surface to either end of the transducer (**Fig. 2**A). The probe is then turned 90°, and the maximum length of the lesion is ascertained. Marks are placed again to either end of the transducer, the depth of the lesion is noted, and the four dots are connected to form a cross hair. The patient's skin is then sterilized, and a needle is inserted through the center of the cross hair at right angles to the original scan planes and passed to the predetermined depth (**Fig. 2**B). The advantage of this technique is that it is less time consuming because the probe requires no special sterile preparation.

Most musculoskeletal procedures, however, can be performed with a free-hand technique, which allows direct, dynamic visualization of the needle tip. The following is the author's method of choice. After planning a safe route of access, a line parallel to the long axis of the transducer face can be drawn on the skin adjacent to the end of the transducer where the needle will be introduced (**Fig. 3**). Once the patient's skin and transducer are sterilized and draped, the probe can be returned quickly to the same location and orientation by aligning the probe to the skin mark. A 1.5-in (3.8 cm) 25-G needle is then used to infiltrate the subcutaneous tissues with local anesthetic such as lidocaine 1% or 2%. The needle is directed toward the intended target under constant observation with the long axis of the needle parallel and in line with the long axis of the transducer face. The angle at which the freezing needle is advanced should be noted mentally because any other needles introduced afterward will follow an identical path. In many cases, it will be possible to advance the freezing needle into the target directly and use the same needle to perform aspiration or injection. This avoids

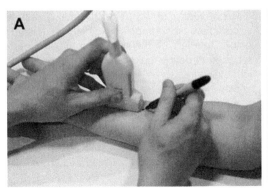

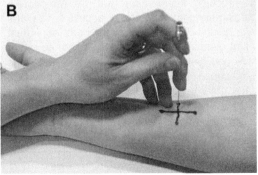

Fig. 2. Safe injection technique. (*A*) Dots are placed on the skin surface to either end of the transducer after determining the maximal length and width of the lesion. (*B*) A cross hair is drawn by connecting the four dots. A needle is then passed through the center of the cross hair to the predetermined depth. (Sterile technique not depicted above.)

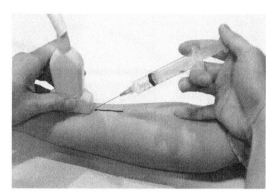

Fig. 3. Freehand technique. Once a safe needle trajectory has been chosen, a line parallel to the transducer face is drawn on the skin at the proposed needle entry site. The needle is introduced to the target along this line under constant ultrasound guidance. (Sterile technique not depicted above.)

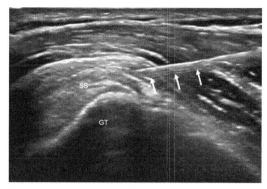

Fig. 4. Reverberation artifact. Coronal sonogram of the distal supraspinatus tendon (SS) upon its insertion onto the greater tuberosity (GT). A 25-G needle introduced for a diagnostic block of the subacromial bursa shows reverberation artifacts (*solid arrows*), which appear as multiple, parallel lines deep to the needle. This artifact, when present, is useful in helping to identify the needle position. Smaller caliber needles tend to produce less, if any, reverberation.

puncturing the patient multiple times and helps to expedite the case. Glenohumeral joints can be accessed routinely with this single-puncture method as can hip joints and hamstring origins in thinner patients. If one intends to perform a procedure with only one needle, it is prudent to securely screw the needle onto the syringe and then unscrew the needle by an eighth turn. This ensures that the syringe can be removed easily from the needle without disturbing the needle's position once at the target site.

It is sometimes difficult to visualize smaller caliber needles, and several strategies are effective in discriminating the needle tip. First, the transducer face should remain as perpendicular to the needle as possible by heel–toe angling and rocking of the probe. When ideally oriented in such a manner, reverberation artifact posterior to the needle is commonly seen, which aids in highlighting the needle (Fig. 4). Another approach is to sweep the transducer from side to side while repeatedly moving the needle in and out, which aids in identifying the tip in real time. Injecting a small amount of local anesthetic will disrupt the adjacent soft tissues and also helps to localize the needle tip. At other times, rotating the transducer 90° to examine the needle in short axis may be useful in determining whether the needle has veered off to one side of the intended course.

Sterile skin preparation and aseptic technique vary tremendously between institutions and radiologists. In our department, sterile coupling gel and disposable sterile drapes are always used. Extra-articular structures are routinely punctured after thorough cleansing of the skin and probe only. Disposable plastic probe covers are used, however, for intra-articular work to minimize the

risk of septic arthritis. Standoff pads are prone to physically interfere with procedures and are, therefore, never used.

The needle size, length, and type should be selected based on the task at hand. Larger needles (18–20 G) are generally required for aspiration of suspected thick material such as pus, ganglia, or organized hematoma. Smaller needles (22–27 G) suffice for most injections but are inappropriate for aspirations unless the aspirate is thin. Specialized needles with cutting tips such as the Westcott biopsy needle (Becton, Dickinson and Company, Franklin Lakes, New Jersey) or core-biopsy needle sets are often required for soft tissue biopsies.

MEDICATIONS

The most common medications used in musculoskeletal intervention are for local anesthesia. Lidocaine 2% (Xylocaine) is the author's drug of choice and has rapid onset with a duration of action of up to 5 hours.[6] Bupivacaine (Sensorcaine, Marcaine) is an alternate slower-onset anesthetic but one which can last up to 12 hours and is available in 0.25%, 0.5%, and 0.75% concentrations. The duration of action of both drugs is shorter with lower concentration formulations.[6]

Corticosteroids have potent anti-inflammatory properties and are commonly prescribed for injection into soft tissues, bursae, tendon sheaths, and joints. At the author's institution, the two corticosteroids used most routinely are triamcinolone acetonide and methylprednisolone acetate (Depo-Medrol). These are generally mixed 1 part lidocaine 2%, 1 part bupivacaine 0.25%, and 2 parts 40 mg/mL corticosteroid before injection.

Several potential side effects of corticosteroids are relevant to musculoskeletal intervention, which practitioners need to be aware of. First, skin atrophy, fat necrosis, and skin depigmentation may develop from corticosteroids applied topically or injected intralesionally, intradermally, or subcutaneously. Methylprednisolone is less prone to causing skin atrophy than triamcinolone[7–11] and, therefore, is preferred when injecting lesions near the skin surface.

Secondly, animal models have shown that the biomechanical properties of tendons are adversely affected by intratendinous corticosteroid administration.[12,13] Corticosteroids may limit formation of granulation and connective tissue, reduce tendon mass, and decrease the amount of load that a tendon can withstand before mechanical failure. Case reports of tendon rupture after intratendinous corticosteroid injection are common in the literature.[14–16] Although corticosteroids have been used to treat tendon degeneration, or tendinosis, inflammation is not a predominant feature of this condition and, when present, may be important in the healing process.[17] Currently, there is no good evidence to substantiate the use of corticosteroids in treatment of chronic tendon lesions.[18] Even peritendinous injections may predispose to tendon rupture[15,19–21] and, therefore, should be performed with caution.

Corticosteroids have also been implicated in cartilage breakdown when injected into synovial joints, particularly weight-bearing articulations.[22–24] Articular surfaces develop multiple cystic defects, which become filled with necrotic debris. Such lesions appear not to develop in similarly injected non–weight-bearing joints. Reduction in cartilage elasticity has also been shown, which may further accelerate cartilage breakdown as the cushioning effect of cartilage is lost. There has been at least one case report of a Charcot-like arthropathy after intra-articular corticosteroid use.[25]

Currently, there is no consensus and no evidence-based guidelines for the number of safe injections at one site or the appropriate interval between injections.[18] As such, many recommendations for the use of locally injected corticosteroids are anecdotal. **Box 1** summarizes some suggestions for corticosteroid use in soft tissues and joints.

INTRA-ARTICULAR INTERVENTION

Eustace and colleagues[27] found that blind injections for shoulder pain, even in the hands of musculoskeletal specialists, are successful only

---

Box 1
Suggestions for corticosteroid injection into soft tissues and joints

- Use methylprednisolone when injecting superficial lesions or superficial joints.
- Mix the corticosteroid with local anesthetic solution to provide immediate but short-term pain relief.
- Avoid intratendinous injections.
- Use caution with peritendinous injections, especially when the adjacent tendon is heavily loaded (such as the patellar and Achilles' tendons) or is torn.
- Avoid intra-articular injections unless there is a specific indication, such as end-stage osteoarthritis.
- Be mindful of injection into structures that communicate with a joint. Examples include the long head of biceps tendon sheath, flexor hallucis longus tendon sheath, and Baker's cysts.
- Advise at least 2 weeks of rest and avoid heavy loading for 6 weeks after peritendinous and intra-articular injections.
- Be careful not to damage the articular cartilage with the needle during injection.
- Allow adequate time between injections to assess its effects, generally a minimum of 6 weeks.
- Be cautious in using more than 3 injections at any one site.
- Do not repeat an injection if at least 4 weeks of symptomatic relief was not achieved after 2 injections.

Data from Speed CA. Fortnightly review: Corticosteroid injections in tendon lesions. BMJ 2001;323(7309):382–6; and Tehranzadeh J, Booya F, Root J. Cartilage metabolism in osteoarthritis and the influence of viscosupplementation and steroid: a review. Acta Radiol 2005;46(3):288–96.

---

in the minority of cases. In their series, only 29% of subacromial injections and 42% of glenohumeral joint injections were performed accurately without image guidance. In another recent study that compared ultrasound-guided and blind aspirations of suspected joint effusions, only 32% of cases returned fluid when performed blindly. In contrast, fluid was aspirated in 97% using ultrasound scan.[28] Indeed, ultrasonography has been shown to be effective in guiding difficult joint aspirations throughout the body.[29,30]

Ultrasound-guided joint aspirations may be performed for diagnosis of conditions such as crystal arthropathy and septic arthritis. In the case of an infected joint, aspiration may be therapeutic as well. Septic joint effusions are commonly hypoechoic with low-amplitude internal echoes but fluid may also be hyperechoic or rarely anechoic (**Fig. 5B**).[31,32] In approximately 0.5% of septic joints, the initial ultrasound examination will find no joint effusion.[33] A repeat ultrasound study should be considered if fever and joint pain persist in these cases. Although septic arthritis may be associated with hyperemia, Doppler ultrasound scan is unreliable in differentiating septic from aseptic joints.[34] Finally, intra-articular injection of local anesthetic should be avoided because lidocaine is bacteriostatic and may contribute to false-negative results.

Ultrasound-guided joint injections are also commonly performed for diagnosis and therapy. Diagnostic blocks are performed by injecting a small amount of anesthetic into a joint and then clinically assessing whether the procedure has improved the patient's symptoms. Several in vitro and animal-based studies have shown chondrotoxic effects resulting from intraarticular exposure to anesthetic solutions, including lidocaine and bupivicaine.[35–41] Although data are preliminary, these results stress the need to perform all intraarticular interventions with caution and only when there is a reasonable clinical indication. The author uses an equal volume mixture of lidocaine and bupivicaine for this purpose, but the total volume of injected solution will depend on the size of the joint. Most hip and shoulder joints easily receive 10 mL, whereas the small joints of the hands and feet may take less than 1 mL. In all cases, injection should be terminated if the patient complains of excessive discomfort. The procedure is useful in confirming or ruling out the source of pain and, in cases of subsequent surgery, helps to predict postsurgical pain relief. Pain response is graded subjectively on a 10-point scale, and the patient is asked to keep a diary of blockade efficacy over the next 24 hours. Patients should be instructed not to overuse the joint because pain relief, although potentially dramatic, will be short-lived.

Therapeutic intra-articular injection of corticosteroid and viscosupplement are useful in treating osteoarthritis[26] and can be performed under ultrasound guidance. Viscosupplementation is a procedure in which hyaluronic acid, or a derivative, is injected directly into afflicted joints and aims to replace what is believed to be an important factor of joint lubrication. Several formulations are commercially available that vary in their duration of effect and treatment schedules. Although the precise mechanism of action is not entirely understood, numerous clinical trials have shown some improvement in pain and joint function.[42,43]

The following section describes potential routes of access to the most commonly injected joints. As already discussed, every precaution should be taken to prevent septic arthritis. Proper sterile preparation and draping of the patient and of the equipment are essential.

Shoulder Joint

The majority of shoulder joints can be injected while the patient is seated. However, if the patient

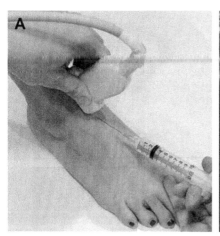
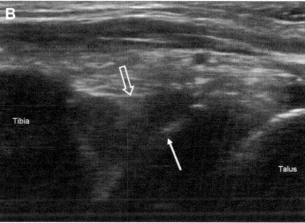

Fig. 5. Ankle joint access from an anterior approach. (*A*) The transducer is aligned in a sagittal plane at the tibiotalar articulation, and the needle is introduced from an anteroinferior approach. Care should be exercised to avoid puncturing the dorsalis pedis artery and extensor tendons. (*B*) Sagittal sonogram of the anterior ankle joint in an intravenous drug abuser. A hypoechoic joint effusion containing low-amplitude internal echoes is interposed between the distal tibia and talar dome and displaces the ankle joint capsule anteriorly (*open arrow*). The needle tip is seen within the joint space (*solid arrow*). (*Sterile technique not depicted above.*)

is known to become faint or is overly anxious, a lateral decubitus position works equally well. Although the glenohumeral joint may be accessed from anteriorly or posteriorly, the preferred approach is the latter. This route is particularly advantageous when performing gadolinium injections before MR imaging because there is less chance of causing interstitial injection of the rotator cuff interval or anterior labrum where misplaced contrast material could simulate disease.

With the patient's hand gently resting on the opposite shoulder, the posterior joint is examined in an axial plane, and the key landmarks of the triangular-shaped posterior labrum, humeral head, and joint capsule are identified (**Fig. 6**). The needle is introduced laterally in an axial plane and is advanced medially. The needle target is between the posterior-most aspect of the humeral head and the posterior labrum. Particular care should be taken to not puncture the labrum or articular cartilage, however. Once the needle tip is felt against the humeral head, a small test injection of anesthetic is performed. With correct intra-articular placement, anesthetic will flow easily into the joint. If there is resistance to injection, gently twirling the syringe or withdrawing the needle by 1 to 2 mm while continuing to inject a small amount of anesthetic will often resolve the problem.

In almost all cases, the 1.5-inch 25-G needle used for local anesthesia will suffice in accessing this joint with a single puncture. In larger patients, the use of a longer 22-G spinal needle may be required.

Elbow Joint

The patient is seated or laid supine with the elbow flexed and the arm placed comfortably across the chest (**Fig. 7A**). The ultrasound probe is then positioned along the posterior elbow and is oriented sagittally such that the triceps tendon is visualized longitudinally. The probe, which remains parallel to the triceps fibers, is then slid laterally until just out of view of the triceps tendon. Key landmarks are the olecranon fossa of the humerus, the posterior fat pad, and the olecranon (**Fig. 7B**). The needle is introduced from a superior approach, passing beside the triceps tendon and through the posterior fat pad to enter the joint space. This joint is easily accessible with a 1.5-inch long needle.

Hip Joint

There are two common approaches to accessing the hip joint and the choice between the two depends on operator preference, the presence of a joint effusion, and body habitus. In both cases, the patient is laid supine and the joint is punctured anteriorly.

When a joint effusion is present or in larger patients, the best approach is often with the probe aligned along the long axis of the femoral neck. The concave transition between the anterior aspect of the femoral head and neck can be visualized clearly, and the joint capsule is seen immediately superficial (**Fig. 8**). The needle is introduced from an inferior approach and passes through the joint capsule to rest on the subcapital femur.

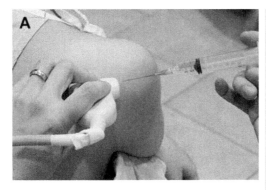
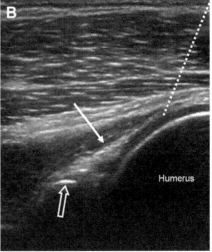

Fig. 6. Shoulder joint access from a posterior approach. (*A*) With the patient seated, the posterior glenohumeral joint is examined in a transverse plane. (*B*) The needle is introduced from a lateral and posterior approach (*dotted line*). Important landmarks include (**1**) the humeral head (Humerus) which is lined by a thin, hypoechoic layer of articular cartilage, (**2**) the bony glenoid rim (*open arrow*), and (**3**) the echogenic, triangular-shaped posterior labrum (*solid arrow*) which arises from the glenoid. (Sterile technique not depicted above.)

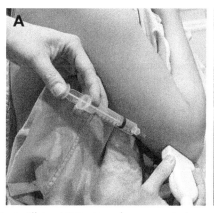
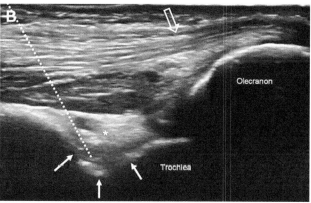

Fig. 7. Elbow joint access from a posterior approach. (*A*) With the patient seated and the affected arm placed across the chest, the posterior joint is examined in a sagittal plane. (*B*) The needle is introduced from a postero-superior approach (*dotted line*), passing adjacent to the triceps tendon (*open arrow*), through the posterior fat pad (*asterisk*) and into the joint. The concave olecranon fossa of the humerus (*solid arrows*) provides a useful landmark. (Sterile technique not depicted above.)

Septic hip arthritis is a frequent clinical concern, particularly in patients with hip arthroplasties. Although a fine needle is useful for joint injections, aspiration for suspected septic arthritis should be performed with an 18-G spinal needle. Not only will purulent material be easier to aspirate, but a 22-G Westcott biopsy needle can be introduced through the larger needle to obtain synovial biopsies, if required.

In thinner patients, it is often easiest to access the hip joint with the ultrasound probe oriented axially. When positioned correctly, the femoral head and acetabular rim will be in view (**Fig. 9**). The needle is introduced from an anterolateral approach, remaining lateral to the femoral neurovascular bundle. The needle tip is advanced until it rests on the femoral head, adjacent to its most anterior aspect. The hip labrum, which arises from the acetabulum, should be avoided.

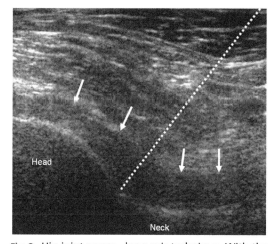

Fig. 8. Hip joint access—long axis technique. With the ultrasound probe aligned along the long axis of the femoral neck, the distinctive concave transition between the femoral head and neck is visualized. In this case, the anterior hip joint capsule (*solid arrows*) is displaced anteriorly by a large joint effusion. The needle is introduced from an inferior and anterior approach (*dotted line*), lateral to the femoral neurovascular bundle (not shown).

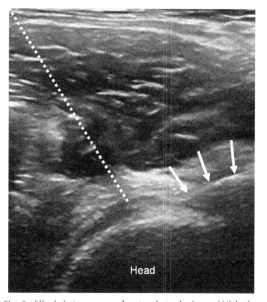

Fig. 9. Hip joint access—short axis technique. With the transducer oriented in a transverse plane, the key landmarks of the femoral head and anterior acetabulum (*solid arrows*) are visualized. The needle is introduced from an anterior and lateral approach (*dotted line*), piercing the anterior joint capsule to rest upon the femoral head. The femoral neurovascular bundle (not shown) is medial to and remote from the needle path.

Knee Joint

A knee joint distended with effusion is most easily injected or aspirated through the suprapatellar bursa with the patient supine and the knee flexed slightly. A small pillow or sponge placed behind the knee is helpful. The probe is placed in a sagittal plane superior to the patella, whereby the fibers of the distal quadriceps tendon are seen in long axis (**Fig. 10**). The probe is kept parallel to the quadriceps tendon but is slid medially or laterally until the quadriceps fibers disappear from view. A needle is then passed directly into the bursa.

For knee joints with no joint effusion, the medial patellofemoral facet affords an excellent target. After palpating the patella and medial patellofemoral joint line, the probe is placed in an axial plane so that the patella and medial femoral condyle are visible. The probe is then turned 90° and oriented along the joint line. The needle is introduced either from an inferior or superior approach directly into the joint.

Ankle Joint

With the patient supine, the anterior tibiotalar joint is examined in a sagittal plane (see **Fig. 5A**). If there is any doubt of correct probe placement, performing plantar flexion and dorsiflexion maneuvers will readily identify the talus moving across the tibia. The position of the dorsalis pedis artery and extensor tendons should be noted and kept away from during needle placement. A needle

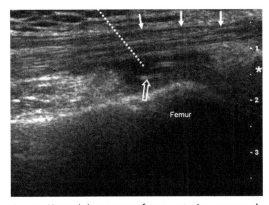

Fig. 10. Knee joint access from anterior approach. Sagittal sonogram of the suprapatellar knee shows the distal quadriceps tendon (*solid arrows*), the distal femur, and the superior patellar pole (*asterisk*). The needle is introduced from an anterior and superior approach (*dotted line*) and is preferably passed to one side of the quadriceps tendon without puncturing it. In this case, synovial plicae (*open arrow*) are present in a mildly distended suprapatellar bursa.

then is introduced into the joint in a sagittal plane using an inferior approach (see **Fig. 5B**).

INTRATENDINOUS INTERVENTION

Calcific and noncalcific tendinosis are two potentially symptomatic diseases that are often refractory to conservative management. The ability of ultrasound scan to accurately depict and localize tendon abnormalities makes ultrasound-guided calcium aspiration and prolotherapy invaluable in treating these conditions.

Treatment of Calcific Tendinosis

Rotator cuff **calcific tendinosis** (also commonly referred to as **calcifying tendinitis**), is caused by the deposition of carbonate apatite crystals,[44] most commonly in the critical zone of the supraspinatus tendon roughly 1 cm proximal to its insertion.[45–47] Uhthoff and Loehr[46] described three distinct stages in the disease process, namely the precalcific, calcific, and postcalcific stages. Depending on the phase of disease, the imaging appearance and physical consistency of the calcification differ significantly as do patient symptoms.

The calcific stage consists of three phases. The **formative** and **resting phases** are chronic and may be associated with varying degrees of pain at rest or with movement. Many patients, however, are asymptomatic.[48] These calcifications tend to be well circumscribed and discrete when examined radiographically[49] and often produce significant acoustic shadowing by ultrasound scan (**Fig. 11**).[50] Attempts at aspirating calcifications in these two phases tend to be difficult because the calcifications are quite hard and chalklike.

The **resorptive phase** is the last phase in the calcific stage and is the most symptomatic. Shedding of calcium crystals into the adjacent subacromial bursa may result in severe pain and restricted range of motion.[51] This phase typically lasts for 2 weeks or longer. These calcifications appear ill-defined on radiographs and produce little or no acoustic shadowing by ultrasonography (**Fig. 12**).[50] When aspirated, these calcified deposits typically are soft with a slurrylike consistency.

Calcific tendinosis is usually a self-limiting condition in which the calcification resorbs after a period of worsening pain.[48] However, in some patients, the condition can lead to chronic pain and functional impairment. The resolution of calcification correlates well with clinical improvement of symptoms[52–57] and, therefore, various treatments have been devised to promote their removal. There is no conclusive evidence that intralesional steroid injection,[58] acetic acid

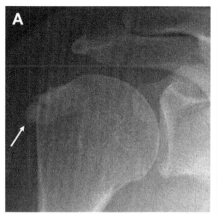
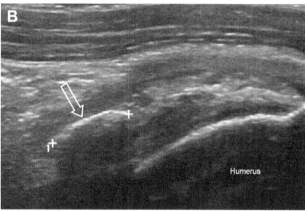

Fig. 11. Hard calcifications in calcific tendinosis. Examples of "hard calcification" that typify the formative phase of calcific tendinosis. (A) The anteroposterior radiograph of patient A shows a large, sharply circumscribed calcification within the infraspinatus tendon (*solid arrow*). (B) In patient B, the supraspinatus tendon is imaged longitudinally. A large intratendinous calcification (*open arrow*) produces significant posterior acoustic shadowing artifact.

iontophoresis,[59,60] or pulsed ultrasound therapy are effective.[48] Extracorporeal shockwave lithotripsy uses acoustic waves to fragment calcium deposits, and substantial or complete clinical improvement has been reported in 66% to 91% of patients.[52,54,61,62] However, access to lithotripter equipment is limited and is less available than ultrasound imaging.

Open or arthroscopic surgery currently provides the greatest long-term relief in terms of substantial or complete clinical improvement with numerous studies reporting between 76.9% and 100% good or excellent results.[49,63–73] However, surgery may be complicated by prolonged postsurgical disability and reflex sympathetic dystrophy.[52,63,74–76] Because conservative

measures are successful in up to 90% of patients,[71] surgery is generally indicated only in those who have progressive symptoms, whose symptoms interfere with activities of daily living, and who have not responded to conservative therapy.[77]

Image-guided needle irrigation and aspiration (**barbotage**) of rotator cuff calcifications has been shown to be an effective minimally invasive technique and was first described three decades ago.[78] In a recent study, del Cura and colleagues[56] reported that 91% of patients experienced significant or complete improvement in range of motion, pain, and disability when aspiration was performed under ultrasound guidance. Given the potential risks of surgery, percutaneous calcium

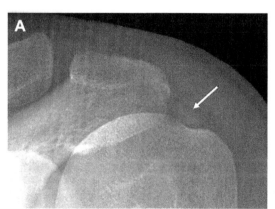
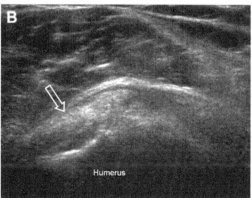

Fig. 12. Soft calcification in calcific tendinosis. Examples of "soft calcification" that characterize the resorptive phase of calcific tendinosis. (A) Faint, ill-defined calcification (*solid arrow*) is seen on the anteroposterior radiograph of patient A who suffers from excruciating shoulder pain. (B) In patient B, a vague, hyperechoic area is seen anteriorly within the supraspinatus tendon, which is scanned in short axis (*open arrow*).

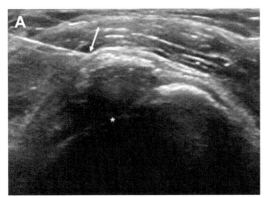
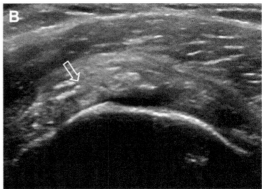

Fig. 13. Incomplete aspiration of supraspinatus calcification. (*A*) Sonogram of the supraspinatus tendon in short axis shows placement of a needle (*solid arrow*) at the edge of a "hard" calcified deposit. There is marked posterior acoustic shadowing that obscures the humeral cortical surface (*asterisk*). Only a small amount of calcification could be aspirated. The calcification instead was gently ground with the needle tip. (*B*) Follow-up sonogram 6 weeks later shows marked change in the appearance of the calcification with loss of the acoustic shadowing seen previously (*open arrow*). The patient's symptoms improved significantly between the two examinations.

aspiration should be considered after failure of medical therapy.[56,79] Successful aspiration may not be possible in cases in which the calcification appears striated because this is thought to represent calcification of the tendon fibers themselves. Also, clinical outcomes when attempting to remove numerous, diffuse, small (<5 mm) calcifications are only fair to poor, even when treated surgically.[80]

Image-guided barbotage techniques vary greatly, and there is no accepted standardized methodology. Needle sizes have ranged from 15 G[81] to 25 G,[58] and some investigators have advocated a two-needle irrigation system,[76,82,83] whereas others have used only one.[56,57,76] In some published results, as many as 15 passes were made through the same calcification,[78,83,84] whereas other researchers opted to limit potential iatrogenic cuff damage by performing a single lesional puncture only.[56,57]

At our institution, we routinely perform a full-shoulder ultrasound examination before any intervention. This is done to ensure that there are no co-existing disorders such as rotator cuff tears. We also ensure a recent set of radiographs has been performed to characterize the calcifications more fully and to act as a baseline for follow-up. The patient is placed into the lateral decubitus position opposite the affected side. Although the procedure can be done sitting, patients have been documented to become syncopal during aspiration.[56] Depending on the location of the calcification in the cuff, the arm is positioned appropriately. In the case of the supraspinatus tendon, a "hand in back pocket" position is used. The calcification is then targeted under ultrasound scan before sterile preparation of the skin

and equipment. A 20-G needle connected to a syringe filled with 2% lidocaine is advanced into the subacromial bursa where a small amount of anesthetic is injected before the needle continues into the calcification. Importantly, lidocaine is injected into the calcification without first aspirating to prevent the needle tip from becoming obstructed. Several short injections, each followed by release of pressure on the plunger, are performed. If successful, lidocaine and calcium fragments will evacuate into the syringe. The syringe should be held below horizontal to prevent re-injection of aspirated material. Also, new lidocaine-filled syringes can be exchanged for when required. Barbotage should be continued until no more calcification can be aspirated. However, it may not be possible to aspirate very hard

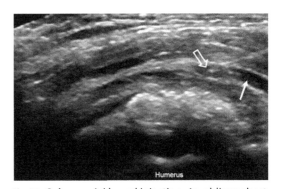

Fig. 14. Subacromial bursal injection. An oblique short-axis sonogram of the supraspinatus tendon shows placement of a needle (*open arrow*) within the subacromial bursa (*solid arrow*). The bursa has been distended partially with injected lidocaine and corticosteroid at the end of a barbotage procedure.

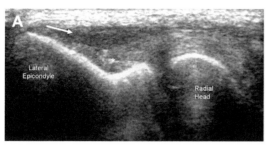
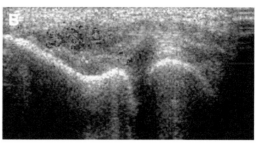

Fig. 15. Common extensor tendinosis. Coronal sonograms of the common extensor tendon origin of the elbow in a patient with lateral epicondylitis clinically. (A) A large, hypoechoic area (*solid arrow*) is seen along the superficial aspect of the tendon, characteristic of tendinosis. Normal tendon is seen immediately deep to the lesion (*asterisk*). (B) The corresponding color Doppler examination of the same area shows marked hypervascularity, which is a common, albeit nonspecific, finding in tendinosis.

calcifications, in which case the calcification can be ground gently with the needle tip by rotating the syringe (**Fig. 13**). This mechanical perturbation of the deposit is hypothesized to stimulate cell-mediated resorption.[57,76,78,85] There is collaborative evidence in the surgical literature that suggests that calcific deposits need not be removed completely to achieve successful outcomes.[72,78] The needle is then withdrawn into the subacromial bursa where a combination of 1 mL 2% lidocaine and 1 mL of 40 mg/mL triamcinolone is injected to mitigate the risk of postprocedural bursitis (**Fig. 14**).

Patients are instructed to rest the shoulder for up to a week and are advised to take nonsteroidal anti-inflammatory medication, as needed, to manage discomfort. A follow-up appointment is made for 6 weeks after barbotage and includes repeat ultrasound and plain film studies.

Treatment of Noncalcific Tendinosis

Tendon degeneration, often referred to as "tendinopathy" or "tendinosis," is not characterized by an inflammatory response but rather infiltration of fibroblasts and vessels.[86] Tendinosis is generally considered to be caused by repetitive microtrauma with an ensuing chronic cycle of tendon degeneration and repair resulting in a weakened tendon. These changes have been shown to appear as hypoechoic areas on sonography (**Fig. 15**).[87] Several techniques have been described to treat tendinosis. Autologous blood, which contains fibroblast growth factors, has been used successfully in treatment of refractory medial and lateral epicondylitis of the elbow.[86,88–90] Ohberg and Alfredson reported significant improvement in chronic achillodynia after obliteration of neovessels using polidocanol as a sclerosing agent.[91]

Prolotherapy is another treatment option that has shown promising results. It is a technique in which injection of an irritant solution (the proliferant) into a ligament or tendon incites a local inflammatory response, which, in turn, induces fibroblast proliferation and collagen synthesis.[92–94] One popular proliferant solution that has been studied

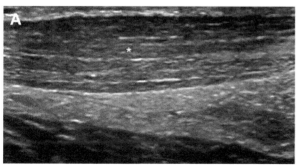
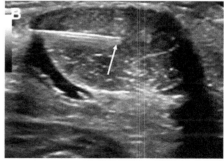

Fig. 16. Achilles tendinosis and prolotherapy. (A) On the initial longitudinal sonogram of the Achilles tendon, marked fusiform swelling of the tendon is present (*asterisk*) in its midportion. There are diffuse echopoor areas within the tendon, and the normal fibrillar echotexture is disrupted, particularly along its superficial aspect. (B) Short axis sonogram of the tendon at the maximal site of swelling shows needle placement (*solid arrow*) before injection of hyperosmolar dextrose. The patient's symptoms nearly completely resolved after five treatments.

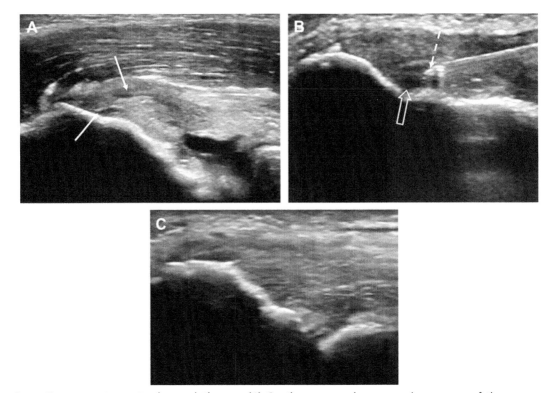

Fig. 17. Common extensor tendon prolotherapy. (*A*) On the preprocedure coronal sonogram of the common extensor tendon of the elbow, two prominent partial tears are present (*solid arrows*). (*B*) A needle is seen within the deeper of the two tears (*dashed arrow*), which has been distended with a small amount of injected dextrose solution (*open arrow*). (*C*) After 10 months (6 injections), the partial tears are no longer seen, and the patient's symptoms had improved subjectively by 90%. However, the tendon continues to be diffusely echopoor and slightly thickened. In the author's experience, even successfully treated tendons often continue to appear quite heterogeneous.

is hyperosmolar dextrose, which has an excellent safety profile and is inexpensive.[95] As little as 0.6% extracellular D-glucose (dextrose) has been shown experimentally to stimulate human cells in producing growth factors within minutes to hours[96] and dextrose concentrations greater than 10% result in a brief inflammatory reaction.[93] In a recent review of the prolotherapy literature, Rabago and colleagues[97] reported positive results compared with controls in both nonrandomized and randomized, controlled studies. Good results have been reported previously after treatment of tendons such as the thigh adductor origins and suprapubic abdominal insertions without image

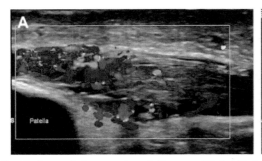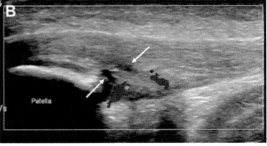

Fig. 18. Jumper's knee and prolotherapy. (*A*) Sagittal sonogram of the patellar tendon origin in a world-class water skier shows a marked amount of hypervascularity and tendon thickening. (*B*) Repeat sonogram after several prolotherapy injections shows significant reduction in the number of vessels present. However, small partial tears are evident along the deep surface of the tendon (*solid arrows*).

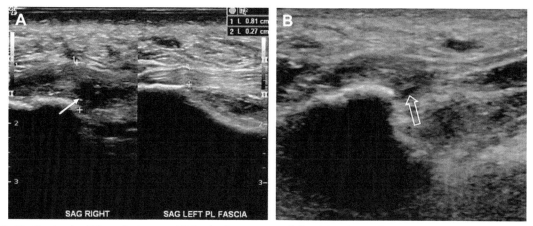

Fig. 19. Plantar fasciitis prolotherapy. (A) Sagittal sonogram of the right plantar fascia origin shows marked thickening and a large partial tear (*solid arrow*) when compared with the asymptomatic left side. (B) After several dextrose injections, the partial tear had decreased substantially in size (*open arrow*), and the patient's symptoms had completely resolved. Despite this, the tendon remains thickened and heterogeneous.

guidance.[98] Intra-articular dextrose administration has also been experimentally used in treatment of osteoarthritis and ACL laxity.[99–101]

Maxwell and colleagues[95] significantly advanced this technique by using ultrasonography to treat chronic Achilles tendinosis. Focal areas of tendinosis and partial tearing were precisely targeted and then injected with 25% dextrose monohydrate solution (**Fig. 16**). In their study, patients showed a significant reduction in tendon pain at rest (88%), with normal activity (84%), and after exercise (78%). The number of intrasubstance tears decreased by 78% and areas of neovascularity diminished by up to 55%. At 1-year follow-up, 67% of patients continued to be asymptomatic, 30% had mild symptoms, and only 3% had moderate symptoms.

As with all interventional procedures, a formal ultrasound examination of the entire area is performed first to characterize the extent and nature of the disease and to exclude other pathology. A 25% dextrose solution is produced by mixing 1 mL of 50% dextrose monohydrate and 1 mL of 2% lidocaine. Once the needle route is planned, and sterile preparation has been performed, a 25-G needle and lidocaine solution are used for local anesthesia. The needle then is advanced directly into the tendon at the site of tendinosis or tearing (**Fig. 17**). Areas of neovascularity are not targeted specifically, but neovessels frequently will coexist in areas of tendinosis and often will decrease with treatment (**Fig. 18**). As advocated by Maxwell and colleagues[95] usually 0.5 mL or less solution is injected into any one

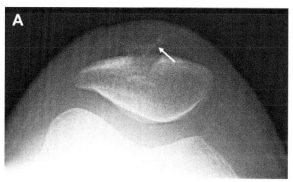

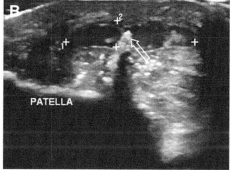

Fig. 20. Frictional bursitis at bone-tendon-bone graft harvest site. (A) Skyline view of the patella in a patient who previously underwent ACL repair. The patellar graft harvest site is surrounded by osseous fragments (*solid arrow*). (B) Sagittal sonogram of the patella shows a fluid collection (indicated by the calipers) centered over one such fragment (*open arrow*). Progressive swelling and pain with knee flexion and extension had developed over several weeks after surgery.

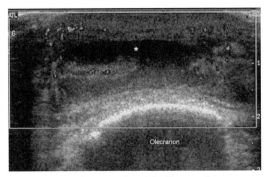

Fig. 21. Septic olecranon bursitis. Short axis sonogram of the olecranon bursa. The synovial-lined bursal walls are markedly thickened and hyperemic, and there is a small amount of anechoic fluid present centrally (*asterisk*). The appearances are nonspecific, and differentiation between septic and aseptic bursitides by ultrasound scan is unreliable.

lesion. However, several lesions may be injected during a single treatment session.

Postprocedure instructions include avoidance of any heavy tendon loading for 2 weeks. Also, nonsteroidal anti-inflammatory medications should not be used for pain relief because they may inhibit the dextrose-stimulated inflammatory reaction. Patients are re-assessed at 6-week intervals, and repeat injections are performed until the patient is asymptomatic or no longer derives any benefit from the treatment. It is worthwhile noting that the tendons in some patients who report complete cessation of symptoms continue to appear thickened and hypoechoic and show hypervascularity (**Fig. 19**). In our series of unpublished results, the majority of patients who derive some benefit from prolotherapy only do so after four or five injections. Prospective patients are made aware of this fact before beginning treatment to circumvent any unrealistic expectations.

INTERVENTION OF GANGLION CYSTS AND BURSAE

Ultrasonography is the ideal modality for image-guided aspiration and injection of most cysts and bursae in the musculoskeletal system. The ability of ultrasound imaging to target even very small collections while avoiding adjacent critical structures in real time is essential in treating these lesions successfully.

Treatment of Bursitis

Bursae are fluid-filled sacs that serve to decrease friction between adjacent structures and may or may not be lined with synovium.[102] Inflammation of a bursa may be caused by repetitive use, infection, systemic inflammatory conditions, and trauma. In treating bursitis, it is important to establish the likely cause. Corticosteroids, which are used commonly to treat bursitis resulting from overuse (**Fig. 20**), would be contraindicated in septic bursitis (**Fig. 21**). Caution should also be exercised when injecting corticosteroids into bursae that communicate with a joint to prevent potential steroid-mediated cartilage damage. Therefore, when treating subacromial-subdeltoid bursitis, rotator cuff tearing should be excluded before injection.

In the case of bursae that are distended with a large amount of fluid, immediate and dramatic improvement in symptoms can be achieved by thorough aspiration (**Fig. 22**). However, if performing a corticosteroid injection into a very small collection, incomplete aspiration of the bursa is sometimes advantageous and will help ensure that the potential space is not collapsed entirely before the medication can be injected intrabursally (**Fig. 23**).

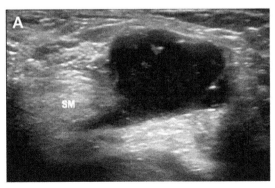
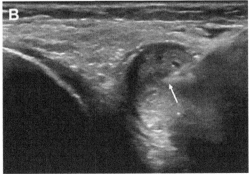

Fig. 22. Semimembranosus bursitis. (*A*) Transverse sonogram of the posteromedial knee. An irregular fluid collection is seen along the medial aspect of the semimembranosus tendon (SM), typical of semimembranosus bursitis. (*B*) A needle (*solid arrow*) has been introduced into the bursa, which has been nearly completely aspirated. The patient experienced immediate relief in his symptoms.

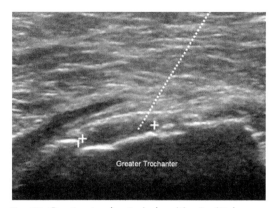

Fig. 23. Greater trochanteric bursitis. Sagittal sonogram of the hip shows a small amount of fluid (indicated by the calipers) adjacent to the greater trochanter. With the patient in a lateral decubitus position, a fine needle can be placed easily into the collection (*dotted line*).

Treatment of Ganglion Cysts

Ganglion cysts are the most common cause of a soft tissue mass in the distal upper extremity.[103] The etiology of ganglia is controversial. One widely held view is that cyst formation occurs as a result of trauma or tissue irritation, whereby mucin is produced by modified synovial cells lining the synovial–capsular interface.[104] The mucin eventually pools behind valvelike structures formed by capsular ducts, resulting in ganglion formation.

Many lesions are asymptomatic and require no treatment. In fact, 40% to 60% of ganglia have been reported to resolve spontaneously.[105,106] However, in other cases, symptoms related to mass effect may mandate intervention (**Fig. 24**). Patients may complain of restricted range of motion, aching, paresthesias, or weakness. Furthermore, cysts that drain externally are at risk of a deep soft tissue or joint infection.

Although surgery has been stated to have success rates of 99%,[107] complications such as joint instability, postoperative stiffness, decreased range of motion, and neurovascular injury make minimally invasive techniques a viable alternative in symptomatic patients. Success rates for blind, percutaneous aspiration vary tremendously from 33%[108] to 85%.[109] In one of the largest published series of wrist ganglia undergoing nonoperative management, 85 patients were randomly assigned to two groups: aspiration alone or aspiration followed by injection of 40 mg of methylprednisolone.[108] The investigators found no difference in the success rate between these two groups. Interestingly, 96% of those ganglia that did not subsequently recur were treated successfully after only one attempt. Of those lesions requiring a second or third aspiration, only 4% eventually resolved. In this series, multiple aspirations were of little benefit. The major limitation of this study was that all punctures were performed without image guidance.

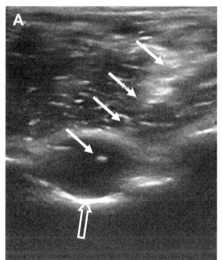
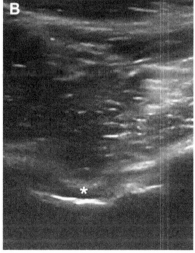

Fig. 24. Spinoglenoid notch ganglion cyst aspiration. (*A*) Transverse sonogram of the spinoglenoid notch (*open arrow*) depicts a small ganglion cyst, presumably impinging upon the suprascapular nerve. An 18-G needle was advanced into the cyst but is only partially visualized along its course (*solid arrows*). (*B*) Transverse sonogram of the spinoglenoid notch after aspirating 2 mL of gelatinous material. The cyst cavity has completely collapsed (*asterisk*). The chronic, dull aching in the posterior shoulder experienced by the patient for months had improved dramatically by the end of the examination.

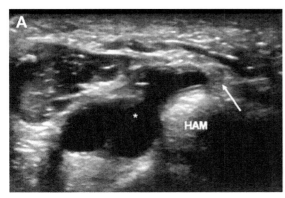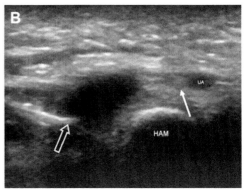

Fig. 25. Aspiration of ganglion cyst causing ulnar nerve palsy. Transverse sonograms of the palmar ulnar wrist. (*A*) A lobulated ganglion cyst (*asterisk*) is seen extending superficial to the hamate (HAM) to abut the ulnar nerve (*solid arrow*). (*B*) A needle (*open arrow*) has partially decompressed the ganglion, which has receded from the ulnar nerve (*solid arrow*) and ulnar artery (UA). The patient's symptoms resolved slowly over the course of several weeks after aspiration.

Breidahl and Adler[110] were the first to describe the use of ultrasound guidance in treatment of ganglia. In their small study population, nine of ten patients derived significant or complete relief after aspiration with a 20-G needle and injection of 40 to 80 mg of triamcinolone. However, the use of corticosteroids in treating ganglia remains controversial.

Ganglia appear as cystic masses by ultrasonography and typically are oval or lobulated in shape (**Fig. 25**).[103,111,112] Internally, a ganglion may be anechoic or contain low-amplitude echoes and septae. An 18-G needle is recommended for aspiration of all suspected ganglion cysts because cyst contents are invariably thick and gelatinous.

SUMMARY

Ultrasound-guided intervention is probably underutilized currently in North America. However, the dynamic, multiplanar capability of ultrasonography makes it an attractive alternative to procedures that might otherwise be performed under fluoroscopic or computed tomography guidance. Indeed, the majority of joints, cysts, and bursae can be accessed routinely under sonographic control. In the cases of barbotage and prolotherapy, ultrasonography has given fresh breath to old concepts and has afforded radiologists new options to treat difficult and chronic tendon problems. It is hoped that this review has served as a springboard for the reader to further investigate the important and diverse role ultrasound imaging is able to play in musculoskeletal intervention.

ACKNOWLEDGMENTS

This article would not have been possible without the outstanding contributions of the medical sonography team at UBC Hospital. In particular, the author wishes to thank Anne Hope, Maureen Kennedy, and Pam Grossman for their unwavering enthusiasm and support. The author also wishes to recognize Paulina Louis for her invaluable help in preparing the manuscript.

REFERENCES

1. Cardinal E, Beauregard CG, Chhem RK. Interventional musculoskeletal ultrasound. Semin Musculoskelet Radiol 1997;1(2):311–8.
2. Dodd GD 3rd, Esola CC, Memel DS, et al. Sonography: the undiscovered jewel of interventional radiology. Radiographics 1996;16(6):1271–88.
3. Rubens DJ, Fultz PJ, Gottlieb RH, et al. Effective ultrasonographically guided intervention for diagnosis of musculoskeletal lesions. J Ultrasound Med 1997;16(12):831–42.
4. Liu PT, Valadez SD, Chivers FS, et al. Anatomically based guidelines for core needle biopsy of bone tumors: implications for limb-sparing surgery. Radiographics 2007;27(1):189–205 [discussion: 206].
5. van Holsbeeck MT, Introcaso JH. Interventional musculoskeletal ultrasound. 2nd edition. St. Louis (MO): Mosby, Inc.; 2001.
6. Repchinsky C, editor. Compendium of pharmaceuticals and specialties. Ottawa (ON): Canadian Pharmacists Association; 2007.
7. Beardwell A. Subcutaneous atrophy after local corticosteroid injection. Br Med J 1967;3:1.
8. Cassidy JT, Bole GG. Cutaneous atrophy secondary to intra-articular corticosteroid administration. Ann Intern Med 1966;65(5):1008–18.
9. Fisherman EW, Feinberg AR, Feinberg SM. Local subcutaneous atrophy. JAMA 1962;179:971–2.

10. Schetman D, Hambrick GW Jr, Wilson CE. Cutaneous changes following local injection of triamcinolone. Arch Dermatol 1963;88:820–8.

11. Goldman L. Reactions following intralesional and sublesional injections of corticosteroids. JAMA 1962;182:613–6.

12. Kapetanos G. The effect of the local corticosteroids on the healing and biomechanical properties of the partially injured tendon. Clin Orthop Relat Res 1982;(163):170–9.

13. Ketchum LD. Effects of triamcinolone on tendon healing and function. A laboratory study. Plast Reconstr Surg 1971;47(5):471–82.

14. Clark SC, Jones MW, Choudhury RR, et al. Bilateral patellar tendon rupture secondary to repeated local steroid injections. J Accid Emerg Med 1995; 12(4):300–1.

15. Ford LT, DeBender J. Tendon rupture after local steroid injection. South Med J 1979;72(7):827–30.

16. Kleinman M, Gross AE. Achilles tendon rupture following steroid injection. Report of three cases. J Bone Joint Surg Am 1983;65(9):1345–7.

17. Wong ME, Hollinger JO, Pinero GJ. Integrated processes responsible for soft tissue healing. Oral Surg Oral Med Oral Pathol Oral Radiol Endod 1996;82(5):475–92.

18. Speed CA. Fortnightly review: corticosteroid injections in tendon lesions. BMJ 2001;323(7309): 382–6.

19. Bickel KD. Flexor pollicis longus tendon rupture after corticosteroid injection. J Hand Surg [Am] 1996;21(1):152–3.

20. Gottlieb NL, Riskin WG. Complications of local corticosteroid injections. JAMA 1980;243(15): 1547–8.

21. Unverferth LJ, Olix ML. The effect of local steroid injections on tendon. J Sports Med 1973;1(4):31–7.

22. MacLean CH, Knight K, Paulus H, et al. Costs attributable to osteoarthritis. J Rheumatol 1998; 25(11):2213–0.

23. McDonough AL. Effects of corticosteroids on articular cartilage: a review of the literature. Phys Ther 1982;62(6):835–9.

24. Moskowitz RW, Davis W, Sammarco J, et al. Experimentally induced corticosteroid arthropathy. Arthritis Rheum 1970;13(3):236–43.

25. Hagen R. [Charcot-like arthropathy following intra-articular injections of corticosteroids]. Nord Med 1971;85(12):381 [in Norwegian].

26. Tehranzadeh J, Booya F, Root J. Cartilage metabolism in osteoarthritis and the influence of viscosupplementation and steroid: a review. Acta Radiol 2005;46(3):288–96.

27. Eustace JA, Brophy DP, Gibney RP, et al. Comparison of the accuracy of steroid placement with clinical outcome in patients with shoulder symptoms. Ann Rheum Dis 1997;56(1):59–63.

28. Balint PV, Kane D, Hunter J, et al. Ultrasound guided versus conventional joint and soft tissue fluid aspiration in rheumatology practice: a pilot study. J Rheumatol 2002;29(10):2209–13.

29. van Holsbeeck MT, Introcaso JH. Musculoskeletal ultrasonography. Radiol Clin North Am 1992; 30(5):907–25.

30. Chhem RK, Kaplan PA, Dussault RG. Ultrasonography of the musculoskeletal system. Radiol Clin North Am 1994;32(2):275–89.

31. Fessell DP, Jacobson JA, Craig J, et al. Using sonography to reveal and aspirate joint effusions. AJR Am J Roentgenol 2000;174(5):1353–62.

32. Shiv VK, Jain AK, Taneja K, et al. Sonography of hip joint in infective arthritis. Can Assoc Radiol J 1990; 41(2):76–8.

33. van Holsbeeck MT, Introcaso JH. Sonography of large synovial joints. 2nd edition. St. Louis (MO): Mosby, Inc.; 2001.

34. Strouse PJ, DiPietro MA, Adler RS. Pediatric hip effusions: evaluation with power Doppler sonography. Radiology 1998;206(3):731–5.

35. Chu CR, Izzo NJ, Papas NE, et al. In vitro exposure to 0.5% bupivacaine is cytotoxic to bovine articular chondrocytes. Arthroscopy 2006;22:693–9.

36. Dogan N, Erdem AF, Erman Z, et al. The effects of bupivacaine and neostigmine on articular cartilage and synovium in the rabbit knee joint. J Int Med Res 2004;32:513–9.

37. Gomoll AH, Kang RW, Williams JM, et al. Chondrolysis after continuous intra-articular bupivacaine infusion: an experimental model investigating chondrotoxicity in the rabbit shoulder. Arthroscopy 2006;22:813–9.

38. Nole R, Munson NM, Fulkerson JP. Bupivacaine and saline effects on articular cartilage. Arthroscopy 1985;1:123–7.

39. Petty DH, Jazrawi LM, Estrada LS, et al. Glenohumeral chondrolysis after shoulder arthroscopy: case reports and review of the literature. Am J Sports Med 2004;32:509–15.

40. Piper SL, Kim HT. Comparison of ropivacaine and bupivacaine toxicity in human articular chondrocytes. J Bone Joint Surg Am 2008;90:986–91.

41. Karpie JC, Chu CR. Lidocaine exhibits dose- and time-dependent cytotoxic effects on bovine articular chondrocytes in vitro. Am J Sports Med 2007;35:1621–7.

42. van den Bekerom MP, Lamme B, Sermon A, et al. What is the evidence for viscosupplementation in the treatment of patients with hip osteoarthritis? Systematic review of the literature. Arch Orthop Trauma Surg 2007 [epub ahead of print].

43. Waddell DD. Viscosupplementation with hyaluronans for osteoarthritis of the knee: clinical efficacy and economic implications. Drugs Aging 2007; 24(8):629–42.

44. Hamada J, Ono W, Tamai K, et al. Analysis of calcium deposits in calcific periarthritis. J Rheumatol 2001;28(4):809–13.

45. Bradley M, Bhamra MS, Robson MJ. Ultrasound guided aspiration of symptomatic supraspinatus calcific deposits. Br J Radiol 1995;68(811):716–9.

46. Uhthoff HK, Loehr JW. Calcific tendinopathy of the rotator cuff: pathogenesis, diagnosis, and management. J Am Acad Orthop Surg 1997;5(4):183–91.

47. Rothman RH, Parke WW. The vascular anatomy of the rotator cuff. Clin Orthop Relat Res 1965;41:176–86.

48. Speed CA, Hazleman BL. Calcific tendinitis of the shoulder. N Engl J Med 1999;340(20):1582–4.

49. Depalma AF, Kruper JS. Long-term study of shoulder joints afflicted with and treated for calcific tendinitis. Clin Orthop 1961;20:61–72.

50. Farin PU. Consistency of rotator-cuff calcifications. Observations on plain radiography, sonography, computed tomography, and at needle treatment. Invest Radiol 1996;31(5):300–4.

51. Neer CS II. Less frequent procedures. Philadelphia: WB Saunders; 1990.

52. Rompe JD, Zoellner J, Nafe B. Shock wave therapy versus conventional surgery in the treatment of calcifying tendinitis of the shoulder. Clin Orthop Relat Res 2001;(387):72–82.

53. Wang CJ, Ko JY, Chen HS. Treatment of calcifying tendinitis of the shoulder with shock wave therapy. Clin Orthop Relat Res 2001;(387):83–9.

54. Wang CJ, Yang KD, Wang FS, et al. Shock wave therapy for calcific tendinitis of the shoulder: a prospective clinical study with two-year follow-up. Am J Sports Med 2003;31(3):425–30.

55. Loew M, Daecke W, Kusnierczak D, et al. Shockwave therapy is effective for chronic calcifying tendinitis of the shoulder. J Bone Joint Surg Br 1999;81(5):863–7.

56. del Cura JL, Torre I, Zabala R, et al. Sonographically guided percutaneous needle lavage in calcific tendinitis of the shoulder: short- and long-term results. AJR Am J Roentgenol 2007;189(3):W128–34.

57. Aina R, Cardinal E, Bureau NJ, et al. Calcific shoulder tendinitis: treatment with modified US-guided fine-needle technique. Radiology 2001; 221(2):455–61.

58. Uhthoff HK, Sarkar K. The shoulder, vol. 2. Philadelphia: WB Saunders; 1990.

59. Leduc BE, Caya J, Tremblay S, et al. Treatment of calcifying tendinitis of the shoulder by acetic acid iontophoresis: a double-blind randomized controlled trial. Arch Phys Med Rehabil 2003; 84(10):1523–7.

60. Perron M, Malouin F. Acetic acid iontophoresis and ultrasound for the treatment of calcifying tendinitis of the shoulder: a randomized control trial. Arch Phys Med Rehabil 1997;78(4):379–84.

61. Daecke W, Kusnierczak D, Loew M. Long-term effects of extracorporeal shockwave therapy in chronic calcific tendinitis of the shoulder. J Shoulder Elbow Surg 2002;11(5):476–80.

62. Maier M, Stabler A, Lienemann A, et al. Shockwave application in calcifying tendinitis of the shoulder–prediction of outcome by imaging. Arch Orthop Trauma Surg 2000;120(9):493–8.

63. Ark JW, Flock TJ, Flatow EL, et al. Arthroscopic treatment of calcific tendinitis of the shoulder. Arthroscopy 1992;8(2):183–8.

64. Ellman H, Kay SP. Arthroscopic subacromial decompression for chronic impingement. Two- to five-year results. J Bone Joint Surg Br 1991;73(3):395–8.

65. Gschwend N, Patte D, Zippel J. [Therapy of calcific tendinitis of the shoulder]. Arch Orthop Unfallchir 1972;73(2):120–35 [in German].

66. Rubenthaler F, Wittenberg RH. [Intermediate-term follow-up of surgically managed tendinosis calcarea (calcifying subacromion syndrome–SAS) of the shoulder joint]. Z Orthop Ihre Grenzgeb 1997; 135(4):354–9 [in German].

67. Tillander BM, Norlin RO. Change of calcifications after arthroscopic subacromial decompression. J Shoulder Elbow Surg 1998;7(3):213–7.

68. Hedtmann A, Fett H. Die sogenannte Periarthropathia humeroscapularis. Z Orthop Ihre Grenzgeb 1989;127:643–9.

69. Huber H. Ist bei der Tendinitis calcarea die operative Kalkentfernung gerechtfertigt. Orthop Praxis 1992;3:179–83.

70. McLaughlin HL. The selection of calcium deposits for operation; the technique and results of operation. Surg Clin North Am 1963;43:1501–4.

71. Rochwerger A, Franceschi JP, Viton JM, et al. Surgical management of calcific tendinitis of the shoulder: an analysis of 26 cases. Clin Rheumatol 1999;18(4):313–6.

72. Seil R, Litzenburger H, Kohn D, et al. Arthroscopic treatment of chronically painful calcifying tendinitis of the supraspinatus tendon. Arthroscopy 2006; 22(5):521–7.

73. Hurt G, Baker CL Jr. Calcific tendinitis of the shoulder. Orthop Clin North Am 2003;34(4):567–75.

74. Wittenberg RH, Rubenthaler F, Wolk T, et al. Surgical or conservative treatment for chronic rotator cuff calcifying tendinitis–a matched-pair analysis of 100 patients. Arch Orthop Trauma Surg 2001;121(1–2):56–9.

75. Rubenthaler F, Ludwig J, Wiese M, et al. Prospective randomized surgical treatments for calcifying tendinopathy. Clin Orthop Relat Res 2003;(410):278–84.

76. Parlier-Cuau C, Champsaur P, Nizard R, et al. Percutaneous treatments of painful shoulder. Radiol Clin North Am 1998;36(3):589–96.

77. Gschwend N, Scherer M, Lohr J. Die tendinitis calcarea des schultergelenks (T. c.). Orthopade 1981; 10:196–205.

78. Comfort TH, Arafiles RP. Barbotage of the shoulder with image-intensified fluoroscopic control of needle placement for calcific tendinitis. Clin Orthop Relat Res 1978;(135):171–8.

79. Normandin C, Seban E, Laredo JD. Aspiration of tendinous calcific deposits. New York: Springer-Verlag; 1988.

80. Resch KL, Povacz P, Seykora P. Excision of calcium deposit and acromioplasty?. Paris. Elsevier; 1997.

81. Lam F, Bhatia D, van Rooyen K, et al. Modern management of calcifying tendinitis of the shoulder. Current Orthopaedics 2006;20:446–52.

82. Farin PU, Jaroma H, Soimakallio S. Rotator cuff calcifications: treatment with US-guided technique. Radiology 1995;195(3):841–3.

83. Farin PU, Rasanen H, Jaroma H, et al. Rotator cuff calcifications: treatment with ultrasound-guided percutaneous needle aspiration and lavage. Skeletal Radiol 1996;25(6):551–4.

84. Pfister J, Gerber H. Chronic calcifying tendinitis of the shoulder-therapy by percutaneous needle aspiration and lavage: a prospective open study of 62 shoulders. Clin Rheumatol 1997;16(3): 269–74.

85. Laredo JD, Bellaiche L, Hamze B, et al. Current status of musculoskeletal interventional radiology. Radiol Clin North Am 1994;32(2):377–98.

86. Connell DA, Ali KE, Ahmad M, et al. Ultrasound-guided autologous blood injection for tennis elbow. Skeletal Radiol 2006;35(6):371–7.

87. Movin T, Kristoffersen-Wiberg M, Shalabi A, et al. Intratendinous alterations as imaged by ultrasound and contrast medium-enhanced magnetic resonance in chronic achillodynia. Foot Ankle Int 1998;19(5):311–7.

88. Edwards SG, Calandruccio JH. Autologous blood injections for refractory lateral epicondylitis. J Hand Surg [Am] 2003;28(2):272–8.

89. Suresh SP, Ali KE, Jones H, et al. Medial epicondylitis: is ultrasound guided autologous blood injection an effective treatment? Br J Sports Med 2006;40(11):935–9 [discussion: 939].

90. Iwasaki M, Nakahara H, Nakata K, et al. Regulation of proliferation and osteochondrogenic differentiation of periosteum-derived cells by transforming growth factor-beta and basic fibroblast growth factor. J Bone Joint Surg Am 1995;77(4): 543–54.

91. Ohberg L, Alfredson H. Ultrasound guided sclerosis of neovessels in painful chronic Achilles tendinosis: pilot study of a new treatment. Br J Sports Med 2002;36(3):173–5 [discussion 176–7].

92. Banks AR. A rationale for prolotherapy. J Orthop Med 1991;13:54–9.

93. Reeves KD. Prolotherapy: basic science, clinical studies, and technique. 2nd edition. Philadelphia: Hanley & Belfus; 2000.

94. Liu YK, Tipton CM, Matthes RD, et al. An in situ study of the influence of a sclerosing solution in rabbit medial collateral ligaments and its junction strength. Connect Tissue Res 1983;11(2–3): 95–102.

95. Maxwell NJ, Ryan MB, Taunton JE, et al. Sonographically guided intratendinous injection of hyperosmolar dextrose to treat chronic tendinosis of the Achilles tendon: a pilot study. AJR Am J Roentgenol 2007;189(4):W215–20.

96. Oh JH, Ha H, Yu MR, et al. Sequential effects of high glucose on mesangial cell transforming growth factor-beta 1 and fibronectin synthesis. Kidney Int 1998;54(6):1872–8.

97. Rabago D, Best TM, Beamsley M, et al. A systematic review of prolotherapy for chronic musculoskeletal pain. Clin J Sport Med 2005; 15(5):376–80.

98. Topol GA, Reeves KD, Hassanein KM. Efficacy of dextrose prolotherapy in elite male kicking-sport athletes with chronic groin pain. Arch Phys Med Rehabil 2005;86(4):697–702.

99. Reeves KD, Hassanein K. Randomized, prospective, placebo-controlled double-blind study of dextrose prolotherapy for osteoarthritic thumb and finger (DIP, PIP, and trapeziometacarpal) joints: evidence of clinical efficacy. J Altern Complement Med 2000;6(4):311–20.

100. Reeves KD, Hassanein K. Randomized prospective double-blind placebo-controlled study of dextrose prolotherapy for knee osteoarthritis with or without ACL laxity. Altern Ther Health Med 2000;6(2):68–74, 77–80.

101. Reeves KD, Hassanein KM. Long-term effects of dextrose prolotherapy for anterior cruciate ligament laxity. Altern Ther Health Med 2003;9(3): 58–62.

102. O'Connor PJ, Grainger AJ. Ultrasound imaging of joint disease. In: McNally EG, editor. Practical musculoskeletal ultrasound. Philadelphia: Churchill Livingstone; 2005. p. 245–62.

103. Miller TT, Potter HG, McCormack RR Jr. Benign soft tissue masses of the wrist and hand: MRI appearances. Skeletal Radiol 1994;23(5):327–32.

104. Angelides AC. Ganglions of the hand and wrist. 4th edition. Philadelphia: Churchill Livingstone; 1999.

105. McEvedy B. The simple ganglion: a review of modes of treatment and an explanation of the frequent failures of surgery. Lancet 1954; 266(6803):135–6.

106. Hvid-Hansen O. On the treatment of ganglia. Acta Chir Scand 1970;136(6):471–6.

107. Angelides AC, Wallace PF. The dorsal ganglion of the wrist: its pathogenesis, gross and microscopic

anatomy, and surgical treatment. J Hand Surg [Am] 1976;1(3):228–35.

108. Varley GW, Needoff M, Davis TR, et al. Conservative management of wrist ganglia. Aspiration versus steroid infiltration. J Hand Surg [Br] 1997; 22(5):636–7.

109. Zubowicz VN, Ishii CH. Management of ganglion cysts of the hand by simple aspiration. J Hand Surg [Am] 1987;12(4):618–20.

110. Breidahl WH, Adler RS. Ultrasound-guided injection of ganglia with corticosteroids. Skeletal Radiol 1996;25(7):635–8.

111. Cardinal E, Buckwalter KA, Braunstein EM, et al. Occult dorsal carpal ganglion: comparison of US and MR imaging. Radiology 1994;193(1):259–62.

112. Bianchi S, Abdelwahab IF, Zwass A, et al. Ultrasonographic evaluation of wrist ganglia. Skeletal Radiol 1994;23(3):201–3.

Ultrasound of the Hindfoot and Midfoot

David P. Fessell, MD[a],*, Jon A. Jacobson, MD[b]

KEYWORDS

- Ultrasound • Hindfoot • Midfoot • Ankle
- Tendons • Ligaments • Masses

Ultrasound (US) is increasingly being used to evaluate musculoskeletal disorders, including foot and ankle pathology.[1–5] Higher frequency transducers and technical advances in recent years have resulted in a higher spatial resolution for sonography compared with MR imaging.[6] Cost saving with US can also be considerable. In many cases the professional and technical cost of an US is approximately 80% less than an MR image of the same anatomy.[7] US has the unique capacity to allow evaluation during dynamic maneuvers which can reveal abnormalities that are not apparent during static imaging. The advantages of an imaging modality that allows visualization during dynamic maneuvers will be highlighted throughout this article. Additional advantages of US include imaging of patients who cannot undergo MR imaging due to pacemakers, hardware, or claustrophobia; direct and real-time evaluation of the site of pain or symptoms with additional history immediately available; flexibility in the field-of-view; ease of contralateral comparison; use of Doppler; and ease of guiding procedures.[8] Disadvantages of US include the learning curve and operator dependence. These disadvantages can be addressed by the simple application of time and effort.

Specialties such as Physical Medicine and Rehabilitation, Rheumatology, and Emergency Medicine are increasingly using US to evaluate musculoskeletal disorders.[9–13] Radiologists, who have years of training in anatomy, pathology, US physics, artifacts, and technical aspects of US imaging, are uniquely suited to apply this versatile modality to foot and ankle pathology. If radiologists are not able to perform musculoskeletal US with great expertise, this business will be taken over by other specialties. If musculoskeletal US is lost, additional modalities such as MR imaging may be lost as well. It is imperative that radiologists continue to be experts in all aspects of musculoskeletal imaging, including US.

The technique for examining the hindfoot and midfoot with US has been described and depicted many recent articles[2,5] and will not be discussed. In this article, normal US anatomy will be shown in all cases before demonstrating the full range of hindfoot and midfoot pathology. Color and power Doppler can aid diagnosis by demonstrating neovascularity in cases of inflammation or fibrosis and will also be discussed.

HINDFOOT AND MIDFOOT TENDONS: GENERAL COMMENTS

Tendon pathology of the hindfoot and midfoot can be difficult to diagnose. In the acute setting, pain and swelling can limit the physical examination. In the setting of chronic injury it may not be possible to differentiate tendon, ligament, or osseous pathology solely on the basis of the physical examination. US is well tolerated in both the acute and chronic settings. Real-time correlation with the site of pain and symptoms aids diagnosis and is a strength of US. Numerous studies have documented the accuracy of US for detecting tendon pathology[14–19] and these studies will be discussed in each tendon section below. US is

This article originally appeared in *Radiologic Clinics of North America* 2008;466:1027–1043

[a] Department of Radiology, University of Michigan Hospitals and Health Centers, 1500 E. Medical Center Drive, Taubman Center, Room 2910Q, Ann Arbor, MI 48109-5326, USA

[b] University of Michigan, 1500 E. Medical Center Drive, TC 2910L, Ann Arbor, MI 48109-5326, USA

* Corresponding author.

E-mail address: dfessell@umich.edu (D.P. Fessell).

Ultrasound Clin 4 (2009) 237–253
doi:10.1016/j.cult.2009.04.008

not limited to three orthogonal planes, as is MR imaging, and is not subject to magic angle artifact, which can limit MR evaluation as the tendons curve along their course. Anisotropy is one artifact which can be seen with US when the transducer is not oriented parallel to the structure being evaluated (**Fig. 1**). However, this artifact is easily avoided by rocking the transducer back and forth to alternately show a normal and anisotropic tendon. Normal ankle tendons are round or ovoid in the transverse plane with a speckled, hyperechoic appearance. In the longitudinal plane they demonstrate a fibrillar pattern or echogenic lines. This classic tendon echo signature is seen in all tendons of the body.

Hindfoot and midfoot tendon pathology is most often due to one or more of the following entities: tenosynovitis, tendinosis, and tendon tear. Subluxation and tendon dislocation are also possible, most commonly with the peroneal tendons. Tendinosis is seen as tendon thickening and may show diffuse or more focal regions of hypoechogenicity and loss of the normal fibrillar echotexture.[1] As with MR imaging, with sonography it may be difficult to distinguish tendinosis from low-grade partial thickness tear in some cases. The more severe the tendon thickening and echogenicity alteration, the more likely partial

tear is present.[20] Tenosynovitis is noted as increased fluid distending a tendon sheath, with or without hypervascular synovium surrounding the tendon. In the setting of an acute or subacute tendon tear, tenosynovitis is usually present and increases the conspicuity of a tear. Tenosynovitis may not be present in cases of chronic tendon tears. Normal fluid, in the range of 1 to 3 mm, can often be seen partially surrounding the tibialis posterior tendon, flexor digitorum longus, and flexor hallucis longus tendons. Such normal fluid is usually located in the dependent portion of the tendon sheath and at the level of the medial and lateral malleoli.[21]

Partial-thickness tears can be in the longitudinal plane ("longitudinal-type split") or in the transverse plane. Longitudinal splits are the more common type affecting the peroneal tendons and are not uncommonly seen affecting the tibialis posterior tendon as well.[17,22,23] Partial-thickness tears appear as a linear and in some cases globular region of hypoechogenicity, without evidence of retraction of the tendon.[16,17] The transverse plane usually provides the most optimal depiction of partial-thickness tears. Complete tendon rupture is seen as complete fiber disruption in the longitudinal plane, often with retraction of the torn tendon margins and absence of the tendon at the level of

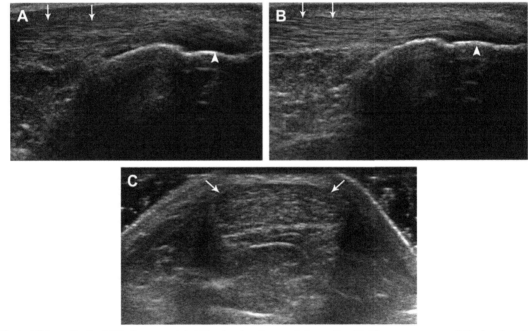

Fig. 1. (*A*) Longitudinal US of a normal Achilles tendon (*arrows*) shows the fibrillar appearance of the tendon. Hypoechogenicity consistent with anisotropy is noted at the insertion on the calcaneus (*arrowhead*). (*B*) Slight angulation of the transducer "fills-in" the hypoechoic region (*arrowhead*), confirming anisotropy. Arrows denote the normal Achilles tendon. (*C*) Transverse US of a normal Achilles tendon (*arrows*) shows the echogenic, fibrillar appearance of the normal tendon.

the defect in the transverse plane. Fluid, debris, and hematoma are often noted in the tendon gap in the setting of an acute tear, with hypoechoic granulation or scar tissue seen at this site in the setting of more chronic tears.

ACHILLES TENDON

Though the Achilles tendon is the strongest tendon in the body, it is also one of the most frequently injured. Often such injuries are sports related, a fitting irony given that the tendon's name is derived from the great Greek warrior, Achilles.[4,24] The Achilles is also unique because it is surrounded by a paratenon, a thin vascular membrane, rather than a synovial sheath as is seen surrounding the other ankle tendons. Therefore normal fluid is never seen adjacent to the Achilles tendon.[21] A spectrum of pathology can affect the Achilles tendon, ranging from acute or chronic peritendinitis, tendinosis, partial tears, and complete rupture. Tears usually occur in a relatively avascular zone located 2 to 6 cm above the calcaneal insertion, and less commonly at the insertion on the calcaneus.[4]

Numerous reports have used US to assess the Achilles tendon for peritendinitis, tendinosis, and tears.[15,20,25] Peritendinitis is demonstrated as ill-defined tendon margins with or without associated fluid and tendinosis (**Fig. 2**).[26] Tendinosis can be diffuse or focal and appears as hypoechogenicity with tendon thickening, usually with a fusiform-appearing tendon in the longitudinal plane (see **Fig. 2**).[20,27] In the transverse plane, tendinosis

may manifest as loss of the normal anterior concavity. Tendon calcifications may also be seen with tendinosis, both by US and radiography.[4] Partial-thickness tears of the Achilles tendon can be diagnosed by a well-defined anechoic or hypoechoic cleft affecting less than the complete cross section of the tendon. As with MR imaging, US may have difficulty distinguishing tendinosis from low- or moderate-grade partial tears; however, all of these entities are usually treated nonoperatively.[15] High-grade partial tears involving more than 50% of the tendon thickness and complete ruptures may be treated operatively or nonoperatively depending on the surgeon and clinical circumstances. Nonoperative treatment of complete ruptures is advocated by some surgeons, especially when the torn tendon ends are approximated or are less than 1 cm separated in plantar flexion (**Fig. 3**). Dynamic evaluation in dorsiflexion and plantar flexion can be easily performed with US and can directly impact patient management and outcome. Power Doppler evaluation showing hyperemia and neovascularization has been shown to correlate with pain severity but not with clinical outcome.[27]

Acute Achilles tendon rupture may be obvious by clinical examination, however it has been reported as missed in more than 20% of cases, likely due to pain and swelling limiting the clinical examination.[15] The gap between the torn tendon ends is often filled with hematoma and debris in the acute setting; and scar or fibrous tissue in more chronic cases.[4] An additional dynamic maneuver, the

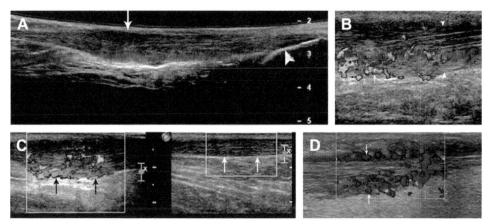

Fig. 2. (A) Longitudinal US of the distal Achilles tendon to the insertion on the calcaneus (arrowhead). The tendon is hypoechoic and enlarged (arrow) consistent with tendinosis. (B) Longitudinal US of the region of tendinosis shows hyperemia (arrows) of the Achilles tendon (between the arrowheads). (C) Split-screen longitudinal US of the hyperemic region of tendinosis with comparison to the contralateral normal Achilles tendon. The region of tendinosis (black arrows) demonstrates thickening and hypernemia compared to the opposite side (white arrows). (D) Longitudinal US of an Achilles tendon with hypoechogenicity (arrows) adjacent to the Achilles. The hypoechoic regions demonstrate hyperemia, consistent with peritendinitis.

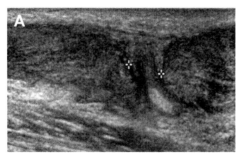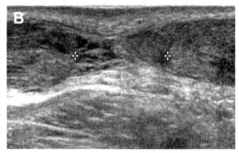

Fig. 3. (*A*) Longitudinal US of a ruptured Achilles tendon during plantar flexion shows less than 1 cm of separation between the torn tendon ends. The patient was successfully treated with casting in plantar flexion. (*B*) Same patient with longitudinal scanning in dorsiflexion shows increased separation and better delineation of the complete tendon rupture.

sonographic Thompson sign, can also be helpful. The calf is gently squeezed as the Achilles tendon is assessed for synchronous tendon movement from proximal to distal. With a complete tear, the proximal torn tendon end will retract proximally but the distal portion of the torn end will not.[4] The foot may also be manually moved from slight dorsiflexion to plantarflexion as an alternate method to show separation of torn tendon ends. Additional helpful signs of a complete tear are herniation of Kager's fat into the site of a tear (**Fig. 4**), refraction artifact (posterior acoustic shadowing) at the site of torn tendon ends (**Fig. 5**), and ease in visualizing the plantaris tendon, which is located medially and may herniate into the site of the tendon tear (**Fig. 6**).[15] An intact plantaris tendon, in the setting of a complete Achilles rupture, should not be mistaken for intact Achilles tendon fibers. Knowledge of the normal anatomy and awareness of this potential pitfall will prevent misdiagnosis.[28] It is also important to assess and report the presence and condition of the plantaris tendon since it may be harvested and used to help reinforce a surgical repair of the Achilles tendon.[29]

The retrocalcaneal bursa is located between the distal Achilles tendon and posterosuperior calcaneal tuberosity. The bursa is reportedly visible in 50% of normal ankles and may contain trace amounts of physiologic fluid, usually less than 3 mm in anteroposterior dimension.[21] This physiologic fluid can be unilateral or asymmetric with the contralateral ankle. Distention of the bursa is consistent with retrocalcaneal bursitis (**Fig. 7**), which may be isolated or seen with rheumatoid arthritis, Reiter's disease, or other seronegative arthritides. Retrocalcaneal bursitis can also be seen with Achilles tendon pathology and with Haglund's syndrome.[30] Much less commonly seen is retro Achilles or infracalcaneal bursitis which is located posterior to the Achilles tendon and may be seen in association with Haglund's syndrome (**Fig. 8**).

PERONEAL TENDONS

In experienced hands, US is highly accurate for imaging peroneal tendon tears and can be used as the first imaging test. A sensitivity of 100%, specificity of 85%, and accuracy of 90% is reported in the orthopedic literature, in comparison to surgical findings.[17] Tears of the peroneal tendons are usually of the longitudinal split type, with complete ruptures much less common. The peroneus brevis is more commonly affected, be it by tear, tenosynovitis, or tendinosis.[17,31] This is likely due to its location between the peroneus longus and the fibula, which allows the tendon to be pinched between these two structures. Longitudinal splits may be acute (most frequently in young patients), or chronic (most commonly in the elderly population). Chronic splits may be asymptomatic.[32] Peroneal splits and tears are usually located

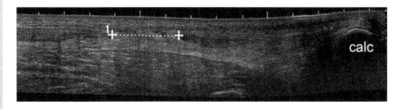

Fig. 4. Longitudinal US of a complete rupture of the Achilles tendon with 2.6 cm of separation between the torn tendon ends and herniation of echogenic Kager's fat into the site of the tear (*dotted line between the crosses*). Calc, calcaneus.

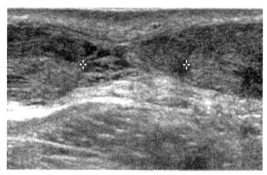

Fig. 5. Longitudinal US of the Achilles tendon with a complete rupture noted between the proximal tendon end (*single arrowhead*) and distal tendon end (*double arrowhead*). Refraction artifact is noted deep to the torn tendon ends (*arrows*).

at the level of the retromalleolar groove and are more frequently, but not exclusively, associated with injury to the superior peroneal retinaculum.[33,34] The axial plane is usually ideal for visualizing longitudinal splits as an anechoic or hypoechoic cleft (**Fig. 9**). The peroneus longus tendon often insinuates into the split, preventing healing.[4]

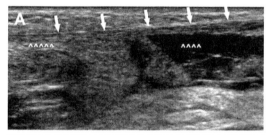

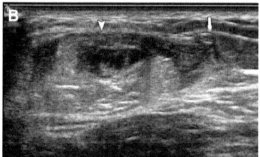

Fig. 6. (*A*) Longitudinal US of a complete rupture of the Achilles tendon. The five small arrowheads denote the proximal tendon end and the four small arrowheads denote debris at the site of the tendon tear. The intact plantaris tendon is noted extending through the site of the Achilles tear (*arrows*). (*B*) Transverse US at the site of the complete Achilles rupture demonstrates the plantaris tendon (*arrow*) and debris at the site of the Achilles tear (*arrowhead*).

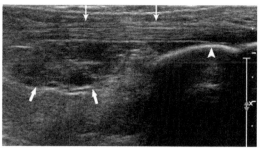

Fig. 7. Longitudinal US shows an intact Achilles tendon (*thin arrows*) to its insertion on the calcaneus (*arrowhead*). The retrocalcaneal bursa is distended and contains debris (*thick arrows*).

As with MR imaging, peroneal tears are more easily visualized when fluid is present distending the tendon sheath, as is usually present in the setting of an acute tear.[4] A potential pitfall that can mimic a peroneal split is the peroneus quartus. This accessory tendon, present in 10% to 20% of individuals, has a variable composition at its insertion, ranging from 100% tendon to predominately or completely muscle. It can be differentiated from a peroneal split by scanning to its distal insertion, usually onto the lateral aspect of the calcaneus (**Fig. 10**).[28,34]

A tear of the peroneus longus can occur in conjunction with a tear of the brevis, or in isolation.[31] Tears of the peroneus longus can occur at the level of the lateral malleolus, at the level of the os peroneum or cuboid groove, or at the level of the midfoot.[4] The os peroneum is located within the peroneus longus tendon. When the ossicle fractures and significantly separates or displaces, the result is usually equivalent to a rupture of the peroneus longus, with retraction of the proximal portion of the fractured os, and often associated peroneal tendon tears.[35]

While tenosynovitis and tendinosis are more common than tendon tears, these entities usually do not require surgical treatment.[4] Tenosynovitis

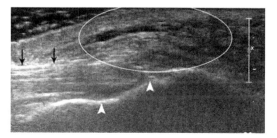

Fig. 8. Longitudinal US shows an intact Achilles tendon (*black arrows*) to its insertion on the calcaneus (*arrowheads*). The retro-Achilles bursa is distended and contains debris (*region within the ellipse*).

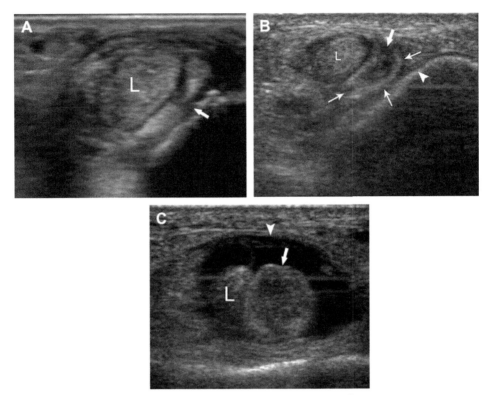

Fig. 9. (A) Transverse US shows a longitudinal split in the peroneus brevis tendon creating two separate portions of the brevis (arrow) at the level of the lateral malleolus. (B) Transverse US from a different patient shows a longitudinal split (thick arrow) in the peroneus brevis tendon (thin arrows) at the level of the lateral malleolus (arrowhead). (C) Transverse US from a different patient shows marked enlargement and internal hypoechogenicity of the peroneus brevis tendon (arrow) with surrounding tenosynovitis (arrowhead). L, peroneus longus tendon.

is noted as fluid which completely surrounds the peroneal tendons, while normal fluid is smaller in amount, dependently located, and not circumferential.[21] Peroneal tenosynovitis is more common in the athletic population, in acute inversion injuries, and ankle instability.[4,36] If peroneal tenosynovitis is identified, special care should be taken to examine the calcaneofibular ligament, since injury to this ligament can permit pathologic communication of joint fluid into the peroneal tendon sheath.[4]

Several factors have been reported to predispose to peroneal tendon pathology, including anatomic variants such as a peroneus quartus muscle or low-lying peroneal muscle belly. Such variants may cause crowding of the peroneal tendons and promote subluxation. Likewise a flat or convex (rather than concave) retromalleolar groove can also promote subluxation. Hypertrophy of the calcaneal peroneal tubercle or retrotrochlear eminence can abrade the peroneal tendons. Acquired conditions can also predispose to peroneal pathology, the most common being injury to the superior peroneal retinaculum.[34]

Additional factors predisposing to peroneal pathology include tarsal coalition, hardware such as orthopedic screws impinging upon the tendons (**Fig. 11**), and fibular or calcaneal osseous spurs.[4,37]

SUBLUXATION AND DISLOCATION OF THE PERONEAL TENDONS

The peroneal tendons may partially displace (subluxate) or completely displace (dislocate) from their normal position posterior to the fibula. In most cases such abnormal tendon movement occurs intermittently and is not directly visualized by static MR imaging. Only dynamic US can directly visualize the tendons as they subluxate or dislocate laterally and anteriorly over the lateral malleolus. Such subluxation or dislocation is most often posttraumatic, due to dorsiflexion and eversion injury. Typically the superior peroneal retinaculum is injured, allowing recurrent dislocation and leading to tendinosis and tendon tear. Dynamic evaluation of the peroneal tendons adds only a few seconds to the standard ankle US

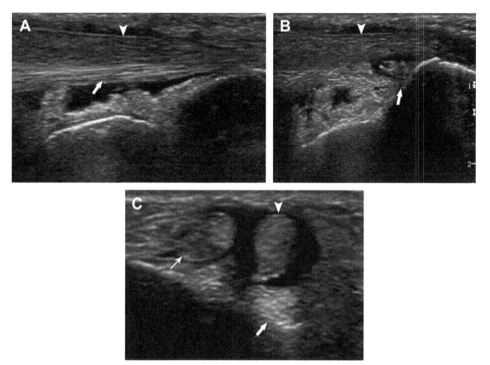

Fig. 10. (A) Longitudinal US shows a peroneus quartus tendon (arrow) deep to the peroneus brevis tendon (arrowhead). Surrounding tenosynovitis is noted. (B) Longitudinal scanning more distally shows the insertion of the peroneus quartus on to the lateral aspect of the calcaneus (arrow) with the peroneus brevis noted more superficially (arrowhead). (C) Transverse US shows the peroneus quartus (thick arrow) deep to the brevis (arrowhead). The peroneus longus is denoted by the thin arrow. Note tenosynovitis.

examination. The probe is placed transverse to the tendons, at the level of the retromalleolar groove and the foot is dorsiflexed and everted.[23] The brevis more commonly dislocates, although one or both of the peroneal tendons can dislocate (Fig. 12).[3,4,23]

The peroneal tendons can also remain behind the fibula, in the retromalleolar groove, but transiently "switch" positions during inversion and eversion (Fig. 13). This entity has been termed "retromalleolar intrasheath subluxation." It may be symptomatic and surgically treated, or

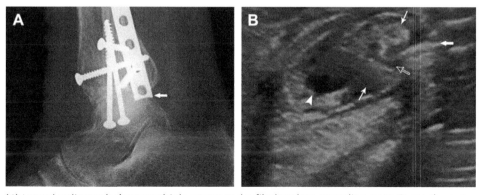

Fig. 11. (A) Lateral radiograph shows multiple screws and a fibular plate extending posterior to the cortex of the fibula (arrow). (B) Transverse US at the level of the lateral fibular plate shows a split (open arrow) creating two portions of the peroneus brevis (thin white arrows) adjacent to the fibular plate (thick white arrow). The arrowhead denotes a small amount of fluid adjacent to the peroneus longus tendon.

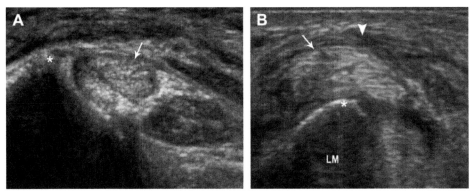

Fig. 12. (A) Transverse US shows the peroneal normal peroneal tendons (arrow) posterior to the distal fibula. Asterisk denotes the lateral aspect of the fibula. (B) Transverse US shows the peroneus longus (arrow) dislocated lateral to the fibula (asterisk) when the ankle is dorsiflexed and everted. Note detached superior peroneal retinaculum (arrowhead). LM, lateral malleolus.

asymptomatic.[23] This entity again requires a dynamic imaging modality which, for all practical purposes, is only possible with US.

MEDIAL TENDONS

The posterior tibialis tendon (PTT) is also a commonly injured tendon. It serves as a primary inverter of the foot and is an important component of the medial longitudinal arch. When the PTT is ruptured or injured, flatfoot deformity can result. Rupture is, however, less common than tendinosis and partial tears. PTT pathology often begins as tenosynovitis, followed by partial tear and then complete rupture. Early diagnosis and treatment is the key to preventing severe disability.[38] The accuracy of US for detecting PTT abnormalities is comparable to MR imaging.[16,18,19,39] The os tibiale externum or os naviculare has been reported to be associated with PTT pathology. This is likely due to mechanical strain from altered tendon mechanics.[40]

As with the peroneal tendons, most pathology involving the PTT is at the level of the malleolus (Fig. 14). Less commonly, pathology is at the level of the navicular insertion since the tendon has multiple strong slips that fan out and insert broadly over the navicular and plantar aspect of the tarsal bones. Dislocation of the PTT is extremely rare.[41] A unique feature of US is the ability to identify small spurs or cortical irregularity in the medial malleolar groove (Fig. 15). Such spurs can abrade the tendon and can be a difficult diagnosis with MR imaging or CT due to their small size and low signal on MR imaging. With US, direct sonographic and clinical correlation is available for pain or symptoms related to a possible tendon abnormality. Normally the axial diameter of the posterior tibial tendon is approximately twice that of the flexor digitorum longus (FDL) tendon.[4] This "rule of

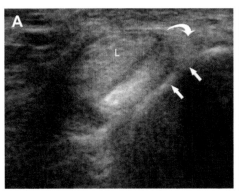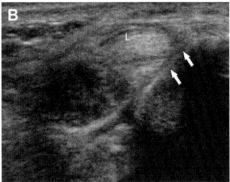

Fig. 13. (A) Transverse US shows the peroneal tendons in their normal location when the ankle is in neutral position. Curved arrow denotes the direction the peroneus longus will move to result in (B). Arrows denote the cortex of the fibular groove. (B) When the ankle is dorsiflexed and everted, the peroneus longus moves anteriorly, adjacent to the fibular cortex (arrows). L, peroneus longus.

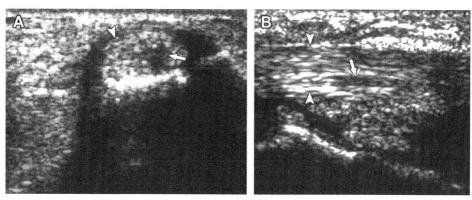

Fig.14. (*A*) Transverse US shows the tibialis posterior tendon (*arrowhead*) with a hypoechoic region extending to the deep surface of the tendon (*arrow*). (*B*) Longitudinal US of the posterior tibial tendon (*between the arrows*) shows a corresponding linear region of hypoechogenicity. Findings are consistent with a longitudinal split of the tibialis posterior tendon.

thumb" allows quick assessment of tendon thickening, as seen with tendinosis, or the thinning that can be seen in some partial tears.

A potential pitfall can occur with a complete rupture of the PTT. In this setting the FDL may be displaced anteriorly and potentially be confused with an intact PTT.[28] Making note that each individual tendon is located in its normal position prevents this potential pitfall. The PTT normally has multiple slips at its navicular and plantar insertion and these should not be mistaken for a longitudinal split. The tendon normally curves as it inserts, and in this region it may look artifactually hypoechoic due to anisotropy. Again, direct correlation with symptoms during scanning of this region aids correct diagnosis.[4]

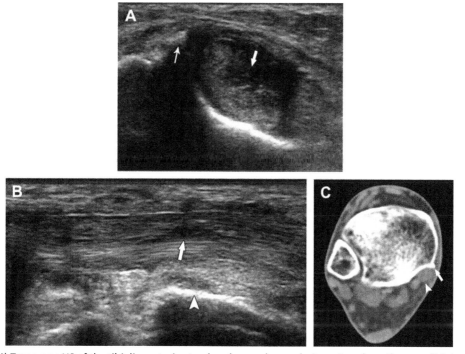

Fig.15. (*A*) Transverse US of the tibialis posterior tendon shows a hypoechoic region along the superficial aspect of the tendon (*thick arrow*) with a spur at the anterior aspect of the medial malleolar groove (*thin arrow*). (*B*) Longitudinal US of the tibialis posterior tendon shows a corresponding linear region of hypoechogenicity (*arrow*) consistent with a longitudinal split. Arrowhead denotes the medial malleolus. (*C*) Axial CT in soft tissue windows demonstrates the osseous spur (*arrow*) at the anterior aspect of the tibialis posterior tendon (*arrowhead*).

While pathology of the FDL is extremely rare, pathology affecting the flexor hallucis longus (FHL) can be seen, especially in individuals involved in ballet, soccer, or basketball.[4] Friction injuries can affect the FHL as it courses beneath the sustentaculum tali and through the fibro osseous tarsal tunnel. Tenosynovitis, stenosing tenosynovitis, and tendinosis can result.[4] An os trigonum and adjacent osseous spurs have been reported to be predisposing factors for FHL pathology. The depth of the FHL can make sonographic evaluation challenging; however, dynamic maneuvers such as actively or passively flexing the great toe can aid in identification and evaluation.[4]

ANTERIOR TENDONS

The anterior tendons are the least commonly involved by pathology compared with the medial, lateral, and Achilles tendons. Of the three extensor tendons, the tibialis anterior tendon (ATT) is the most commonly involved by pathology. Though tears of the ATT are uncommon, they classically present with a history of "mass" and evaluation reveals not a mass but rather a torn and retracted tendon (**Fig. 16**). ATT tears typically occur within 3 cm of its insertion.[42] Causes of ATT injury include abrasion by impinging osteophytes from the first tarsal metatarsal joint or talonavicular joint, or from impinging hardware after surgery.[42,43] Impingement may only be noted during dynamic maneuvers such as plantar flexion. US is well suited for such dynamic evaluation. Tendon laceration can occur from penetrating trauma and very rarely from fracture.[44] Discontinuity of the tendon fibers and retraction of the torn tendon ends are noted with US when an ATT rupture is present. A longitudinal "split" of the distal ATT has been noted on MR imaging in asymptomatic volunteers and may be a normal variant as the tendon inserts, similar to the PPT insertion onto the navicular and plantar midfoot.[42]

Tendinosis of the anterior tibial tendon is noted as thickening of the tendon less than or equal to 5 mm at the level of the tarsal bones.[42] Pathology of the extensor hallucis longus and extensor digitorum longus tendons is less common, compared with the ATT and has been described secondary to ill-fitting shoes or impinging osteophytes. The extensor digitorum longus tendon may be abraded by an osseous ridge at the dorsal aspect of the talus.[37] This can also be the site of a ganglion cyst (see *Masses* below).

LIGAMENTS

Injury to ankle ligaments is by far the most common type of ankle pathology. A traumatic inversion force is the typical mechanism of injury. The lateral ligaments are most frequently torn; among the components of the lateral collateral ligament complex, the anterior taloficular ligament is most commonly torn. In most cases, ankle ligament ruptures can be diagnosed with high accuracy by physical examination alone.[45] In acute cases with equivocal diagnosis, or in chronic

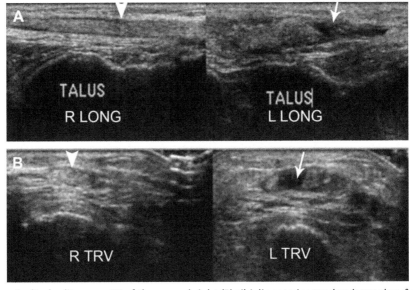

Fig. 16. (*A*) Longitudinal split screen US of the normal right (R) tibialis anterior tendon (*arrowhead*) and ruptured left (L) tibialis anterior tendon (*arrow*). (*B*) Transverse split screen US of the normal right tibialis anterior tendon (*arrowhead*) and ruptured left tibialis anterior tendon (*arrow*).

cases with persistent symptoms, US can play a role. In some cases surgical treatment may be needed, with reconstruction of the ligaments to stabilize the ankle and restore pain-free function.[4]

Normal ankle ligaments have a fibrillar echotexture and are sharply marginated, (**Fig. 17**).[46] Anisotropy can be seen with ankle ligaments. As with tendon imaging, this potential artifact is avoided by scanning with the ultrasound beam perpendicular to the ligament. Mild sprain is noted as slight thickening or loss of the normally fibrillar echotexture (**Fig. 18**). With partial tear there is discontinuity of the ligament but it remains taut with dynamic maneuvers that place the ligament under tension. With complete tear, a hypoechoic gap is noted and the ligament fibers do not become taut with any maneuver (**Fig. 19**).[47] Osseous avulsion at a ligament attachment site denotes a severe ligament injury.[47] Chronic tears that have undergone scarring may demonstrate thickening of the ligament. Ossification may also be noted within such ligaments.[4] Using a 13-MHz transducer, the reported sonographic accuracy for evaluating the status of the anterior talofibular ligament is 90% to100%; calcaneofibular ligament, 87% to 92%; and anterior tibiofibular ligament, 85% when compared with MR imaging.[46]

When the anterior talofibular ligament is injured, the calcaneofibular ligament should be carefully assessed since sequential injury of the lateral ligaments, from anterior to posterior, is almost always the norm. The anterior talofibular ligament is examined dynamically during plantar flexion and during inversion stress, or using the anterior drawer test.[4] Lateral talar process fracture can also be assessed when scanning the anterior talofibular ligament by sweeping the probe clockwise to assess the lateral aspect of the talus.[48] The calcaneofibular ligament can be examined dynamically during dorsiflexion with inversion. The peroneal tendons are located immediately

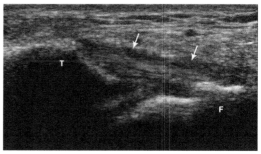

Fig. 18. Longitudinal US of a hypoechoic and thickened anterior talofibular ligament (*arrows*) consistent with sprain. F, fibula; T, talus.

superficial to the calcaneofibular ligament (**Fig. 20**). As noted previously, fluid in the peroneal tendon sheath should prompt careful assessment of the calcaneofibular ligament since ligament injury can allow communication with the peroneal tendon sheath. Visualization of the proximal attachment of the calcaneofibular ligament may be limited by sonography secondary to its position deep to the lateral malleolus.[4]

The anterior tibiofibular ligament is injured in cases of "high ankle sprain." For dynamic imaging, the ankle is placed in dorsiflexion and varus.[4] The deltoid ligament is much less commonly injured but can be examined dynamically with dorsiflexion and eversion stress (**Fig. 21**).[46] If acute deltoid ligament injury is suspected, the lateral malleolus should be assessed for associated fracture and the anterior tibiofibular ligament for associated injury.[47]

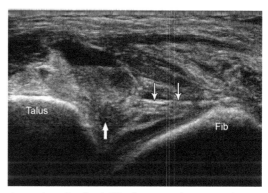

Fig. 19. Longitudinal US of an acutely ruptured anterior talofibular ligament. Thick arrow denotes the site of rupture, at the talar attachment with surrounding hematoma. Thin arrows denote the more normal portion of the ligament at its fibular attachment. Fib, fibula.

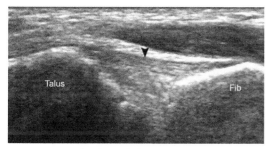

Fig. 17. Longitudinal US of the normal anterior talofibular ligament (*arrowhead*). The normal ligament is echogenic and of uniform thickness. F, fibula.

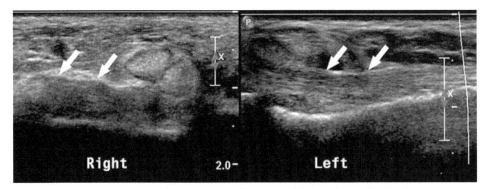

Fig. 20. Longitudinal split screen US of a patient with a normal left calcaneofibular ligament (*arrows*) and a ruptured right calcaneofibular ligament (*arrows*). Note the calcaneofibular ligament is located immediately deep to the round, echogenic peroneal tendons.

ANKLE JOINT PATHOLOGY

US is well suited for rapid evaluation of joint fluid and can also guide aspiration.[49] It has been reported that static US can detect as little as 2 mL of ankle fluid, versus 1 mL for MR imaging of the ankle.[50] Dynamic maneuvers, such as scanning during dorsiflexion and plantar flexion may aid detection of smaller amounts of fluid. Simple joint fluid appears as anechoic distention of the anterior joint capsule (**Fig. 22**). More complex joint fluid may appear sonographically similar to synovitis. Dynamic maneuvers, including scanning during dorsiflexion and plantar flexion and during compression of the joint capsule by the transducer, can aid evaluation. With dynamic maneuvers, collapse of the joint capsule and visualization of swirling hypoechoic fluid, and joint recess compressibility favors complex joint fluid rather than synovitis. If the complex intra-articular region demonstrates internal flow on Doppler evaluation, the findings are consistent with synovitis or an intra-articular mass such as pigmented villonodular synovitis. Intra-articular bodies can be accurately detected with US and appear as hyperechoic foci, usually with surrounding fluid. The sonographic sensitivity and specificity for detection of intra-articular bodies has been reported to be 100% and 95% respectively.[51]

PLANTAR FASCIITIS

While plantar fasciitis is often diagnosed clinically, US can be helpful, especially in chronic cases or those recalcitrant to conservative therapies. Plantar fasciitis is the most common cause of heel pain and can be found in young athletes as well as obese and elderly patients.[4,52] The reported sensitivity and specificity of sonography is 80% and 89% compared with MR imaging.[53] The high prevalence of this condition, combined with the expense of MR imaging, may favor US imaging in many cases.

The normal plantar fascia appears as a fibrillar band measuring 3 to 4 mm in thickness. With plantar fasciitis, fascia is hypoechoic and greater than 5 mm in thickness at the calcaneal attachment (**Fig. 23**).[54,55]

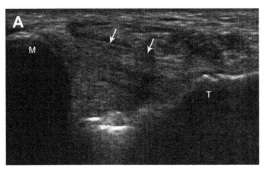
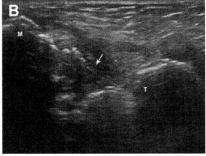

Fig. 21. (*A*) Longitudinal US of a normal deltoid ligament (*arrows*) with components noted coursing from the medial malleolus to the talus. (*B*) Longitudinal US of a torn deltoid ligament with wavy, echogenic fibers retracted from the talar insertion (*arrow*). M, medial malleolus; T, talus.

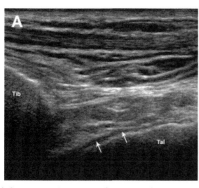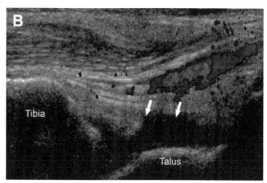

Fig. 22. (*A*) Longitudinal US of a normal anterior tibiotalar joint without detectable fluid. Arrows denote the hypoechoic cartilage of the talus. Tal, talus; Tib, tibia. (*B*) Longitudinal US of a joint effusion at the anterior tibiotalar joint (*arrows*). Note Doppler flow in the more superficial dorsalis pedis artery.

Rupture of the plantar fascia is much less common but occurs in a similar patient population.[4] Location of these entities is different, with fasciitis at the calcaneal attachment and plantar fascial ruptures at the proximal or middle portion of the fascia. Acute fascial tears are noted as disruption of the fibers with surrounding or intervening fluid. The plantar fascia can be dynamically assessed by extending the toes dorsally, potentially aiding conspicuity of fascial tears.[4] The differential diagnosis of plantar heel pain also includes a foreign body, which is well assessed with US (see foreign bodies below).

MASSES

US can diagnostically evaluate the most common ankle masses, such as a ganglion cyst, nerve sheath tumor, abscess, and aneurysm; and aid diagnosis of other masses. Specific features which aid diagnosis of a mass include location, relationship to adjacent vessels, nerves, joints and tendons, internal blood flow with Doppler evaluation, and compressibility.[43] Dynamic evaluation

during joint motion can also be helpful in some cases, such as differentiating joint fluid, which moves with joint motion, from an adjacent ganglion which does not.

Ganglion cysts are often multiloculated and my have internal septations. A neck or communication with an adjacent tendon sheath or joint may be seen and should be searched for diligently to aid surgical resection. Ganglia can be anechoic or, in some cases, hypoechoic and may contain internal debris (**Fig. 24**).[56,57] They are well defined, with no internal Doppler flow.[56,58] An adventitial "medial malleolar bursa" can be seen at the medial malleolus, most commonly seen in ice skaters or hockey players, and thought to be due to poorly fitting footwear.[59]

Infection of the soft tissues of the hindfoot and midfoot ranges from cellulitis to abscess. Subcutaneous edema is noted as a reticular pattern of hypoechogenicity in the subcutaneous tissues. Clinical correlation is required to separate edema from cellulitis. Soft tissue gas can be seen with an infectious process, sinus tract, or secondary to surgery or intervention. Gas is noted as a focus

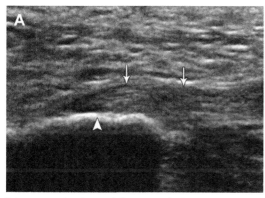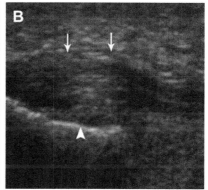

Fig. 23. (*A*) Longitudinal US of the normal plantar fascia (*arrows*) at the calcaneal origin (*arrowhead*). (*B*) US of plantar fascitis shows the hypoechoic and thickened plantar fascia (*arrows*) at the calcaneal origin (*arrowhead*).

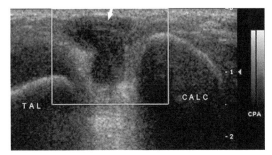

Fig. 24. Transverse US at the lateral ankle shows a hypoechoic ganglion cyst between the calcaneus (calc) and talus (tal). Note the absence of internal Doppler flow.

of hyperechogenicity which may also show comet-tail artifact.[43] An abscess can appear hyperechoic or hypoechoic, often with an echogenic rim and overlying skin thickening. An abscess may demonstrate surrounding hyperemia but does not have internal Doppler flow. Swirling of complex fluid may be seen with transducer pressure. US can also aid aspiration.[49]

Nerve sheath tumors appear as a well-defined fusiform mass, with hypoechoic or mixed echogenicity. They may demonstrate internal hyperemia. Schwannomas and neurofibromas may exhibit a sonographic "target sign" with central hypoechogenicity and peripheral hypoechogenicity.[58] An entering or exiting nerve is a key discriminator and can separate a nerve sheath tumor from other more nonspecific masses.

Lipomas can have characteristic US imaging features including a well-defined ovoid shape parallel to the skin surface, relative hyperechogenicity, and absence of internal blood flow on Doppler evaluation.[58] While the sonographic appearance overlaps with that of other masses,

in the context of a long-standing, stable, and pliable mass, the diagnosis can be inferred with follow-up to assure stability. MR imaging is diagnostic for a lipoma and can be obtained for corroboration as needed.

An aneurysm, while rare in the hindfoot or midfoot, has also been described.[43] Ultrasound is well-suited to evaluate an aneurysm and can easily and rapidly identify the mass as originating from a vessel. Doppler evaluation should be used and can demonstrate a focal or fusiform enlargement of the vessel. Several additional uncommon ankle masses have been described by ultrasound including a glomus tumor, epidermal inclusion cyst, and subcutaneous granuloma annulare.[58] Like many masses which are evaluated with MR imaging, these masses have a nonspecific sonographic appearance.

FOREIGN BODIES

Foreign bodies are relatively common in the foot. Ultrasound has shown sensitivity and specificity of 90% to100% for detection of foreign bodies in multiple cadaveric and clinical studies.[60–63] The smallest reported foreign body detected by US is 0.5 mm.[64] False negatives are unusual but can potentially occur if the foreign body is very small, located adjacent to a bone or ligament, or is obscured by soft tissue gas. False positives are also rare but can potentially be seen secondary to echogenic gas bubbles, calcifications, or echogenic scar tissue.[62] Whenever possible, radiographs should be reviewed before US to assess for associated osseous and soft tissue findings. It is optimal to perform US before surgical exploration since soft tissue gas can cause an artifact that limits the sonographic evaluation by obscuring or simulating a foreign body. Tissue harmonics, an

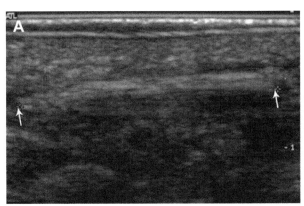
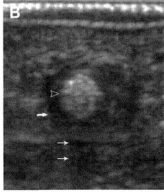

Fig. 25. (A) Longitudinal US of a wooden foreign body (between the arrows) in the foot. (B) Transverse US of the foreign body (arrowhead) with a surrounding hypoechoic halo (thick arrow) and posterior acoustic shadowing (thin arrows).

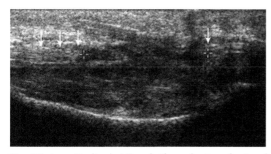

Fig. 26. Longitudinal US of the plantar foot of a patient who stepped on a piece of glass. The flexor hallucis longus tendon has been lacerated and is retracted proximally. The three arrows denote the proximal end of the ruptured tendon and the single arrowhead the distal end of the tendon. The tendon was surgically repaired.

optimal scanning mode used in abdominal ultrasound, may decrease the conspicuity and shadowing of the foreign body and should be used with caution when assessing for a foreign body.[65] In general, we do not find tissue harmonics to be of great utility in musculoskeletal ultrasound.

All foreign bodies appear echogenic, regardless of their composition.[66] A hypoechoic surrounding halo[62] may be noted, as well as variable posterior shadowing (Fig. 25). These features can aid

detection and diagnosis, especially of small foreign bodies. Doppler interrogation should always be used when evaluating foreign bodies and can aid detection of the foreign body which may be seen as an echogenic structure surrounded by hyperemia. Low-velocity Doppler settings should be used.[62] Doppler evaluation can help differentiate fluid (no Doppler flow) from phlegmonous tissue (may demonstrate Doppler flow). The presence of a foreign body should prompt a diligent search for associated complications such as tendon or neurovascular injury (Fig. 26). Associated findings such as tenosynovitis, joint effusion, abscess (Fig. 27), and periostitis should prompt immediate notification of the referring clinician so that timely treatment for infection can be instituted.

SUMMARY

US offers several advantages for imaging the hind and midfoot, including its unique capacity to allow evaluation during dynamic maneuvers. This feature can reveal abnormalities that are not apparent during static imaging. US permits imaging of patients who cannot undergo MR imaging and provides real-time evaluation of the symptomatic site. Additional history can be obtained from the patient during US evaluation and the contralateral anatomy can be quickly assessed as needed. US has demonstrated great utility and accuracy for imaging the hindfoot and midfoot, including tendon, ligament, joint, and soft tissue pathology. It is imperative that radiologists provide expertise in all aspects of musculoskeletal imaging, including US.

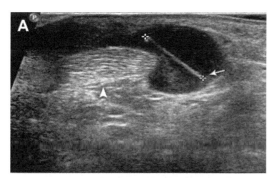

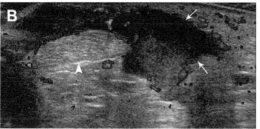

Fig. 27. (A) US performed transverse to the Achilles tendon (arrowhead) shows an abscess superficial to the Achilles with a linear echogenic foreign body (arrow, between the cursors). (B) Transverse US performed at an adjacent level with Doppler demonstrates hyperemia surrounding the abscess (arrows). Arrowhead denotes the Achilles tendon.

REFERENCES

1. Jacobson JA. Ultrasound clinics. Philadelphia: W.B. Saunders Company; 2007. p. 765.
2. Jacobson JA. Fundamentals of musculoskeletal ultrasound. Philadelphia: Saunders Elsevier; 2007. 345.
3. Khoury V, Cardinal E, Bureau NJ. Musculoskeletal sonography: a dynamic tool for usual and unusual disorders. AJR Am J Roentgenol 2007;188:W63–73.
4. Khoury V, Guillin R, Dhanju J, et al. Ultrasound of ankle and foot: overuse and sports injuries. Semin Musculoskelet Radiol 2007;11:149–61.
5. Bianchi S, Martinoli C, Gaignot C, et al. Ultrasound of the ankle: anatomy of the tendons, bursae, and ligaments. Semin Musculoskelet Radiol 2005;9:243–59.
6. Erickson SJ. High-resolution imaging of the musculoskeletal system. Radiology 1997;205:593–618.

7. Parker L, Nazarian LN, Carrino JA, et al. Musculoskeletal imaging: medicare use, costs, and potential for cost substitution. J Am Coll Radiol 2008;5:182–8.

8. Nazarian LN. The top 10 reasons musculoskeletal sonography is an important complementary or alternative technique to MRI. AJR Am J Roentgenol 2008;190:1621–6.

9. Lew HL, Chen CP, Wang TG, et al. Introduction to musculoskeletal diagnostic ultrasound: examination of the upper limb. Am J Phys Med Rehabil 2007; 86:310–21.

10. Chew K, Stevens KJ, Wang TG, et al. Introduction to diagnostic musculoskeletal ultrasound: part 2: examination of the lower limb. Am J Phys Med Rehabil 2008;87:238–48.

11. Brown AK, O'Connor PJ, Roberts TE, et al. Recommendations for musculoskeletal ultrasonography by rheumatologists: setting global standards for best practice by expert consensus. Arthritis Rheum 2005;53:83–92.

12. Grassi W, Filippucci E. Ultrasonography and the rheumatologist. Curr Opin Rheumatol 2007;19:55–60.

13. Legome E, Pancu D. Future applications for emergency ultrasound. Emerg Med Clin North Am 2004;22:817–27.

14. Rawool NM, Nazarian LN. Ultrasound of the ankle and foot. Semin Ultrasound CT MR 2000;21:275–84.

15. Hartgerink P, Fessell DP, Jacobson JA, et al. Full-versus partial-thickness Achilles tendon tears: sonographic accuracy and characterization in 26 cases with surgical correlation. Radiology 2001;220: 406–12.

16. Waitches GM, Rockett M, Brage M, et al. Ultrasonographic-surgical correlation of ankle tendon tears. J Ultrasound Med 1998;17:249–56.

17. Grant TH, Kelikian AS, Jereb SE, et al. Ultrasound diagnosis of peroneal tendon tears. A surgical correlation. J Bone Joint Surg Am 2005;87:1788–94.

18. Chen YJ, Liang SC. Diagnostic efficacy of ultrasonography in stage I posterior tibial tendon dysfunction: sonographic–surgical correlation. J Ultrasound Med 1997;16:417–23.

19. Gerling MC, Pfirrmann CW, Farooki S, et al. Posterior tibialis tendon tears: comparison of the diagnostic efficacy of magnetic resonance imaging and ultrasonography for the detection of surgically created longitudinal tears in cadavers. Invest Radiol 2003;38:51–6.

20. Astrom M, Gentz CF, Nilsson P, et al. Imaging in chronic Achilles tendinopathy: a comparison of ultrasonography, magnetic resonance imaging and surgical findings in 27 histologically verified cases. Skeletal Radiol 1996;25:615–20.

21. Nazarian LN, Rawool NM, Martin CE, et al. Synovial fluid in the hindfoot and ankle: detection of amount and distribution with US. Radiology 1995;197:275–8.

22. Diaz GC, van Holsbeeck M, Jacobson JA. Longitudinal split of the peroneus longus and peroneus

23. Neustadter J, Raikin SM, Nazarian LN. Dynamic sonographic evaluation of peroneal tendon subluxation. AJR Am J Roentgenol 2004;183:985–8.

24. Kannus P, Natri A. Etiology and pathophysiology of tendon ruptures in sports. Scand J Med Sci Sports 1997;7:107–12.

25. Paavola M, Paakkala T, Kannus P, et al. Ultrasonography in the differential diagnosis of Achilles tendon injuries and related disorders. A comparison between pre-operative ultrasonography and surgical findings. Acta Radiol 1998;39:612–9.

26. Kainberger FM, Engel A, Barton P, et al. Injury of the Achilles tendon: diagnosis with sonography. Am J Roentgenol 1990;155:1031–6.

27. Zanetti M, Metzdorf A, Kundert HP, et al. Achilles tendons: clinical relevance of neovascularization diagnosed with power Doppler US. Radiology 2003;227:556–60.

28. Patel S, Fessell DP, Jacobson JA, et al. Artifacts, anatomic variants, and pitfalls in sonography of the foot and ankle. AJR Am J Roentgenol 2002;178: 1247–54.

29. Lui TH. Endoscopic-assisted Achilles tendon repair with plantaris tendon augmentation. Arthroscopy 2007;23:556.e551–5.

30. Lee JC, Calder JD, Healy JC. Posterior impingement syndromes of the ankle. Semin Musculoskelet Radiol 2008;12:154–69.

31. Saxena A, Cassidy A. Peroneal tendon injuries: an evaluation of 49 tears in 41 patients. J Foot Ankle Surg 2003;42:215–20.

32. Sammarco GJ. Peroneal tendon injuries. Orthop Clin North Am 1994;25:135–45.

33. Sobel M, Geppert MJ, Olson EJ, et al. The dynamics of peroneus brevis tendon splits: a proposed mechanism, technique of diagnosis, and classification of injury. Foot Ankle 1992;13:413–22.

34. Wang XT, Rosenberg ZS, Mechlin MB, et al. Normal variants and diseases of the peroneal tendons and superior peroneal retinaculum: MR imaging features. Radiographics 2005;25:587–602.

35. Brigido MK, Fessell DP, Jacobson JA, et al. Radiography and US of os peroneum fractures and associated peroneal tendon injuries: initial experience. Radiology 2005;237:235–41.

36. Gray JM, Alpar EK. Peroneal tenosynovitis following ankle sprains. Injury 2001;32:487–9.

37. Shetty M, Fessell DP, Femino JE, et al. Sonography of ankle tendon impingement with surgical correlation. AJR Am J Roentgenol 2002;179:949–53.

38. Johnson KA, Strom DE. Tibialis posterior tendon dysfunction. Clin Orthop Relat Res 1989;239: 196–206.

39. Nallamshetty L, Nazarian LN, Schweitzer ME, et al. Evaluation of posterior tibial pathology: comparison

brevis tendons with disruption of the superior peroneal retinaculum. J Ultrasound Med 1998;17:525–9.

of sonography and MR imaging. Skeletal Radiol 2005;34:375–80.

40. Schweitzer ME, Caccese R, Karasick D, et al. Posterior tibial tendon tears: utility of secondary signs for MR imaging diagnosis. Radiology 1993;188:655–9.

41. Ouzounian TJ, Myerson MS. Dislocation of the posterior tibial tendon. Foot Ankle 1992;13:215–9.

42. Mengiardi B, Pfirrmann CWA, Vienne P, et al. Anterior tibial tendon abnormalities: MR imaging findings. Radiology 2005;235:977–84.

43. Fessell DP, Jamadar DA, Jacobson JA, et al. Sonography of dorsal ankle and foot abnormalities. AJR Am J Roentgenol 2003;181:1573–81.

44. Din R, Therkilsden L. Rupture of tibialis anterior associated with a closed midshaft tibial fracture. J Accid Emerg Med 1999;16:459.

45. van Dijk CN, Mol BW, Lim LS, et al. Diagnosis of ligament rupture of the ankle joint. Physical examination, arthrography, stress radiography and sonography compared in 160 patients after inversion trauma. Acta Orthop Scand 1996;67:566–70.

46. Peetrons P, Creteur V, Bacq C. Sonography of ankle ligaments. J Clin Ultrasound 2004;32:491–9.

47. Morvan G, Busson J, Wybier M, et al. Ultrasound of the ankle. Eur J Ultrasound 2001;14:73–82.

48. Copercini M, Bonvin F, Martinoli C, et al. Sonographic diagnosis of talar lateral process fracture. J Ultrasound Med 2003;22:635–40.

49. Fessell DP, van Holsbeeck M. Ultrasound guided musculoskeletal procedures. In: Jacobson JA, editor. Ultrasound clinics. Philadelphia: W.B. Saunders Company; 2007. p. 737–57.

50. Jacobson JA, Andresen R, Jaovisidha S, et al. Detection of ankle effusions: comparison study in cadavers using radiography, sonography, and MR imaging. AJR Am J Roentgenol 1998;170:1231–8.

51. Frankel DA, Bargiela A, Bouffard JA, et al. Synovial joints: evaluation of intraarticular bodies with US. Radiology 1998;206:41–4.

52. Schepsis AA, Leach RE, Gorzyca J. Plantar fasciitis. Etiology, treatment, surgical results, and review of the literature. Clin Orthop Relat Res 1991;266: 185–96.

53. Sabir N, Demirlenk S, Yagci B, et al. Clinical utility of sonography in diagnosing plantar fasciitis. J Ultrasound Med 2005;24:1041–8.

54. Kane D, Greaney T, Shanahan M, et al. The role of ultrasonography in the diagnosis and management of idiopathic plantar fasciitis. Rheumatology 2001; 40:1002–8.

55. Cardinal E, Chhem RK, Beauregard CG, et al. Plantar fasciitis: sonographic evaluation. Radiology 1996;201:257–9.

56. Ortega R, Fessell DP, Jacobson JA, et al. Sonography of ankle Ganglia with pathologic correlation in 10 pediatric and adult patients. AJR Am J Roentgenol 2002;178:1445–9.

57. Wang G, Jacobson JA, Feng FY, et al. Sonography of wrist ganglion cysts: variable and noncystic appearances. J Ultrasound Med 2007;26:1323–8 [quiz: 1330–21].

58. Pham H, Fessell DP, Femino JE, et al. Sonography and MR imaging of selected benign masses in the ankle and foot. AJR Am J Roentgenol 2003;180: 99–107.

59. Brown RR, Sadka Rosenberg Z, Schweitzer ME, et al. MRI of medial malleolar bursa. AJR Am J Roentgenol 2005;184:979–83.

60. Jacobson JA, Powell A, Craig JG, et al. Wooden foreign bodies in soft tissue: detection at US. Radiology 1998;206:45–8.

61. Schlager D, Sanders AB, Wiggins D, et al. Ultrasound for the detection of foreign bodies. Ann Emerg Med 1991;20:189–91.

62. Davae KC, Sofka CM, DiCarlo E, et al. Value of power Doppler imaging and the hypoechoic halo in the sonographic detection of foreign bodies: correlation with histopathologic findings. J Ultrasound Med 2003;22:1309–13 [quiz: 1314–6].

63. Crawford R, Matheson AB. Clinical value of ultrasonography in the detection and removal of radiolucent foreign bodies. Injury 1989;20:341–3.

64. Failla JM, Holsbeeck Mv, Vanderschueren G. Detection of a 0.5-mm-thick thorn using ultrasound: a case report. J Hand Surg 1995;20:456–7.

65. Gibbs TS. The use of sonography in the identification, localization, and removal of soft tissue foreign bodies. Journal of Diagnostic Medical Sonography 2006;22:5–21.

66. Horton LK, Jacobson JA, Powell A, et al. Sonography and radiography of soft-tissue foreign bodies. AJR Am J Roentgenol 2001;176:1155–9.

Index

Note: Page numbers of article titles are in **boldface** type.

A

Ultrasound Clin 4 (2009) 255–260
doi:10.1016/S1556-858X(09)00044-9
1556-858X/09/$ see front matter © 2009 Elsevier Inc. All rights reserved.

Printed and bound by CPI Group (UK) Ltd, Croydon, CR0 4YY

14/10/2024

01774165-0001